YOGA
for EVERYONE

A COMPLETE STEP-BY-STEP GUIDE TO YOGA AND MEDITATION, FROM GETTING STARTED TO ADVANCED TECHNIQUES

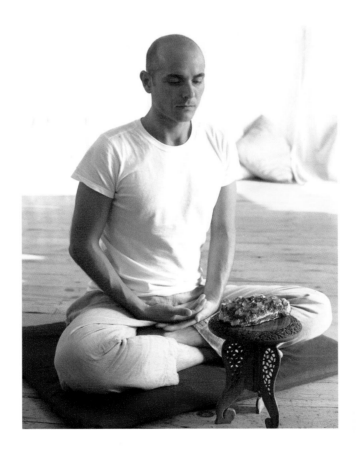

JUDY SMITH, DORIEL HALL, BEL GIBBS

LORENZ BOOKS

This edition is published by Lorenz Books
Lorenz Books is an imprint of Anness Publishing Ltd
Hermes House, 88–89 Blackfriars Road, London SE1 8HA
tel. 020 7401 2077; fax 020 7633 9499
www.lorenzbooks.com; info@anness.com
© Anness Publishing Ltd 2004

UK agent: The Manning Partnership Ltd, 6 The Old Dairy
Melcombe Road, Bath BA2 3LR; tel. 01225 478 444
fax 01225 478 440; sales@manning-partnership.co.uk

UK distributor: Grantham Book Services Ltd
Isaac Newton Way, Alma Park Industrial Estate
Grantham, Lincs NG31 9SD; tel. 01476 541080
fax 01476 541061; orders@gbs.tbs-ltd.co.uk

North American agent/distributor: National Book Network
4501 Forbes Boulevard, Suite 200, Lanham, MD 20706
tel. 301 459 3366; fax 301 429 5746; www.nbnbooks.com

Australian agent/distributor: Pan Macmillan Australia
Level 18, St Martins Tower, 31 Market St, Sydney, NSW 2000
tel. 1300 135 113; fax 1300 135 103; customer.service@macmillan.com.au

New Zealand agent/distributor: David Bateman Ltd
30 Tarndale Grove, Off Bush Road, Albany, Auckland
tel. (09) 415 7664; fax (09) 415 8892

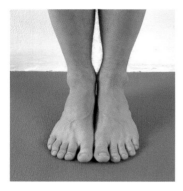

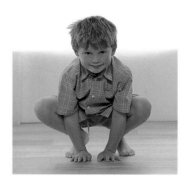

A CIP catalogue record for this book is available from the British Library.

10 9 8 7 6 5 4 3 2 1

Publisher Joanna Lorenz
Editorial Directors Judith Simons and Helen Sudell
Senior Editor Sarah Ainley
Project Editors Katy Bevan and Ann Kay
Designer Anita Schnable
Photography Clare Park, John Freeman and Michelle Garrett
Additional Photography Bonieventure Bagalue
Photography Stylist Sue Duckworth
Photographer's Assistant Lisa Shalet
Illustrator Lucy Grossmith
Production Controller Pedro Nelson
Yoga Positions Juliet Byrne, Laura Dymock,
David Johnston, Peter Oakley, Jenny Roche, Judy Smith

Previously published in three separate volumes: **Iyengar Yoga**,
Meditation and **Yoga for Children**

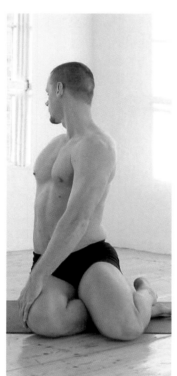

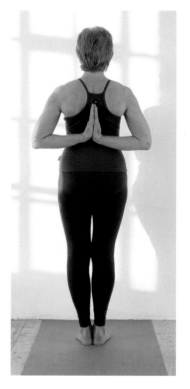

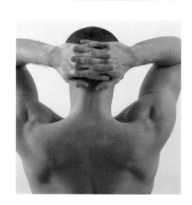

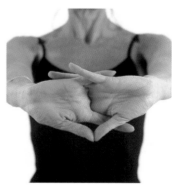

YOGA

for EVERYONE

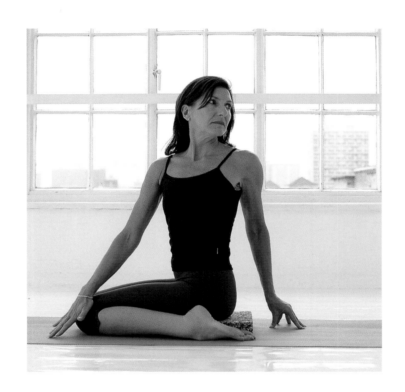

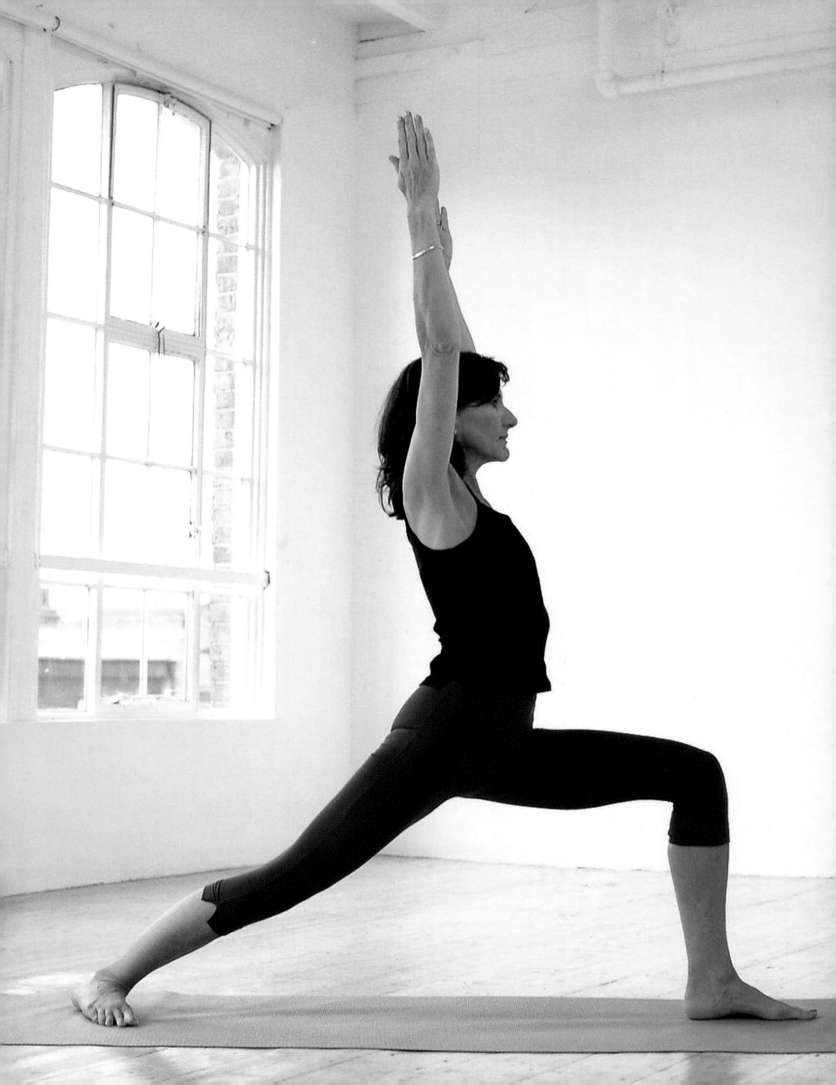

Contents

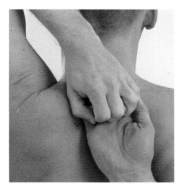

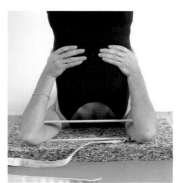

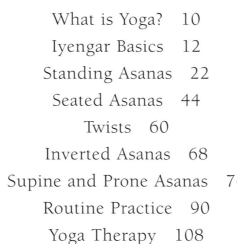

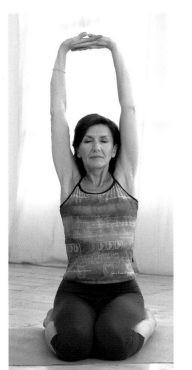

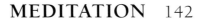

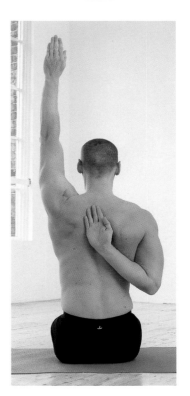

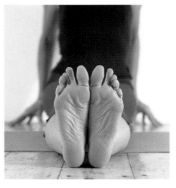

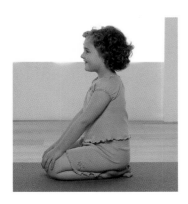

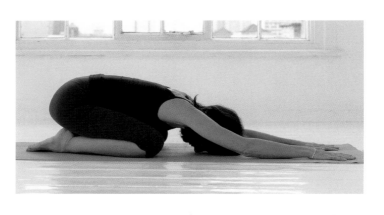

Introduction

We exist on many levels, in body, mind and spirit, but in the modern world it is all too easy for our lives to become fragmented. We may lay too much emphasis on mental processes, for example, neglecting our physical well-being or the fostering of caring relationships and our spiritual development. Imbalances like this can lead to stress and dissatisfaction: what is needed is a means of unifying and balancing all aspects of life.

Balance and harmony are the essence of yoga. For most people in the West, the most familiar and accessible aspect of yoga is the practice of asanas, or postures, which develop a strong, toned and flexible physique. But in Hindu philosophy these exercises are only the beginning of a journey that leads all the way to spiritual enlightenment. As the postures stretch and relax the body they deepen the breathing, relieving tension and stress. The ceaseless chatter of the mind is stilled, and freed from the turmoil of everyday concerns it is able to turn inwards to find spiritual wisdom in a state of expanded awareness. It is this state of meditation that lies at the heart of yoga.

Most of the yoga taught today is based on the *Yoga Sutras*, a set of texts on yoga meditation traditionally attributed to the ancient Indian sage Patanjali. He is thought to have lived around 300BC, but it is certain that yoga itself is far older than this. Patanjali's texts fused the

many yogic traditions that existed in his time to create a coherent philosophical system. The Sutras were then handed down orally from teachers to students for generations, before being written down in Sanskrit.

All the practices described by Patanjali are steps leading to the ultimate goal of enlightenment, the state of universal understanding that lies beyond the thinking mind and is achieved through meditation. In addition to this main purpose, however, the practice of hatha, or physical, yoga offers many other benefits for health and stress relief.

The classical postures of Iyengar yoga slow and deepen the breathing, allow energy to flow freely and bring a "feel-good" factor to the body, while also relaxing and resting the mind. They are designed to promote strength, balance,

below left and right Students of Iyengar yoga practising seated and standing postures.
opposite Namaste is the traditional greeting among yogis.

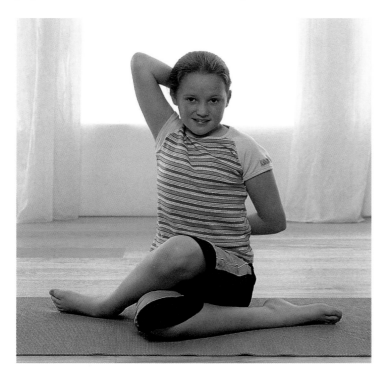

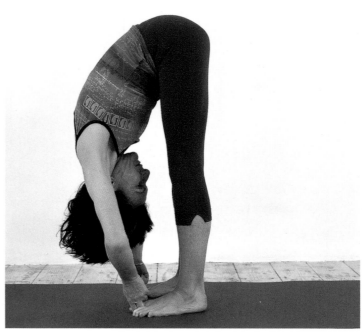

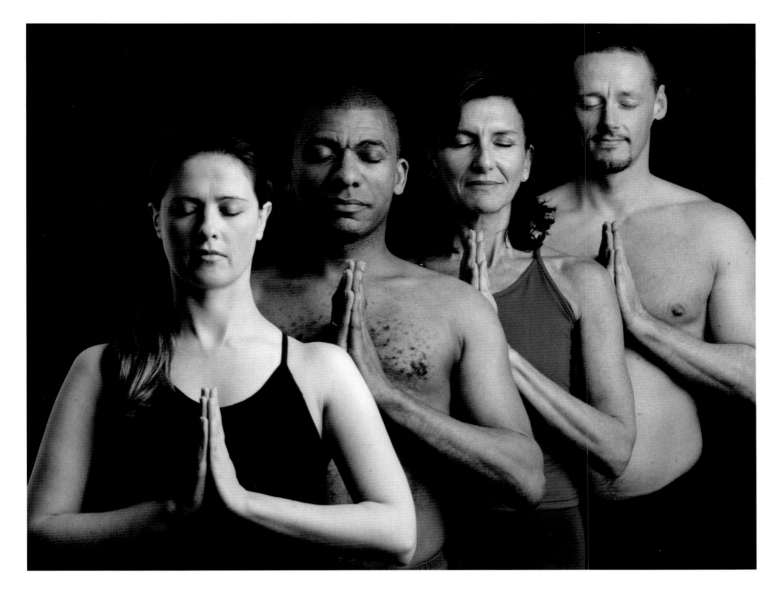

flexibility and relaxation. When you begin to practise them regularly, you will be amazed at how quickly your body begins to shed the tightness and tension that have been restricting it, leading to a wonderful sense of well-being.

It's important to make sure that you are achieving the right alignments when you first take up yoga, so there is no substitute for attending a class where your movements can be observed and checked by a qualified teacher. This book is designed for use in conjunction with regular classes. In the first section, the classical asanas are presented in order of their importance in practice. Step-by-step photographs show clearly how to approach each posture and provide a useful reference for practice at home. There are also suggestions for ways of modifying the movements for beginners and those who are less flexible.

By linking movement with the subtle control of the breath, yoga works from within. Performing the postures is not just about moving the body into the correct "shapes"; the gentle stretches and movements, working with the

breath, both release muscular tension and allow energy to flow freely. The lungs are strengthened and the circulation improved, supporting the functions of all the organs. The first part of the book concludes with a chapter outlining ways in which specific yoga postures can be used therapeutically to heal or alleviate a range of common ailments and problems.

Making yoga part of your daily routine will bring a clearer mind and a more open-hearted acceptance of life, opening the way to the state of meditation. A brief introduction to meditative practice is included here to help you approach this transformative expansion of consciousness.

Yoga is indeed a way of life, and it's never too soon to begin. If you have children, you can involve them in your practice too – in doing so you will be bestowing a gift whose benefits will last them all their lives. The final part of the book shows how to capture young imaginations with adaptations of the asanas, creating easy animal postures, group activities and games that everyone can join in.

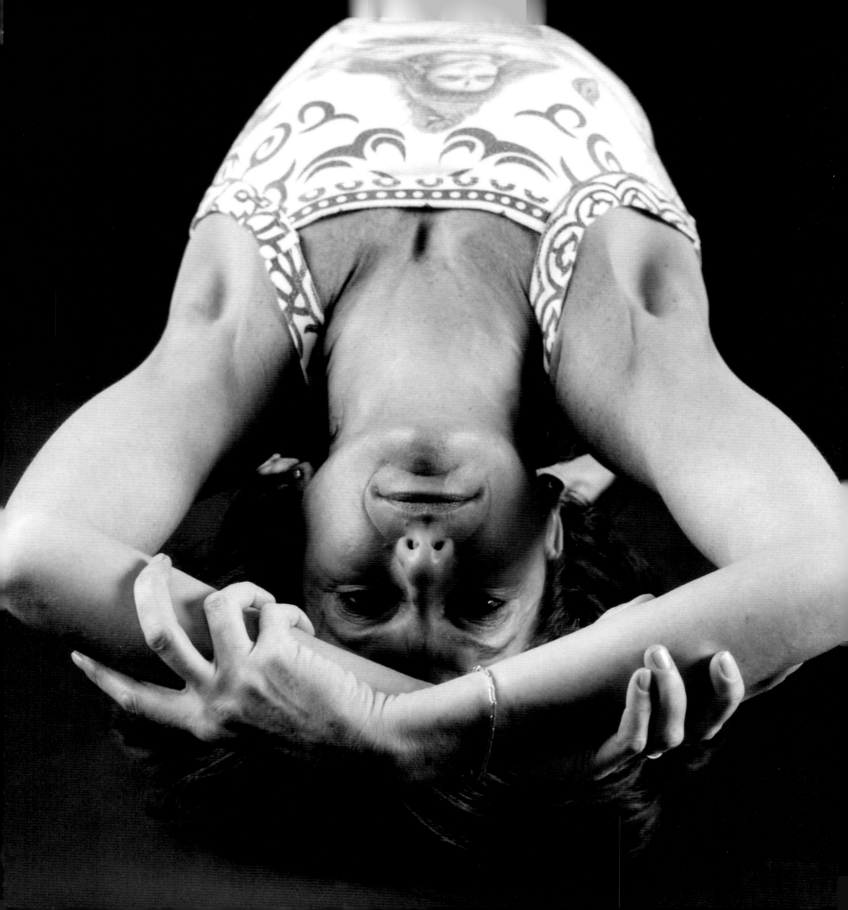

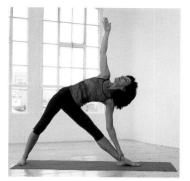
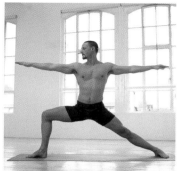
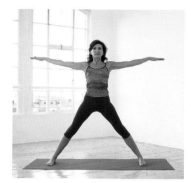
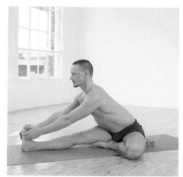

Iyengar Yoga

Here are classic yoga postures that are suitable for all levels of fitness and flexibility, as well as different age groups. The benefits include a calmer mind and supple body.

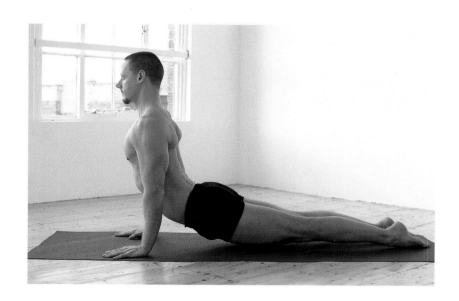

Judy Smith

What is Yoga?

Yoga is a practical philosophy, not a religion, and requires no allegiance to any particular system of belief. The word "yoga" comes from the Sanskrit word "yug", meaning to join, yoke or unite. It is a traditional Indian philosophy that involves the integration of the physical and spiritual in order to achieve a sense of well-being. This synthesis and inseparability of the body and mind leads to a greater connection to one's consciousness.

In the practice of yoga, the body is linked to the movement, mind and breath to bring about a feeling of balance, relaxation and harmony. The practitioner uses the physical self to refine the mind. Through this thorough training of the body and thought, one is taught to awaken every cell of one's self and one's soul.

The practice of physical postures (asanas) improves a variety of ailments, strengthens and tones muscles and develops flexibility. Various movements in the postures result in blood saturating, nourishing and cleansing the remotest parts of the body. Psychologically, yoga increases concentration, stills the mind and promotes a feeling of balance, tranquillity and contentment.

There is a difference between yoga and other physical exercises. Yoga asanas are psycho-physiological, while physical jerks are purely external. Asanas develop body awareness, muscles and flexibility, as well as generating internal awareness and stabilizing the mind. In physical exercises, body movements may be done with external precision, whereas in yoga, together with the precision, a deeper awareness is awakened, which brings about balance in body and spirit.

Mr B.K.S. Iyengar has systematized over 200 classical yoga asanas, the result of which is Iyengar yoga. This version of yoga practice is methodical and progressive, and emphasizes precision, detailed correctness and absolute safety. The postures have been structured and categorized to allow students of all levels of fitness and ability to progress surely and safely from basic to more challenging postures and, by so doing, to gain flexibility, strength and sensitivity in mind, body and spirit.

Iyengar yoga, with its attention to detail, challenges both the head and the physical frame, and enables those who practise it to exercise control and discipline in all aspects of life. It is advisable to practise every day, but it is easy to tailor the routines suggested in this book to suit the amount

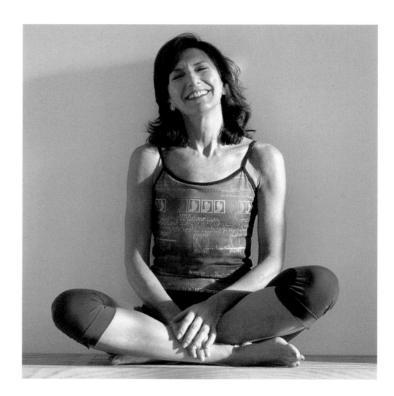

above Regular yoga practice benefits all aspects of your being, strengthening your body, renewing your energy, calming your mind and brightening your spirit.

of time available. It is best to set aside a similar time each morning or evening to practise and to make this part of your daily routine. Not only will your posture and flexibility improve, but you will became physically stronger, calmer and a more balanced and centred human being.

If you have not practised yoga before, the advice in this book should be used in conjunction with the expert guidance of a trained teacher. Joining a class is a motivating and enjoyable way to learn the postures and ensures that you are practising correctly.

Everyone can be helped by yoga, from the elderly and children to people with minor complaints and various problems, both physical and mental. When they begin, their

right When first learning the more challenging postures, it is a great support to have an attentive teacher.
below The constant practice of yoga brings flexibility, freedom from tension and peace of mind.

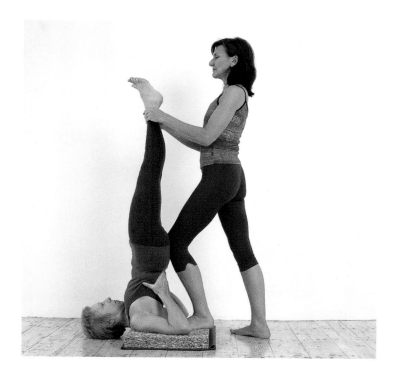

bodies and minds may be stiff and unyielding, but they will walk out of the class taller and with their entire beings radiating serenity and peace.

Practising the asanas and pranayama (breathing) with honesty and diligence, intelligence and awareness, will bring about clarity, energy and serenity in all aspects of your life. The asanas and programmes offered in this book are suitable for both beginners and more experienced practitioners and should be repeated and practised as often as circumstances allow, anything from an hour a week to several hours a day. Practised regularly, Iyengar yoga will bring you joy, light and happiness as you travel along your path to enlightenment.

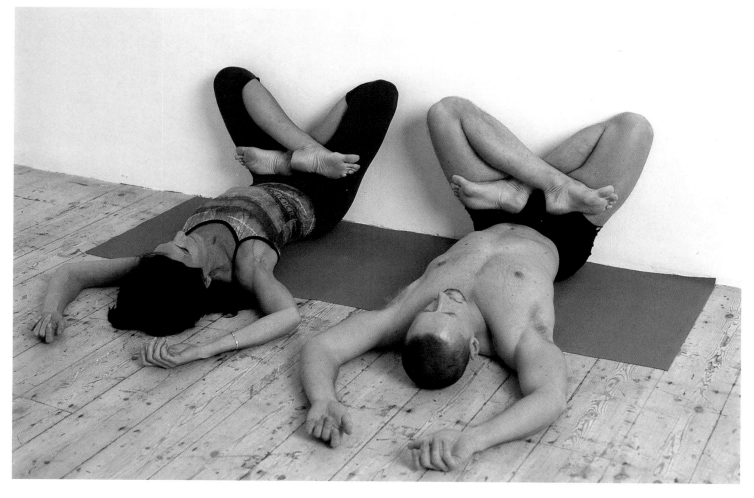

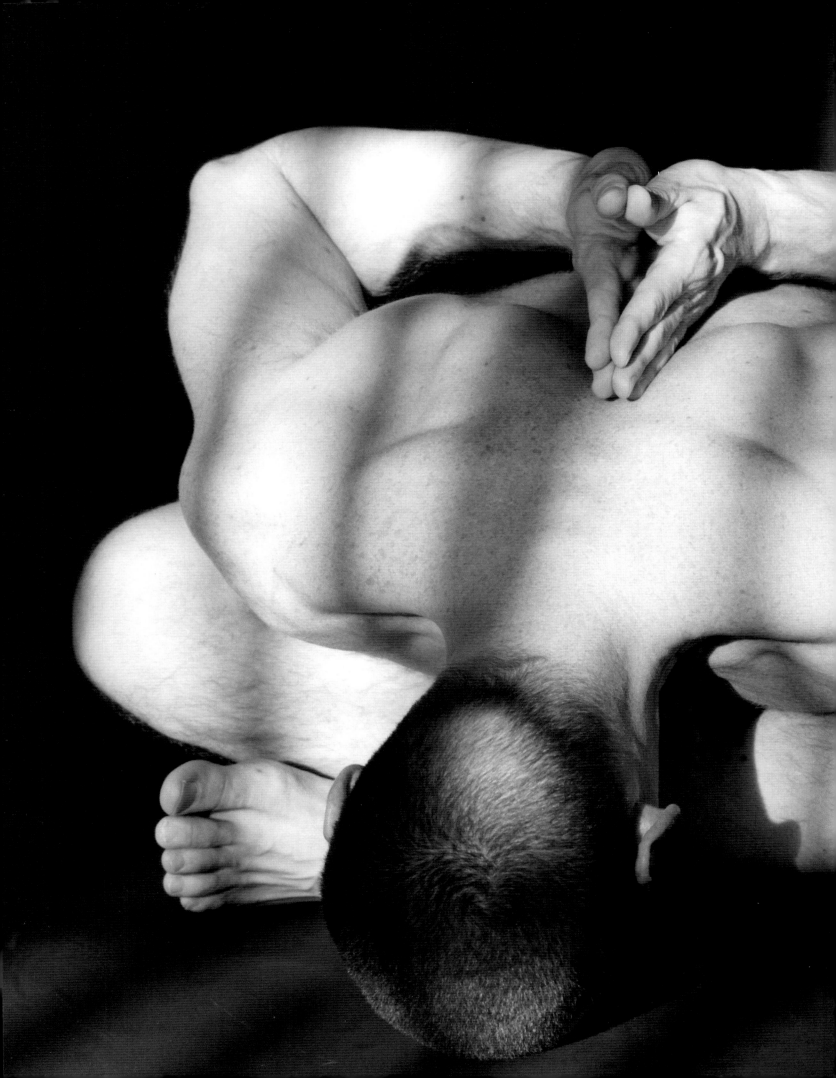

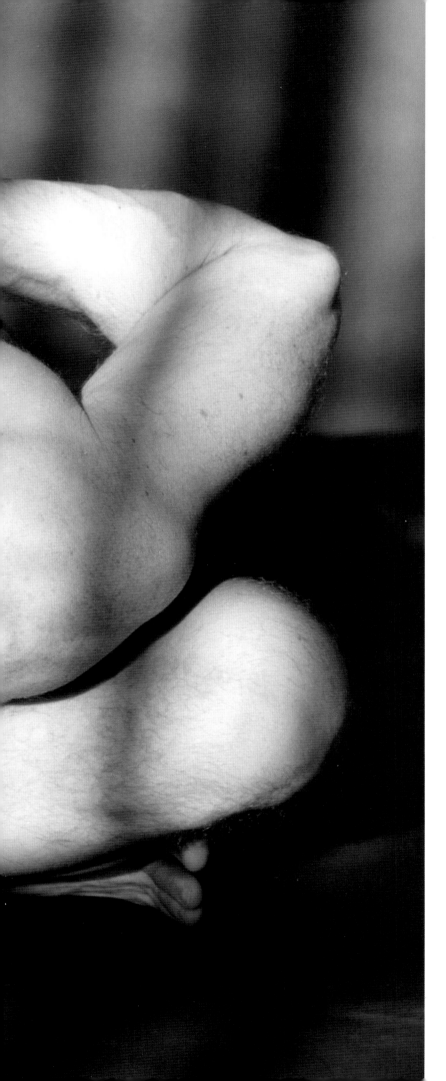

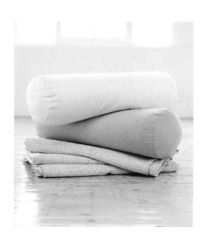

Iyengar
basics

"Yoga is a practical philosophy. It shows, from moment to moment, the way to face the world and at the same time to follow a spiritual path. Yoga strikes a balance between the happiness of the world, that is self-centred happiness, and the happiness which extends beyond one's own self." B.K.S. Iyengar

History and Philosophy

Iyengar yoga focuses on correct alignment of the body so that it can develop harmoniously and anatomically perfect. If the student practises with intelligence and awareness, there is little chance of injury or pain. As all bodies are different and people have specific weaknesses and difficulties, Iyengar yoga makes use of props to help students achieve the best possible poses within their limited capacity.

The Iyengar method, which is renowned for its precision and attention to detail, involves the practice of asanas (postures) and pranayama (breathing). Because of the intense concentration required to position parts of the body, both skeletally and muscularly, the mind becomes focused and sharp, and this results in a form of "meditation in motion". Practitioners strive for this state of total physical awareness, mental clarity and ultimate serenity.

A vital aspect of Iyengar yoga is the sequencing of postures. There is a cumulative effect when poses are practised in a particular order, and when this is adhered to there is less chance of injury and incorrect practice. Iyengar yoga can also be used therapeutically to treat a variety of ailments.

There are numerous styles of yoga, of which Iyengar is one. It was developed by Yogacharya B.K.S. Iyengar, one of the world's most respected experts on yoga. As a child he suffered from various illnesses, and at the age of 16 was introduced to yoga by his sister's husband, Sri T. Krishnamacharya,

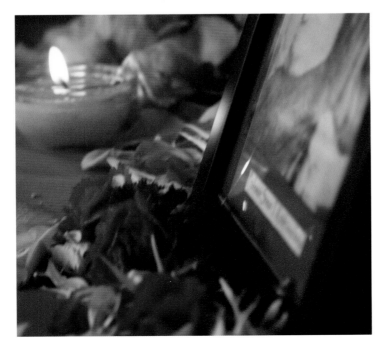

who was a teacher in Mysore. Iyengar began practising yoga to regain his health and strength, and in 1936 his guru sent him to Pune for six months to teach.

The precision and perfection in his practice was reflected in his teaching, and the number of students grew. He became recognized and respected as a yoga teacher, and in 1952 he met Yehudi Menuhin. This encounter was instrumental in introducing yoga and Mr Iyengar to the Western world. Menuhin was a dedicated student and invited Mr Iyengar to England to teach him. Many people joined in these classes, and soon a large number of Westerners became his students and invited him back the following year.

Back in Pune, he decided that he wanted the masses to experience yoga but was restricted by the size of the rooms and halls in which he taught. In 1975 he opened his own institute, the Ramamani Iyengar Memorial Yoga Institute, named in memory of his wife, who died just before his dream was realized. Students from all over the world regularly visit Pune and spend a month being taught by his daughter, Geeta, and son, Prashant, with their father keeping a watchful eye on everybody. Mr Iyengar is in his mid-80s, and to see him carry out some of the asanas is a real inspiration to his devoted followers. There are hundreds of Iyengar yoga institutes training students in his method of yoga around the world, including Europe, America, Japan, Israel, Australia, New Zealand, South Africa and Canada, as well as Bombay, Bangalore, Delhi, Madras and Rishikesh.

Mr Iyengar's comprehensive book *Light on Yoga* was published in 1966. This work has been acknowledged as the Bible of yoga and has been widely translated. Other books written by Mr Iyengar are *Light on Pranayama*; *The Art of Yoga*; *The Tree of Yoga* and *Light on Yoga Sutras of Patanjali*.

left The founders of yoga and gurus past and present are venerated and admired.
opposite It is through the dedication and hard work of B.K.S. Iyengar himself that Iyengar yoga has become such a popular form of yoga.

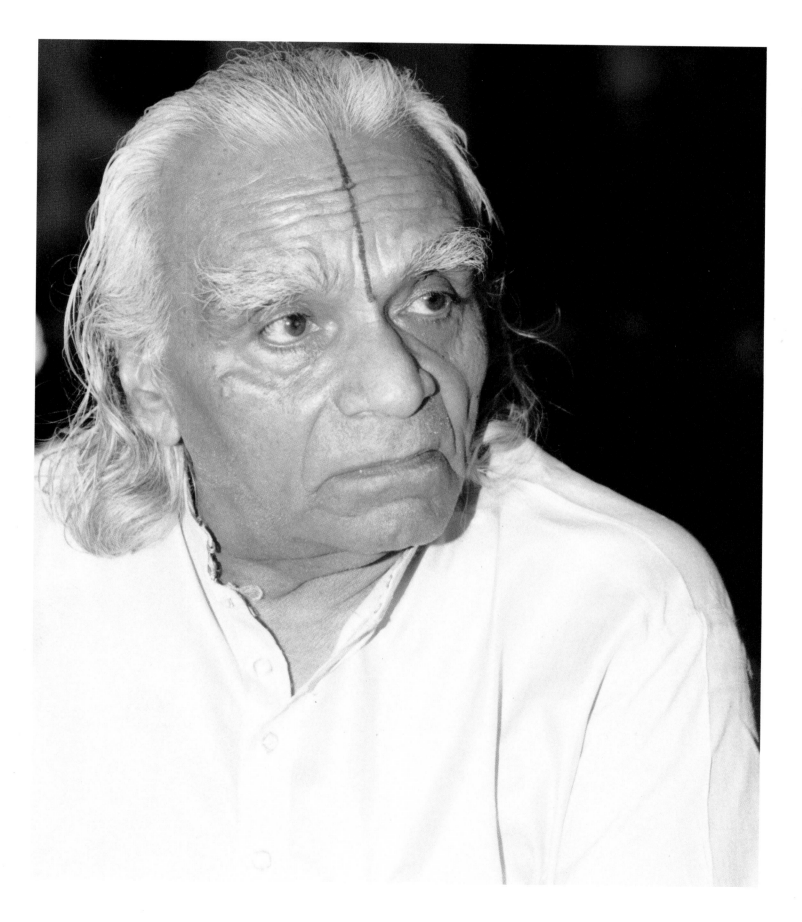

The Yoga Sutras

The philosophy followed by B.K.S. Iyengar is that of Patanjali, a sage who lived in India around 300BC. Patanjali is depicted as a statue with a man's torso and the coiled tail and seven-headed crown of a serpent. In the traditional symbolism of ancient India, this represents infinity. Two of his hands are folded in prayer, representing a meditative state, while the other two hands are holding a conch and discus of light. The conch reminds us of our yoga practice and the discus represents the wheel of time or the law of cause and effect. One half of his face is smiling, the other is serious.

Patanjali is known as the founder of yoga and he codified a set of 196 aphorisms called the Yoga Sutras. This work systematizes the principles and practices of yoga by bringing together all the various strands of the theory and practice, and presenting them in one concise, comprehensive text. These aphorisms cover all aspects of life, beginning with a code of conduct and ending with man's vision of his true self. Patanjali shows how, through the practice of yoga, we can transform ourselves, gain control over the mind and emotions, overcome obstacles hindering our spiritual enlightenment and attain the goal of yoga.

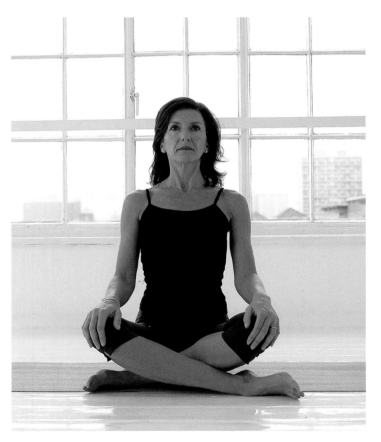

The eight limbs of yoga

According to Patanjali, yoga consists of eight limbs. Each of these limbs has its own separate identity, but all form part of a whole, and when they are integrated, the eight stages become true yoga. The eight aspects of yoga are:

1 **Yama** (Social discipline)
These five universal laws include: non-violence; truthfulness; non-stealing; sexual restraint; and freedom from desire. As codes of ethical behaviour, they should be followed in everyday life to promote harmony and understanding in society.

2 **Niyama** (Individual discipline)
These five principles of personal conduct are cleanliness; contentment; austerity; study of one's own self; and devotion to God. While the yamas apply to universal morals, the niyamas are rules of behaviour that apply to one's physical and mental discipline.

3 **Asana** (Postures)
According to Patanjali's Sutras, "Postures bring about stability of the body and poise of the mind." Practising asanas improves flexibility, vitality and health, and activates the organs (heart, lungs, kidneys, liver, spleen and pancreas). However, the true importance of postures is the connection between body and mind, so the two become interwoven, initiating the path from physical to spiritual awareness.

4 **Pranayama** (Breath control)
Patanjali states that pranayama should be practised only after a firm foundation in asana has been established. Practising pranayama releases tension in the body, calms the nervous system and keeps the mind tranquil.

5 **Pratyahara** (Withdrawal and control of the senses)
This withdrawal of the senses from objects of desire is the link between the first four limbs and the last three. After following the rules for universal and personal ethics (yama and niyama) and practising asanas and pranayama, one can turn one's senses inwards and achieve complete tranquillity.

left Simple cross legs position, or Sukhasana, is a comfortable pose in which to meditate. Choose a posture you will be able to stay in for a long time.

6 **Dharana** (Concentration)

After work on the body in asanas, refinement of the mind though pranayama and internalization of the senses of perception in pratyahara, the sixth stage, dharana, is reached. Here the mind is in a state of total absorption and is concentrated on a single point or task in which it is totally engrossed. The longer the mind remains in this state of focus, the more powerful it becomes.

7 **Dhyana** (Meditation)

When the practitioner maintains uninterrupted focus of attention in dharana, it becomes dhyana. In this state of deep concentration and undisturbed meditation, the mind, body and breath become one and merge into a single state of being.

8 **Samadhi** (Self-realization)

This is the culmination of yogic achievement – a true sense of communion and peace. This settling of the mind is the essence of yoga, where one has risen above the senses as a result of the complete refinement of both body and mind. The body and senses are at rest as if asleep, the mind and reason are alert as if awake, yet everything has gone beyond consciousness.

The first five limbs (yama, niyama, asana, pranayama and pratyahara) are known as the disciplines of yoga. They prepare the body and clear the mind and senses in readiness for the next three limbs (dharana, dhyana and samadhi), which are known as the attainments of yoga. Patanjali says, "The study of the eight limbs of yoga leads to the purification of the body, the mind and the intellect; the flame of knowledge is kept burning and discrimination is aroused."

The demands of modern life can bring about stress, which leads to illness as well as mental anguish. Good health is the harmony between body, mind and soul. It is a result of a balanced diet, exercise and a mind that is stress-free. In yoga, the asanas revitalize the body and pranayama brings about a sense of calmness. This helps to free the mind of negative thoughts caused by the fast pace of today's world. It is encouraging to know that in this age of pressure, there are well-established techniques in yoga to restore health and help contribute to a life of happiness and harmony.

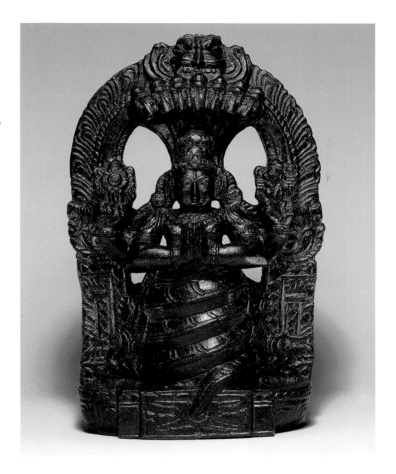

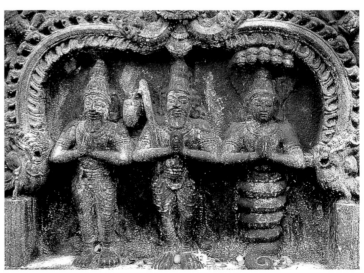

top This is a statuette representing Patanjali, the ancient Indian sage acknowledged as the founder of yoga. His sutras, or writings, have been translated from Sanskrit and interpreted by many.
bottom Here on the right is Patanjali as the serpent god, and one of a trinity of devotees witnessing the dance of the god Natajara at his temple in Chidambaram. The other figures are Vyaghrapada, a rishi or sage, with the feet of a tiger, and Simhavarman, an early king.

How to Practise the Asanas

The first part of this book presents a basic introduction to Iyengar yoga. It offers a selection of postures from each of the asana groups – standing postures for vitality; seated postures for serenity; twists, which are cleansing; inverted poses for developing mental strength; supine poses, which are restful; and prone poses, which are energizing. There is also a section on relaxation and pranayama (breathing).

Generally, the asana groups and the individual postures within each group are listed in the order in which they should be learned and practised as outlined in the system devised by Mr Iyengar.

Instructions are given for each posture, and photographs show the final posture, as well as the various stages leading to it. Students who already have some experience of yoga practice will find the sequences of photographs useful reminders, while the instructions are clear enough for beginners to follow. There are also tips on how to improve the posture and how props can help less flexible students. (See overleaf for details of props and how to use them.)

The Routine Practice chapter provides over 20 suggested programmes that vary in degree of difficulty and duration. Students should begin with Sequence 1 and proceed at their own pace, remembering to consolidate and not be in too much of a hurry to get to the last routine. It is not about how fast you work, but about the quality, understanding and proficiency of your practice.

The Yoga Therapy chapter provides programmes and advice for students with minor medical conditions. Props are used in most of these sequences to help less able students attain the best pose possible within their personal physical constraints.

Approaching yoga practice

"An asana is not a posture which you assume mechanically. It involves thought, at the end of which a balance is achieved between movement and resistance." B.K.S. Iyengar

Practice is essential for improving both physical and mental discipline. There are no rules for when, how often or how long you should do this, but obviously the more regular the practice, the greater the benefit to the practitioner. Practice must be adapted to suit one's circumstances, and the intensity and level of each session should reflect this. For example, if you feel tired after a long day at the office,

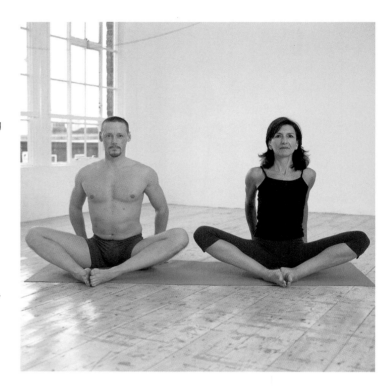

above Baddhakonasana, a seated posture. Practising yoga in company, or in an organized class with a qualified teacher, is a motivating way to begin, and continue, to learn.

practise restful/calming postures; if you feel stiff and lethargic, practise standing poses. Listed below are some general guidelines for practice:

• This book should be used in conjunction with, not instead of, attending classes. It is important to be instructed and corrected by a teacher.

• Wear light, loose, comfortable clothing that allows free and uninhibited movement.

• Practise with bare feet on a non-slip mat or floor. A carpet is not good as the feet slide and cannot grip the surface.

- The best time to practise is on an empty stomach. If possible, wait at least 4–5 hours after a heavy meal and 2–3 hours after a snack.

- Practise in a warm, airy room out of direct sunlight.

- Remove hard contact lenses.

- In each group of asanas, first practise the easier version before attempting the more difficult one. It is advisable to gain proficiency in the simpler version over a period of a few days before progressing to the final pose.

- Practise with full concentration and awareness of the parts of the body involved in each asana. The postures should be done slowly, smoothly and with full understanding.

- Pay attention to accuracy and alignment. When the body is correctly aligned, the flow of energy is uninterrupted.

- It is important to breathe while in the postures. Where no specific instructions are given, breathe normally. Generally you should inhale on upward movements, where the chest and abdomen are expanded and broad, and exhale on downward/forward movements, where the chest and abdomen may be compressed.

- Maintain the pose for as long as is possible without causing any physical or mental strain. Keep the eyes, mouth, throat and abdomen relaxed throughout.

- The eyes should be kept open and the mouth shut in all postures, unless otherwise instructed.

- If adverse physical or mental effects are felt during or after practice, seek the advice of a qualified Iyengar teacher.

- Each practice session should be followed by 5 minutes relaxation in Corpse pose (Savasana).

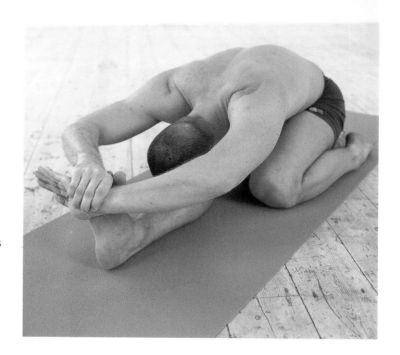

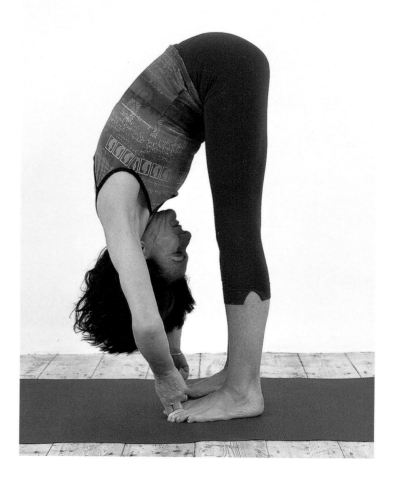

above right One of the five basic forward bending postures, Trianga Mukhaikapada Pascimottanasana.
right Finger to Toe pose, or Padangusthasana, strengthens the legs and makes the spine more flexible. Both standing and sitting forward bends aid digestion and tone the abdominal organs.

Equipment

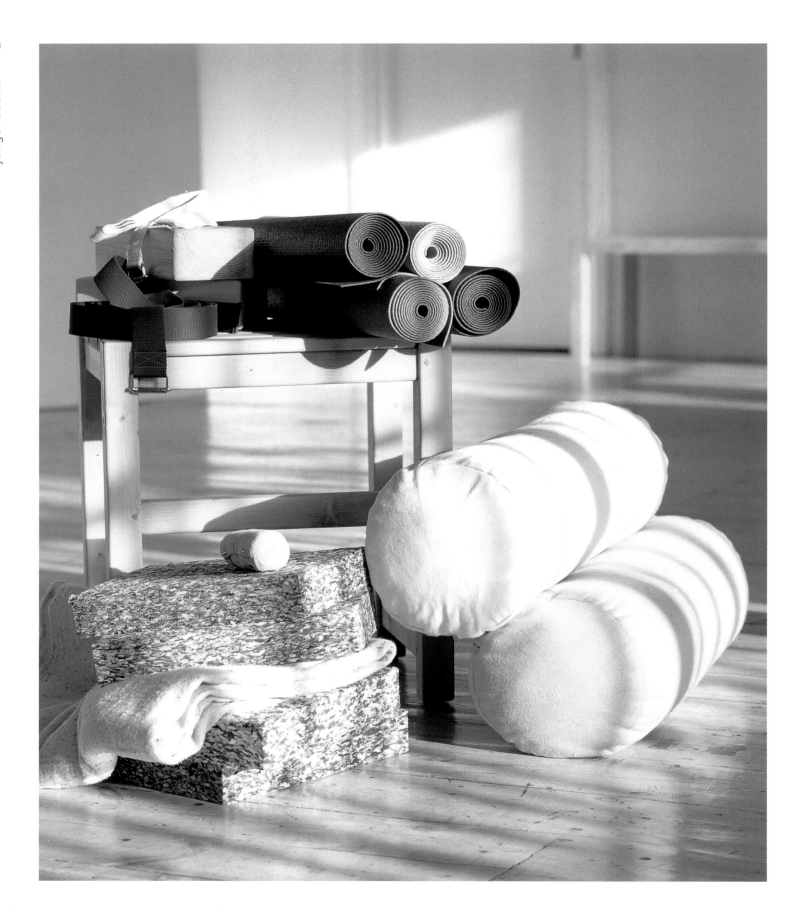

Historically, yogis used logs of wood, stones and ropes to help them practise asanas effectively. Mr Iyengar has invented a variety of props that allow the postures to be held easily and for longer, without strain. The use of props makes the asanas more accessible to all yoga students, whether they are stiff or flexible, young or old, weak or strong, beginners or advanced. Props may also be used by those who wish to conserve their energy because of fatigue or injury. They allow muscular extension to take place while the brain remains passive. Mr Iyengar refers to this as practising "with effortless effort".

Non-slip mats These prevent the feet from sliding during standing poses. It is helpful to draw or fold a line down the centre of the mat to assist with alignment.

Chair A chair is used for easy twisting postures, e.g. Chair pose (Bharadvajasana), or as a support for the body in Chair Sarvangasana and Ardha Halasana.

Wooden blocks These are used when stiffer students find that they cannot reach the floor with their hands. In sitting and standing postures, they can be used to support the legs or hands and to help with twisting poses.

Foam blocks Many students find it difficult to lift the spine in seated poses. Sitting on one or two foam blocks helps to achieve this spinal lift. Blocks are used to support the neck and shoulders in Salamba Sarvangasana, and in restorative poses the blocks are used to support the student's head.

Bolsters Used mainly in restorative and recuperative postures, bolsters support the head or the spine. A couple of cushions or rolled-up blankets can be substituted.

Eyebags These are small bean bags used to calm the eyes in recuperative poses. Also used is the traditional crêpe bandage, that should be lightly wrapped around the head and eyes, helping to release tension around the eye area.

Straps Use straps around the feet in straight-legged postures where the hands cannot catch the toes or foot. The strap is used in Salamba Sarvangasana to prevent the arms sliding apart, and in Supta Baddhakonasana to secure the feet together, close to the pelvis.

opposite A selection of props used to help students. Furniture and other objects in the home can be adapted and used as props, or they can be purchased from yoga centres.
right Bolsters and blankets are useful. You may already have similar items at home.
far right Blocks are made of wood, cork or foam.

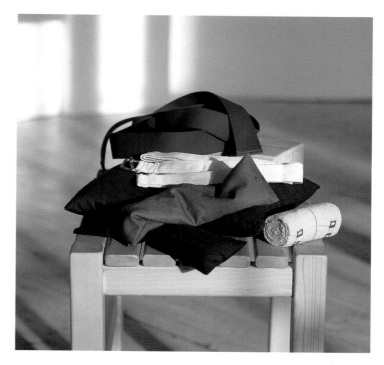

above Halasana stools come in different heights for all shapes of body. Bandages and bean bags are useful aids to calm the eyes and keep the mind quiet.

Halasana stool This stool is used to support the thighs in Ardha Halasana. In standing twists, the raised foot is supported on a stool or chair. The head may be supported on the Halasana stool in restorative poses.

Blankets Folded blankets may be used instead of foam blocks. They are used to support the head in Savasana, pranayama and restorative postures. They give additional lift to the spine in seated and twisting asanas. A rolled-up blanket can be used to support the feet in Virasana. On a practical note, in Savasana the body temperature is lowered, so cover up and use the blanket for warmth.

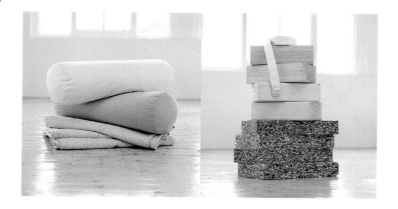

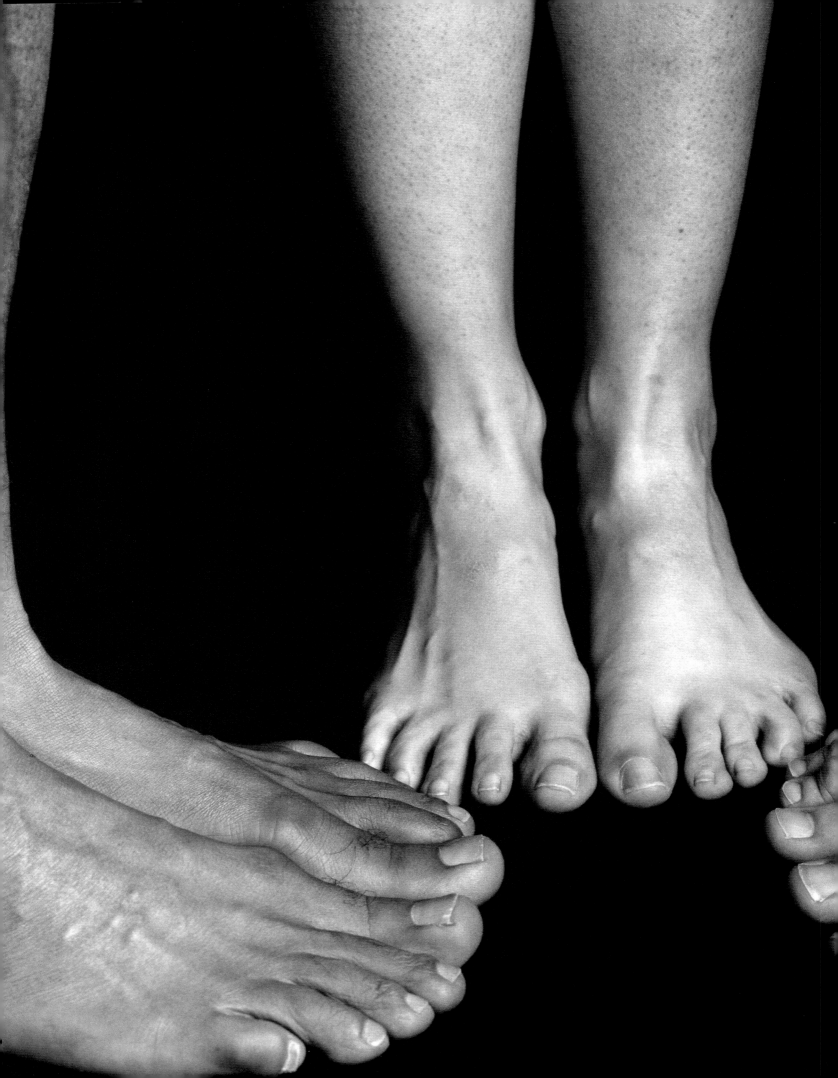

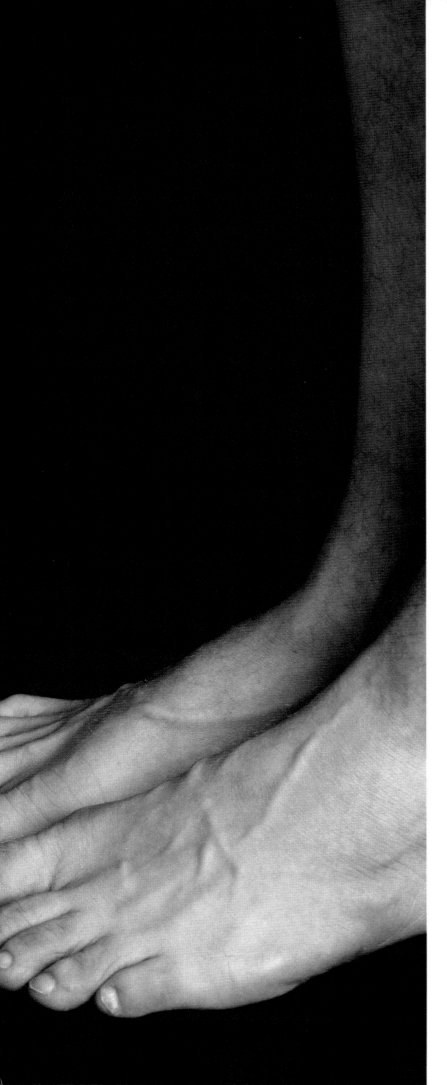

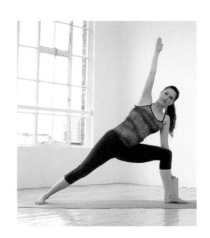

standing
Asanas

Standing postures are dynamic and energizing and form the basis of all other postures. Through them practitioners become familiar with various parts of the skeletal and muscular body and learn to use their intelligence to bring action and awareness to these parts. Standing postures develop strength, stamina and determination.

Mountain pose
TADASANA

This pose teaches you how to stand correctly. It brings attention to posture and makes you aware of how the legs and feet have to work in order to stand up straight. All standing poses begin and end with Tadasana.

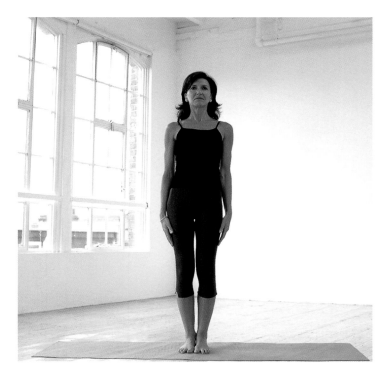

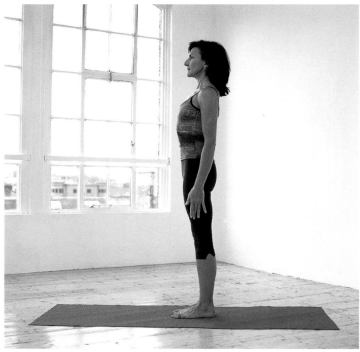

1 Stand with the feet together – big toes, inner ankles and inner heels touching. Spread the body weight evenly over the feet, keeping the inside edges of the feet parallel.

Tighten/lift the kneecaps and pull up the thigh muscles so the legs stretch strongly. Feel the spine extending upwards and the lift in the front of the body. Roll the shoulders back and take the shoulder blades into the body to open the chest.

2 Allow the arms to hang down the sides of the body with the palms facing the legs.

Extend the neck up, relax the face and look straight ahead. Hold for 30–60 seconds.

Focus on Tadasana
• Although relatively simple, this posture is crucial as it teaches awareness of the body and the recognition of any postural difficulties. Try to perfect this posture before moving on to the next pose.
• Press the feet firmly into the floor and extend the crown of the head towards the ceiling.
• Extend the sides and back of the neck, balancing the head on the top of the spine.
• Feel the front body "opening" from pubis to chin.
• Project the breastbone towards the front of the chest.
• Ensure that the body is stretching evenly on all sides – front, back, left and right. Strain is caused to the body by leaning habitually to one side or the other.

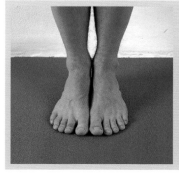

Focus on feet
• It is important to keep the inside edges of the feet parallel, and the big toes and ankle bones together Weight should be evenly spread over the heels and soles of the feet.

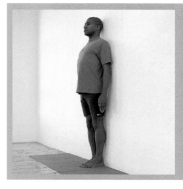

Modification
• If you find it hard to balance, try Tadasana standing against a wall. This is also helpful to ensure that you are standing straight, and not leaning forwards or backwards.

Tree Pose
VRKSASANA

This posture tones and stretches the leg muscles and teaches balance. Consistent practice of the balancing postures will improve your concentration and increase muscle tone and general poise.

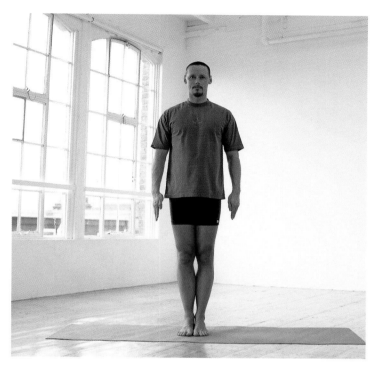

1 Stand in Tadasana – feet together, eyes still.

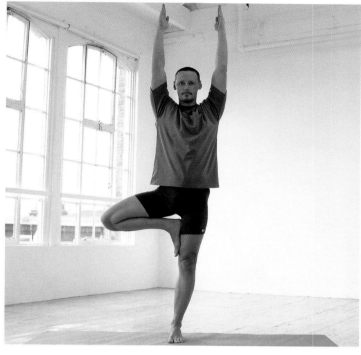

3 Inhale and stretch the arms over the head with palms facing one another. Straighten the elbows and extend the arms and trunk up.

Join the palms if you can do so without bending the elbows, otherwise keep them apart. Hold for 30–60 seconds. Exhale, then lower the arms and the right leg and repeat on the other side.

Focus
• To help maintain balance, try to focus the eyes on an object in the middle distance. Balancing poses such as Vrksasana can contribute to improving concentration in the long term.

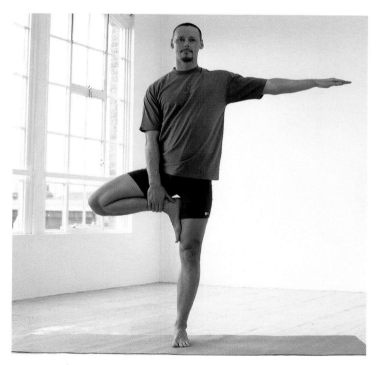

2 Bend the right knee to the side (without disturbing the left leg). Hold the ankle and place the sole of the right foot high on the left inner thigh with the toes pointing towards the floor. Keep the bent (right) knee back in line with the left leg and keep the left leg steady.

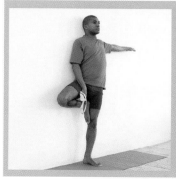

Modification
• To help with balance, use the wall for support and hold the foot up with a strap.
• Keep the grounded foot pressing firmly into the floor.
• Don't allow the left leg to bow to the side.

Extended Triangle Pose
UTTHITA TRIKONASANA

This pose strengthens the legs, makes the hips more flexible and relieves backache. In this posture, when turning the feet, it is important not to turn the hips as well. Start on the right side, then repeat the posture to the left.

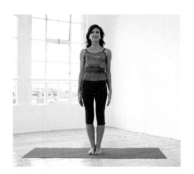 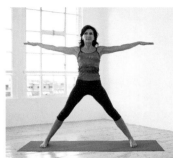

1 Stand in Tadasana.

2 Inhale deeply, jump or step* your feet 1–1.2m/3–4ft apart and extend the arms out to the side, keeping the palms facing the floor (* students with back problems should step their feet apart).

Ensure that both feet are level with one another, legs extended and straight, knees lifted.

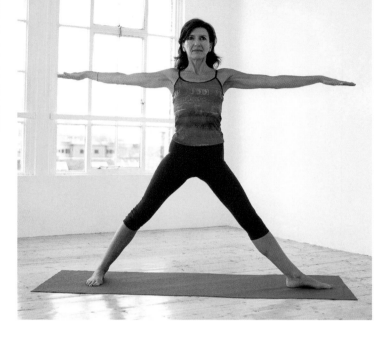

3 Turn your left foot out about 90 degrees (so that it is parallel to the side of your mat), and turn your right foot slightly inwards (about 15 degrees). The left heel should be in line with the instep of the right foot. As you turn the right foot in, rotate the right leg outwards, and as you turn the left foot outwards, rotate the whole leg to the left, so that the legs are rotating away from one another. Keep the left knee pulled up and facing in the same direction as the left foot.

Modification
• The final aim is to reach the floor, with the palm face down. If you cannot reach, place the hand on the ankle. If you need more help, use a brick standing on its end under the left hand to get more extension in the spine and to allow the chest to turn towards the ceiling.
• Students who are less flexible can do this posture with the back against the wall to aid balance. In this case, place the brick next to the wall to keep it steady, or try the posture with the back foot against the wall.
• If the neck aches when turning the head, either look straight ahead or look towards the left foot.

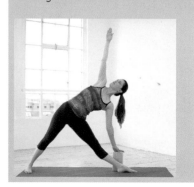 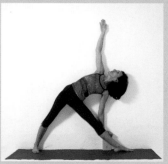

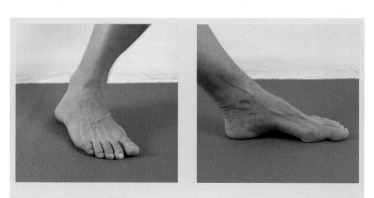

Focus
• Turn the back foot in 15 degrees. Press the corners of both feet into the floor and lift the instep.
• Stretch the toes forwards and the heels back to lengthen the soles of the feet.

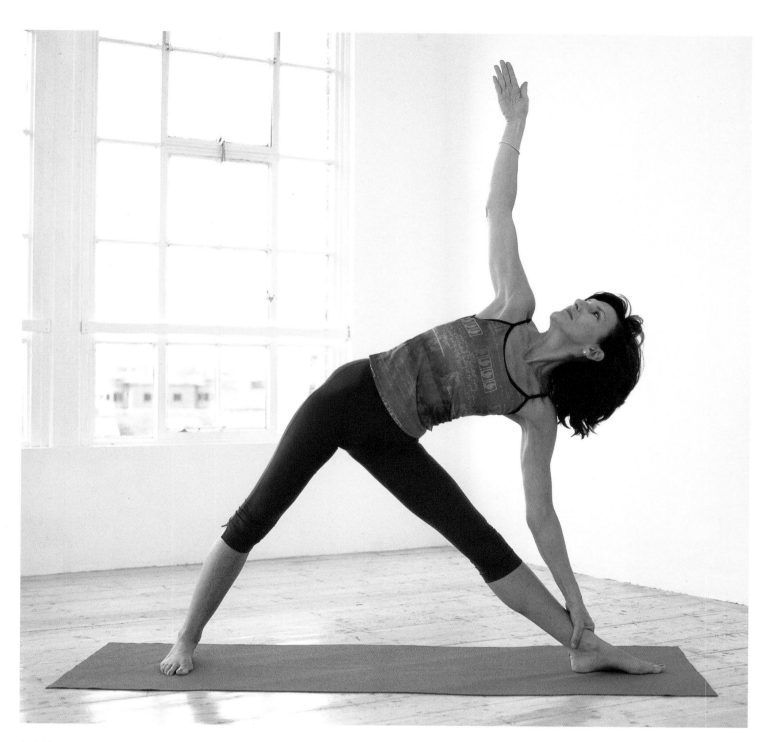

4 Lift the trunk, extend the arms further and then exhale and stretch the trunk sideways to the left. Hold the left ankle with the left hand.

Extend the right arm upwards, keeping the palm facing forwards and keeping it in line with the left arm. Turn the head and look towards the right thumb.

Extend both legs strongly and rotate the navel forwards and upwards.

Hold for 30–40 seconds, inhale and come up, then turn the right foot out and the left foot inwards and repeat on the other side. After doing both sides, come back to the centre of the mat in Tadasana.

Extended Lateral Angle Pose
UTTHITA PARSVAKONASANA

This posture strengthens legs and spine, and helps to open the chest. The full lunge twists the body, stimulating the organs inside the body and aiding digestion and the elimination of toxins.

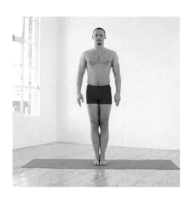 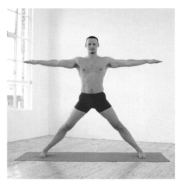

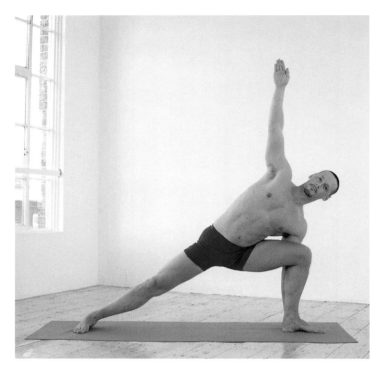

1 Stand in Tadasana.

2 Inhale deeply, jump or step your feet 1.3m/4.5ft apart and extend the arms out to the sides, keeping the palms facing the floor. Next, turn the right foot inwards 15 degrees and the left foot outwards 90 degrees. Broaden the palms and extend the whole of each arm from the top of the shoulder to the fingertips. Move the shoulders away from the ears.

3 Keep the right leg firm and straight, and bend the left knee to 90 degrees – keeping the shin perpendicular and the thigh parallel to the floor. Exhale and extend the trunk sideways, placing the fingertips of the left hand on the floor by the outer edge of the left foot. Keep the right leg stretched and firm – to do this press the outer edge of the right foot into the floor.

Focus
• As with all directional postures, begin with the right side, then continue with the left for balance.
• If the neck is uncomfortable, look straight ahead, not towards the ceiling.
• Move the buttock of the left (bent) leg forwards towards the left inner thigh and, at the same time, keep the left knee moving back slightly, thus keeping the groin open.
• Keep the top arm pointing towards the ceiling, as this will help to keep the chest open and lifted.
• Make sure that the back foot is turned in by 15 degrees and the instep is in line with the heel of the front foot.

Modification
• Use a wooden block under the left hand to open the chest more.
• Do the posture with the back against the wall to improve the alignment.
• This posture can be done at right angles to the wall, with the back foot against the wall for support.

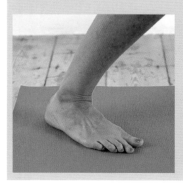 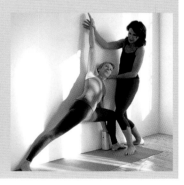 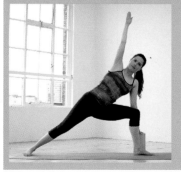 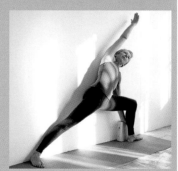

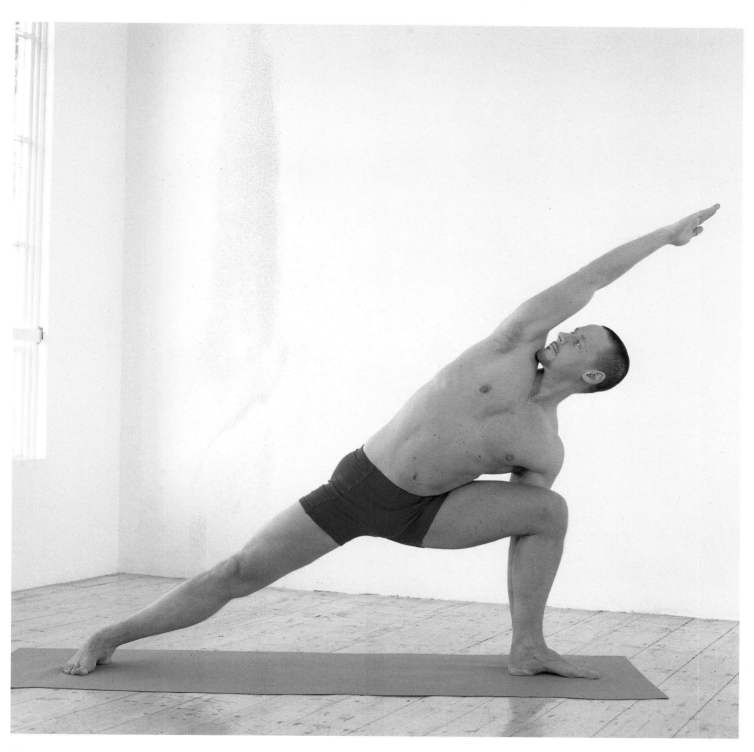

4 Turn the right arm towards the head and extend this arm over the head with the palm facing the floor. Turn the head to look towards the ceiling.

Fully extend the right leg and arm and turn the navel towards the ceiling.

Breathe normally and hold for 30–40 seconds. Inhale and come up, turn both feet forwards, rest hands on hips and then repeat the posture on the right side.

After finishing both sides, come back to Tadasana in the centre of your mat.

Warrior Pose II
VIRABHADRASANA II

This pose strengthens the legs, brings flexibility to the spinal muscles and tones the abdominal muscles. Although this is called the second posture it is practised first as it is less challenging.

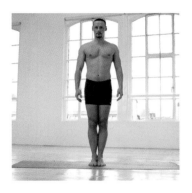
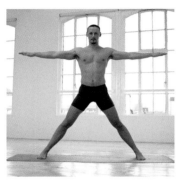

1 Stand in Tadasana.

2 Inhale deeply, jump or step your feet 1–1.2m/3–4ft apart and extend the arms out to the side, palms facing the floor.

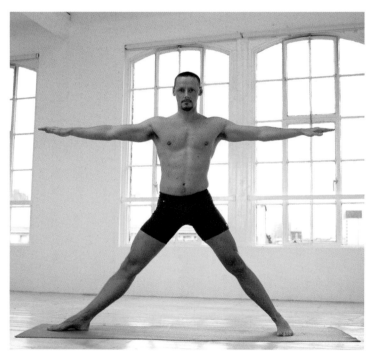

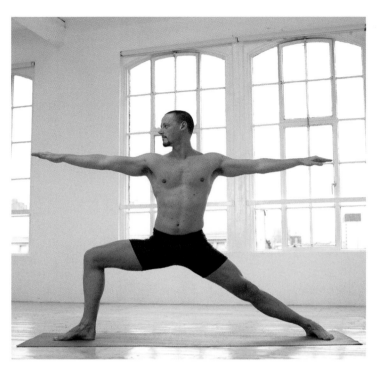

4 Extend the trunk up from the hips and, as you exhale, bend the right leg to 90 degrees, keeping the left leg firm and straight. Extend the arms strongly to the right and left with the palms facing the floor, stretch the trunk upwards, open the chest, turn the head and look along the right arm.

Extend the left arm more to the left so that the trunk doesn't lean towards the right. The crown of the head should be extending straight up towards the ceiling.

Open the chest, relax the face and breathe normally. Hold for 30–40 seconds, inhale and come up. Turn the feet forwards and repeat on the other side.

3 Turn the right foot out and the left foot in 15 degrees.

After completing both sides, come back into Tadasana.

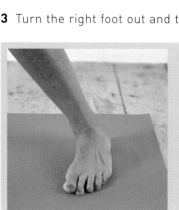

Focus
- Make sure that the back foot is turned in 15 degrees.
- Firmly press the outer edge and the heel of the back foot into the floor to create strength and stability in the back leg.

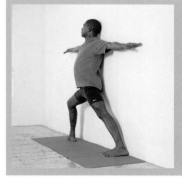

Modification
- Lean the back of the body against the wall for better alignment.
- Alternatively, place the back heel against the wall, with the fingertips of the back hand touching the wall.

Warrior Pose I
VIRABHADRASANA I

This is a challenging pose in which the chest is well expanded, which in turn improves breathing. It also helps with stiffness in the shoulders, back and neck.

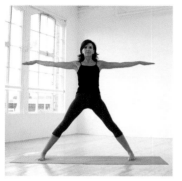 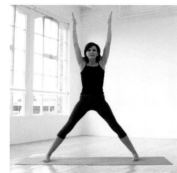

1 Stand in Tadasana, inhale deeply, jump or step the feet 1–1.2m/3–4ft apart and raise the arms to shoulder level.

2 Turn the palms upwards and extend the arms towards the ceiling, keeping the elbows straight and the palms facing one another. If your lower back aches when taking the arms up, then keep your hands on your hips.

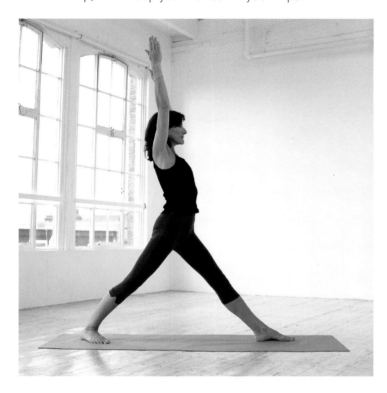

3 Turn the right foot and leg in deeply, about 40 degrees, and the left foot out 90 degrees. Simultaneously turn the hips, trunk and shoulders to the left.

Both sides of the trunk should be parallel – so bring the right hip forwards, while taking the left hip slightly back, to keep them even.

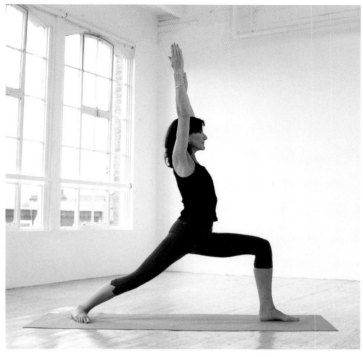

4 Exhale and bend the left leg to form a 90-degree angle. Extend the trunk upwards, as if it were being lifted out of the hips. Move the shoulder blades into the body to open the chest. Extend the chin towards the ceiling and look up. Maintain the full extension on the back leg and keep the hips, shoulders and trunk rotating to the left. Hold for 20–30 seconds, inhale, come up and lower the arms. Repeat on the other side, coming back to Tadasana.

Focus
• Don't strain or hold the breath in this posture. Breath is energy, so breathe evenly.
• If the lower back is uncomfortable in this pose, do it with the hands on the hips.

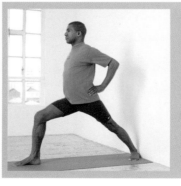

Modification
• If difficulty is experienced in turning the back foot inwards, either work with the back heel against a wall, or support the back heel with a foam block used as a raise.

Half Moon Pose
ARDHA CHANDRASANA

This pose strengthens the legs and helps improve balance. Regular practice will improve concentration and co-ordination. Because of the strong extension of the spine, it helps correct alignment and makes the back supple.

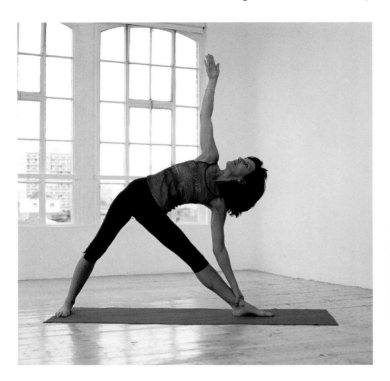

1 Start in Tadasana, then move into the full pose for Utthita Trikonasana.

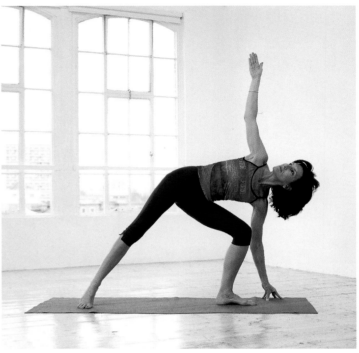

3 Exhale and draw the right foot slightly in towards the left leg. Straighten the left leg and the right leg will lift up.

Focus
• Keep the top hip (the one facing the ceiling) directly above the bottom hip (of the standing leg).
• If the neck is stiff, look ahead, not towards the top hand and the ceiling.

Modification
• If balancing is difficult, do the posture with the back of the body against the wall.
• Use a wooden block as support for the left hand.
• Alternatively, rest the foot of the lifted leg on a ledge or stool, using blocks to achieve the correct height.

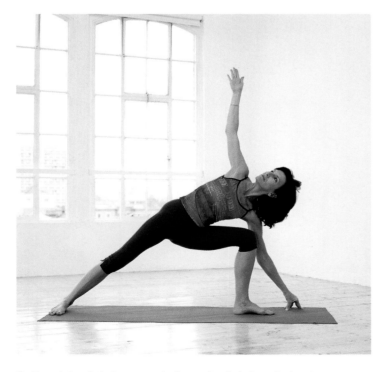

2 Bend the left knee and place the left hand about 30cm/1ft beyond the outer edge of the left foot. Bring the weight of the body on to this foot, using the hand to maintain balance.

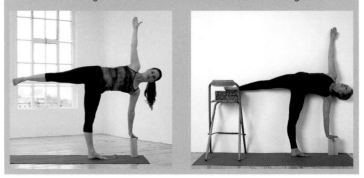

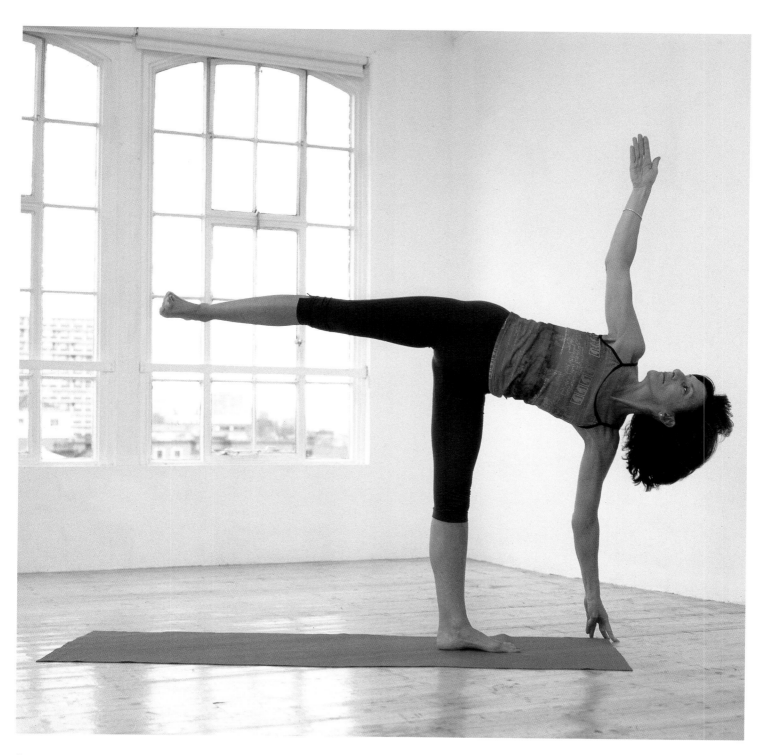

4 Raise and extend the right leg – keeping it parallel to the floor. Keep the left leg firm and pulled up and ensure that it is perpendicular to the floor.

If you are confident with the balance, extend the right arm up towards the ceiling, keeping it in line with the left arm.

Slowly turn the head to look at the right hand and open the chest, lifting the ribs upwards by twisting the waist.

Hold for 20–30 seconds, breathing normally, then come up and repeat on the second side. After finishing both sides, come back to Tadasana.

Extended Leg Raises
UTTHITA HASTA PADANGUSTHASANA I & II

This pose tones the muscles of the lower spine and strengthens the legs. It is done by standing on one leg, extending the other leg, to the front or the side, and catching the big toe with the fingers.

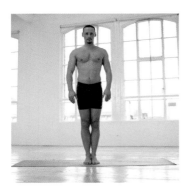
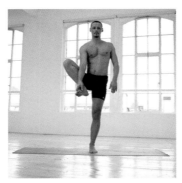

1 Stand in Tadasana.

2 Bend the right knee and clutch the big toe with the first and second finger of the right hand.

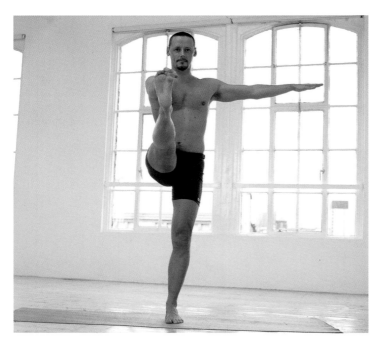

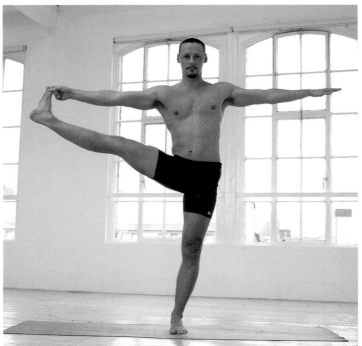

3 Utthita Hasta Padangusthasana I – Straighten the right leg forwards. Keep the knee of the extended leg pointing upwards, and the standing leg vertical.

4 Utthita Hasta Padangusthasansa II – Sideways Extended Leg Raise – keep the left foot pointing forwards and bend the right knee to the side. Hold the big toe with the fingers of the right hand. Stretch the right leg out to the side. Ensure that the right knee faces the ceiling. Straighten the right arm. Extend the spine upwards. Stretch the left arm out to the side. Look ahead, breathing normally, and hold for 20–30 seconds. Stretch the trunk up, open the chest, moving the shoulder blades into the back, keep the left leg firm and straight.

Focus
• As the right leg is raised and straightened, ensure that the left foot (on the floor) does not turn out. Keep the toes on this foot pointing forwards.
• Keep the trunk upright, not leaning towards the raised leg. If you lean, support the lifted foot on a ledge.
• Balancing poses improve concentration and poise.

Modification
Initially holding the toes may prove to be too challenging, especially if you have tight hamstrings, so using a strap around the foot or resting the foot on a chair is recommended.

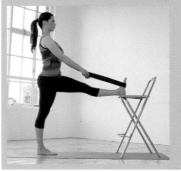
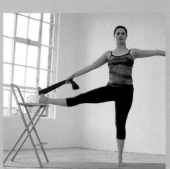

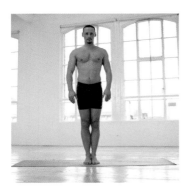

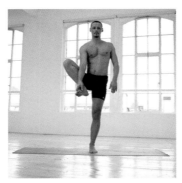

Warrior Pose III
VIRABHADRASANA III

This posture is an intensified continuation of Virabhadrasana I. It tones the abdominal organs, strengthens the legs, makes the spine more flexible and improves balance. It gives the practitioner agility in both body and mind.

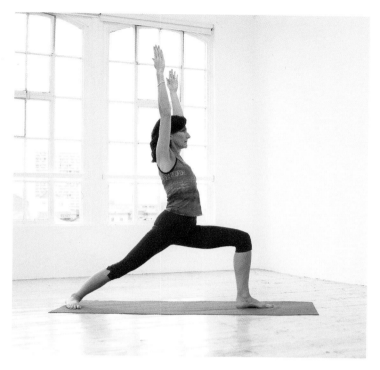

1 Follow the instructions for Virabhadrasana I.

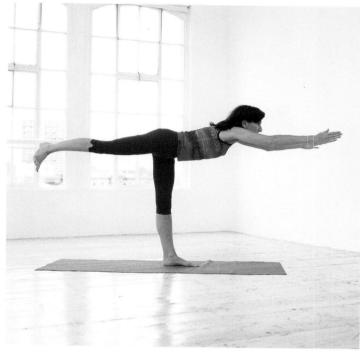

3 Extend the trunk more, straighten the left leg and lift the right leg up so that it is parallel to the floor. With the right leg, trunk, head and arms parallel to the floor, extend the fingertips away from the head and extend the right inner heel away from the head. Hold this position for 20–30 seconds.

Come down by bending the left leg, lowering the right foot to the floor and raising the trunk up – this is Virabhadrasana I. Repeat on the other side, and then come back to Tadasana.

If the lower back is painful, support the lifted leg on a ledge and the hands on a chair. Do not strain or compress the back of the neck.

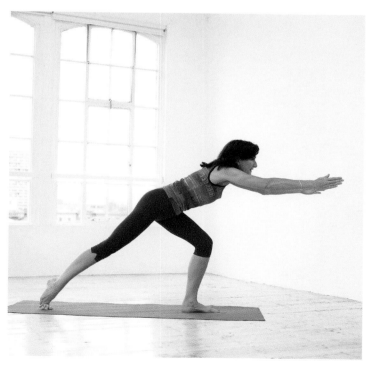

2 Exhale and extend the trunk and arms forwards over the left thigh.

Keep the hips level by pulling the right hip forwards if necessary.

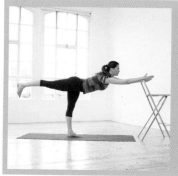

Modification
• The fingertips of the extended hands can press into the wall, or rest on a chair or ledge to extend the spine more.
• The hips must be level and the raised leg straight.

Reverse Triangle Pose
PARIVRTTA TRIKONASANA

This pose increases the flow of blood to the lower back region and therefore improves the flexibility of the spine. It also strengthens the legs and hips and invigorates the abdominal organs.

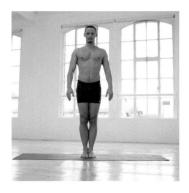

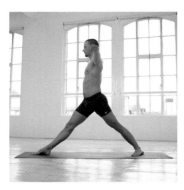

1 Stand in Tadasana, inhale and spread feet and arms apart.

2 Turn the right foot out 90 degrees and the left foot in 45 degrees. Exhale and rotate the trunk and head to the right.

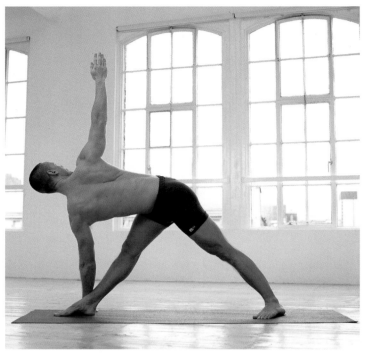

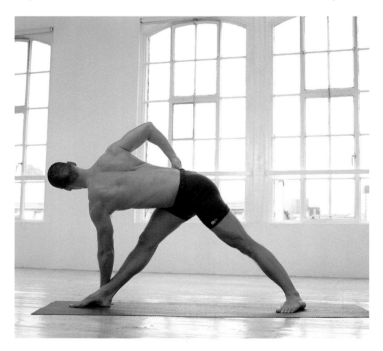

3 Extend the left arm over the right leg and place the fingertips of the left hand on the outside of the right foot.

4 Turn the trunk towards the right and extend the right arm strongly upwards in line with the right shoulder. Extend the spine and open the chest. Keep the head in alignment with the tailbone. Hold for 30–40 seconds. Inhale, rotate the trunk back to its original position and come up. Repeat on the other side and then come back to Tadasana.

Modification
• Less-flexible students can do this posture with the back against the wall.
• Use a wooden block under the right hand to get more extension in the spine and to allow the chest to turn towards the ceiling.
• Do the posture with the back foot against the wall.
• Put a foam block under the right heel to allow the chest to rotate farther.

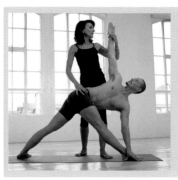

Focus
• Keep the right hip pointing upwards, so it does not collapse down into the body.
• Keep the head in line with the tailbone when looking up, maintaining a straightness in the spine.

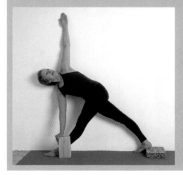

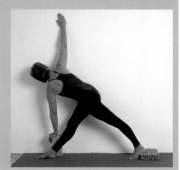

Revolving Lateral Angle Pose
PARIVRTTA PARSVAKONASANA

This posture is a more intense version of Parivrtta Trikonasana and therefore the effects are greater. The abdominal organs are more constricted, thus aiding digestion and helping to eliminate toxins from the colon.

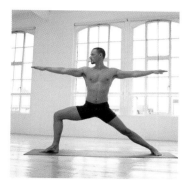
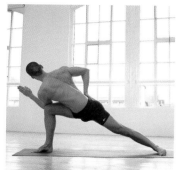

1 Begin in Virabhadrasana II, with the right leg bent and the arms extended out to the sides, keeping the palms facing the floor.

2 Rotate the trunk, pelvis, abdomen and chest towards the bent right leg. Take the left side of the trunk over the right thigh, bend the left elbow and hook it over the right thigh.

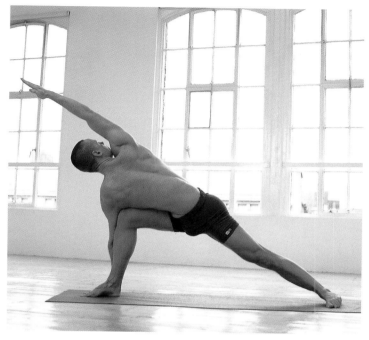

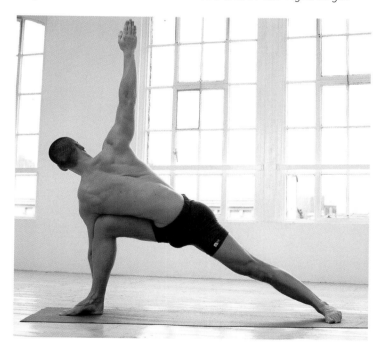

3 Rotate the trunk and chest more, and place the fingertips of the left hand on the floor on the outside of the right foot. Extend the right arm up towards the ceiling.

4 Turn the right palm towards the head, extending the arm over the head in line with the ear. Keep the left leg strong and straight. Turn the chest towards the ceiling more and, if possible, look up.

Hold for 20–30 seconds, then inhale, lift the left hand from the floor, raise the trunk, and come up. Repeat on the other side, and then come back to Tadasana.

Focus
• Throughout this posture, make sure the back (left) leg is straight.
• Keep the right shin perpendicular to the floor.

Modification
• Work parallel to the wall, supporting the lower hand on a block and the back heel on a raise.
• Work with the back heel against the wall. The heel is lifted on the wall while the toes are on the floor.
• This is a strenuous postition, so if it is too much, try keeping the top hand resting on the waist.
• Assistance in stretching the arm fully can help.

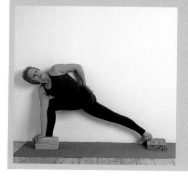
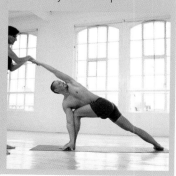

Intense Side Chest Stretch
PARSVOTTANASANA

This helps to maintain mobility in the neck, shoulders, elbows and wrists, and strengthen the abdominal muscles. It improves flexibility in the spine and hips and, once the head is down, calms the brain.

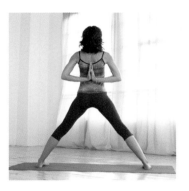 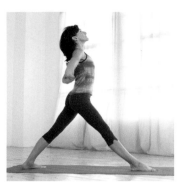

1 Stand in Tadasana, and join the hands behind in Namaste. Inhale and jump or step the feet 1–1.2m/3–4ft apart.

2 Turn the right foot out 90 degrees and the left foot in 45 degrees. Turn the hips, trunk and shoulders to the right.

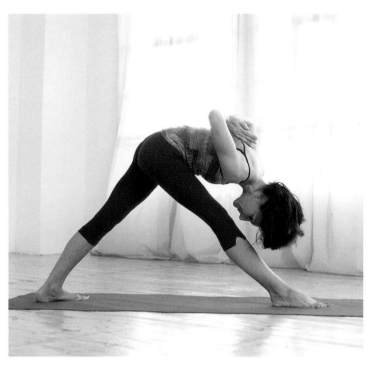

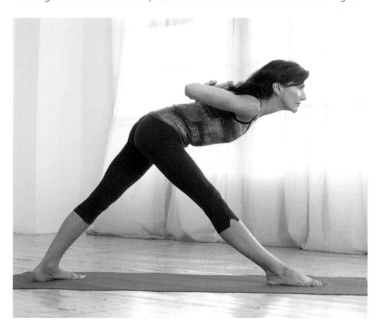

3 Extend the spine forwards. Lift the chin towards the ceiling and look up to make the back concave.

4 Exhale and extend the trunk over the right leg, taking the head towards the right foot. Keep both legs poker straight, the hips level and the weight evenly distributed between both feet. Hold for 30–40 seconds, raise the trunk, turn the feet forwards, release the hands and repeat on the other side. Come back to Tadasana.

Modification
• Until stability is learned, do the posture with the hands on the waist and, after coming forwards, place the hands on the floor on either side of the front foot.
• Don't allow all the weight to collapse on to the front leg. Press both feet equally into the floor.
• If the back is painful, place each hand on a wooden block after coming forwards, and then extend down.

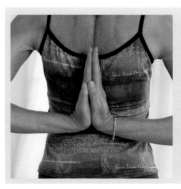

Focus
• Keep the palms flat together behind the back. This will increase flexibility in the wrists and shoulders. If the hands cannot go into Namaste, however, hold the elbows behind the back.

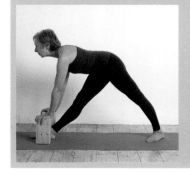 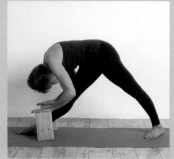

Forward Extension Legs Wide Apart
PRASARITA PADOTTANASANA

This pose is usually practised towards the end of the standing poses. Increased blood flows to the trunk and head, quietening the body and mind and promoting a feeling of tranquillity and serenity.

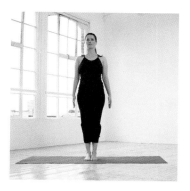
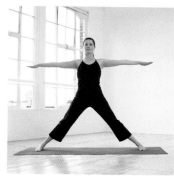

1 Stand in Tadasana.

2 Inhale and jump or step the feet 1.2–1.5m/4–5ft apart. Make sure the toes of each foot are level and the feet are parallel.

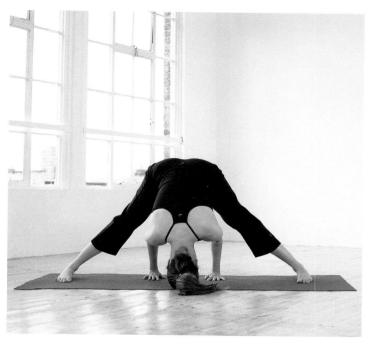

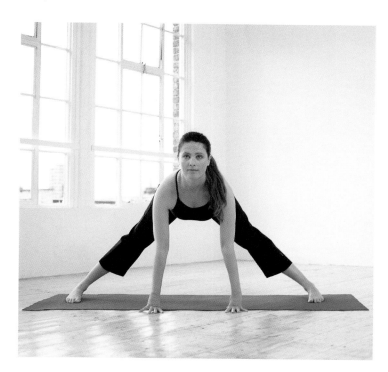

3 Straighten the legs by pulling up the knees and thigh muscles. Exhale and extend the trunk forwards from the hips, stretching the spine.

Place the fingertips on the floor, shoulder-width apart, directly under the shoulders.

Straighten the arms, stretch the legs and extend the trunk forwards, making the back concave and extending the front of the body from the pubis to the chin. Look up.

4 Bend the elbows back, extend the trunk to the floor and place the crown of the head on the floor. Lift the shoulders to release the head nearer to the floor, breathe normally and hold for 20–30 seconds. Inhale, lift the head and trunk and make the back concave. Place the hands on the hips and come back to Tadasana.

Focus
• Move the inner thigh muscles away from each other, i.e. inner thighs move towards outer thighs.
• Press the outer edges of both feet into the floor without letting the outer ankle bones bulge down.
• Even though the trunk moves forwards and then down, keep both legs stretching up towards the ceiling.
• This pose stretches the hamstring muscles.

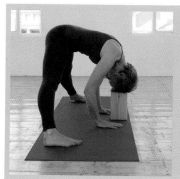

Modification
• If the hands don't reach the floor, support each hand with a wooden block.
• If the head doesn't reach the floor, support the crown of the head with foam or wooden blocks.

Forward Extension
UTTANASANA I

In this pose the spine is given an intense stretch. The abdominal organs are toned and, because the head is down, the increased flow of blood soothes the brain cells. It also relieves fatigue.

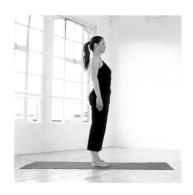
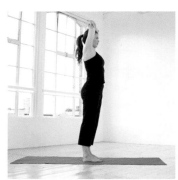

1 Stand in Tadasana with the feet 30cm/1ft apart. The inner edges of the feet should be parallel to one another and the toes level. Keep the legs and knees straight.

2 Fold the arms, catching the left elbow with the right hand and the right elbow with the left hand. Inhale and extend the folded arms above the head in line with the ears. Lift and extend the entire body upwards.

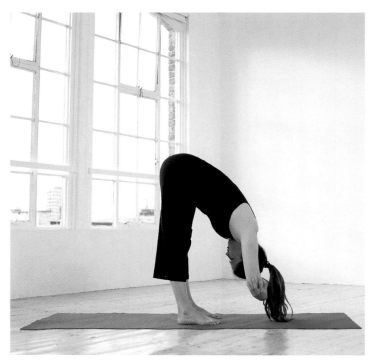

4 Extend the trunk down to the floor, keeping the legs straight, and extend the trunk and arms nearer to the floor. Inhale, lift the trunk, release the elbows and come back to Tadasana.

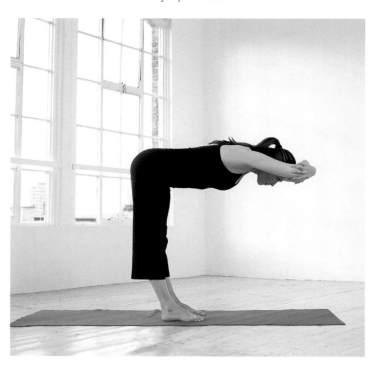

3 Exhale and extend the trunk forwards.

Focus
• This is a relaxing forward bend, although the legs remain strong, with the knees lifted. Allow gravity to do the rest of the work for you.

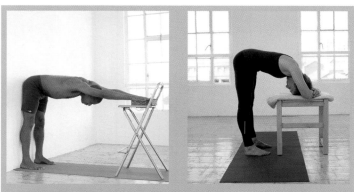

Modification
• For students with a stiff or painful back and tight hamstring muscles, do supported Uttanasana I – put the hands on a support at hip level, and extend the spine forwards. An alternative is to rest the head on a support, such as a Halasana stool softened with a blanket.
• If the back is uncomfortable in the final posture, take the feet wider apart and turn the toes slightly inwards.
• Keep the legs extending strongly upwards to elongate the spine and to protect the lower back.

Finger to Toe Pose
PADANGUSTHASANA

This posture strengthens the legs, makes the spine more flexible and also activates and tones the abdominal organs, improving digestion. Students who cannot catch their toes can hold their ankles.

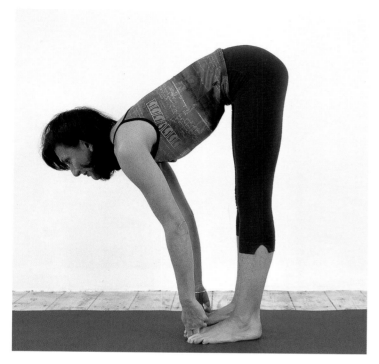

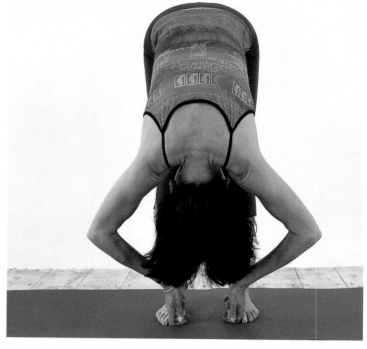

1 Stand in Tadasana with the feet 30cm/1ft apart. Bend the trunk forwards and down, then catch the big toes with the thumbs, index and middle fingers. Stretch the legs up and extend the trunk forwards. Straighten the arms, inhale, make the back concave, lift the chest and look up.

3 On the next exhalation, bend down farther by pulling on the toes, and take the head towards the feet.

Hold for 20–30 seconds, inhale and come up into Tadasana.

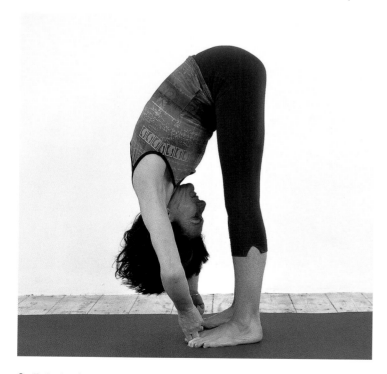

2 Exhale, bend the elbows out and extend the trunk down.

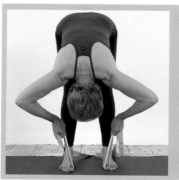

Modification
• If you are unable to reach the feet, use two straps wrapped around the toes, or rest the hands on blocks.
• If the back hurts, take the feet slightly wider apart and turn the toes inwards.

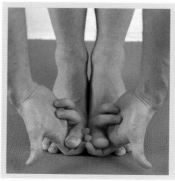

Focus
• Use the first two fingers on each hand to wrap firmly around the big toe so you can use the leverage to pull your top half down. Move further into the posture with each exhalation.

Eagle Pose
GARUDASANA

This is a balancing posture that keeps both ankles and shoulders flexible and is recommended for preventing cramps in the calf muscles. Concentration and balance are also improved.

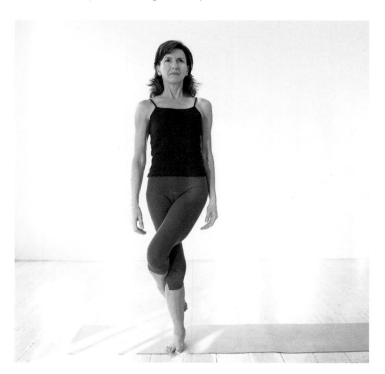

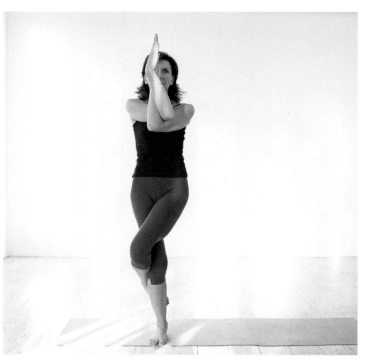

1 Stand in Tadasana. Exhale and slightly bend the right knee and cross the left thigh and knee over the right thigh. Take the left shin behind the right calf, and hook the left foot behind the right calf muscle.

Balance on the right foot, spreading out the foot, with the weight evenly distributed between the toes and heel. Ensure that both hips are level and face forwards. If the knees are painful, practise the pose with the legs in Tadasana and intertwine the arms only.

When first learning this posture, it is necessary to separate out the hand and foot movements, but eventually these will become one flowing movement.

2 Bend the elbows and lift them to shoulder level with the thumbs towards the face. Cross the right elbow over the left, intertwining the forearms, placing the palms together.

Hold for 15–20 seconds, release the arms and legs, come back to Tadasana and repeat on the other side, crossing right thigh over left and left elbow over right.

Modification
• To help with balance, do the posture with the back against the wall.
• To practise the leg work only, push the fingertips against a wall to hold you upright.
• In full posture, keep both knees facing forwards and extend the trunk upwards.

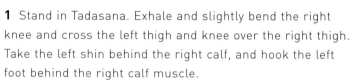

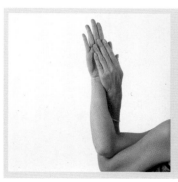

Focus
• Cross the right arm over the left, and touch palms.
• If you find it hard to balance, it may help to keep the eyes still, focusing on an object or a spot in the distance in front of you.

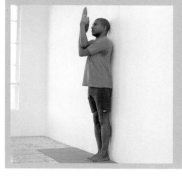

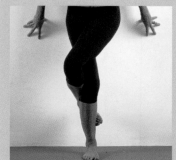

Fierce Pose
UTKATASANA

This pose is like sitting on an imaginary chair. It makes the shoulders and ankles more flexible and strengthens the legs. The abdominal organs and spine are toned and the chest is fully expanded.

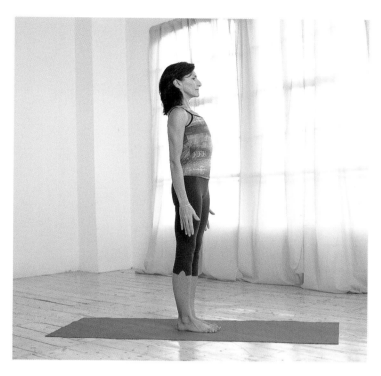

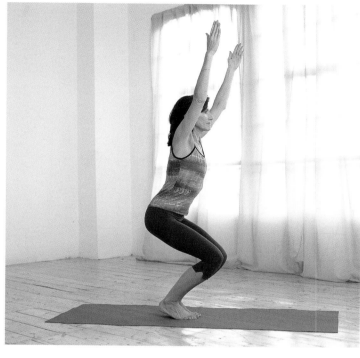

1 Stand in Tadasana – feet together, chest lifted, shoulders relaxed and down.

3 Exhale, bend the knees and lower the trunk down – as if you were going to sit on a chair.

Bend strongly in the ankle joints, press the heels down, bend in the knees, bend in the hips and stretch the arms strongly up. Keep the chest as far back as possible. If the elbows are straight, then join the palms.

Focus
• Bend more at the ankle and knee joints.
• Move the thighs down towards the floor while lifting the hips and trunk away from the legs.
• Although the trunk leans forwards, try to draw it back towards the vertical.

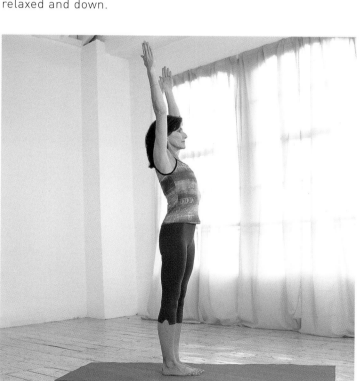

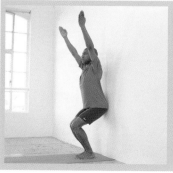

Modification
• It may be easier, at first, to rest against the wall to help with balance. Regular practice will help with stiff shoulders and ankles, strengthening the legs and activating the spine.

2 Inhale and extend the arms up towards the ceiling with the palms facing one another. Straighten the elbows and extend the palms and fingers up.

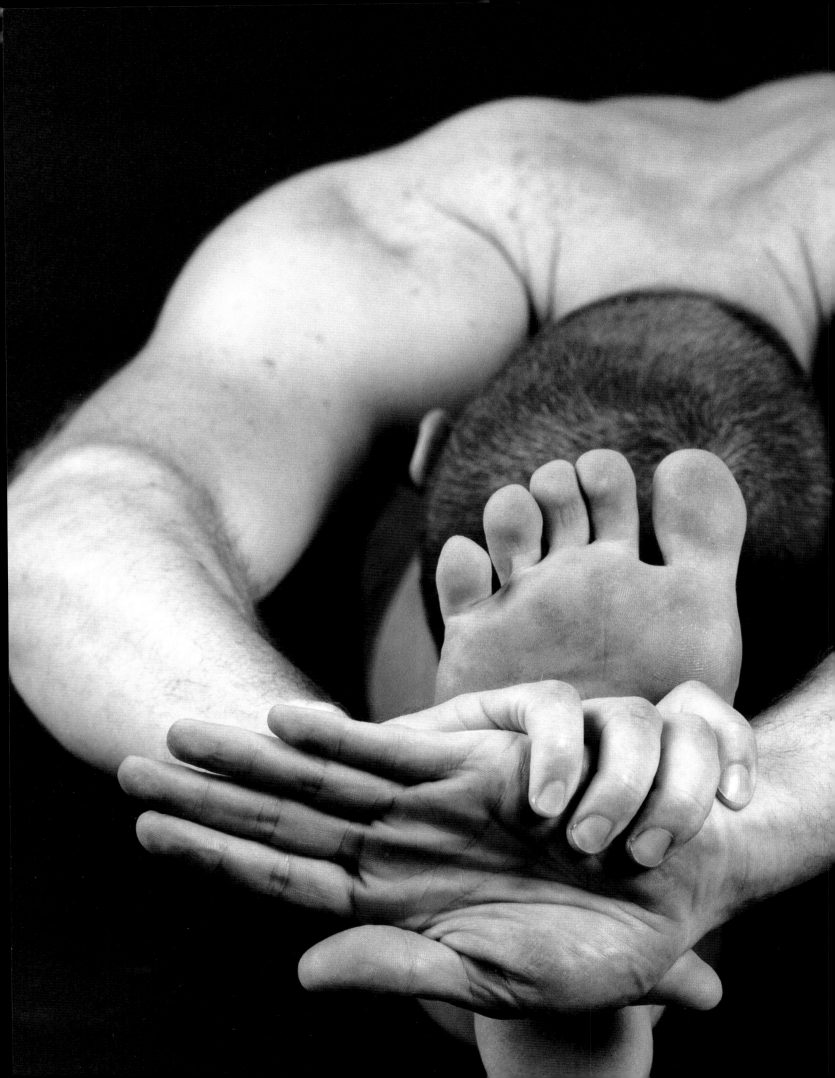

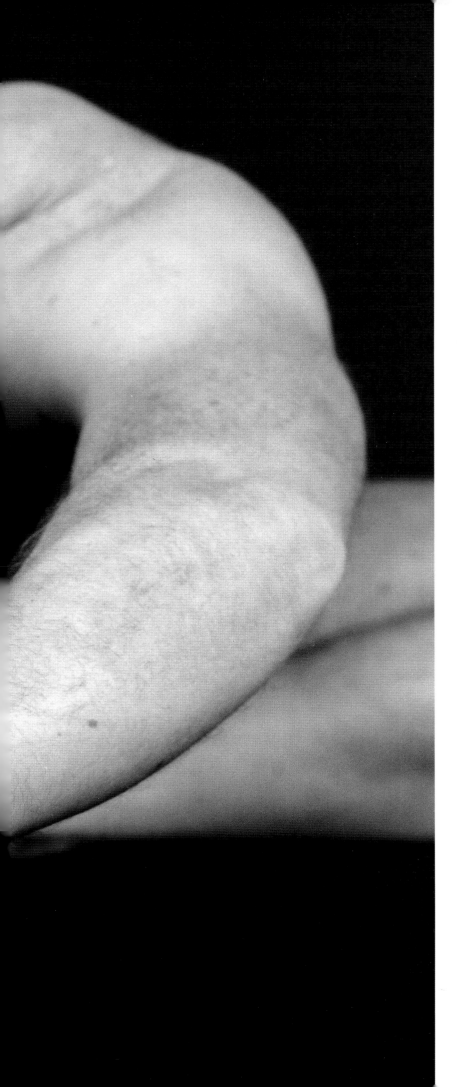

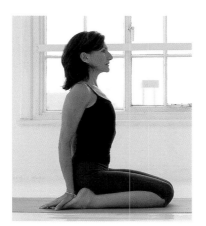

seated
Asanas

All seated postures improve flexibility to the hips, knees and ankles. They reduce tension in the diaphragm and throat, making breathing smoother and easier. They keep the spine firm, pacify the brain and stretch the muscles of the heart.

Simple Cross Legs
SUKHASANA

This posture keeps the knees and ankles flexible and nourishes the abdominal organs by encouraging blood circulation. Since the spine is erect in this pose, the mind stays alert and attentive.

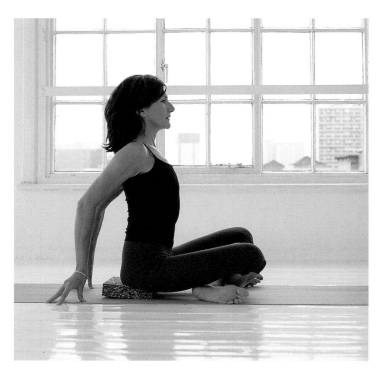

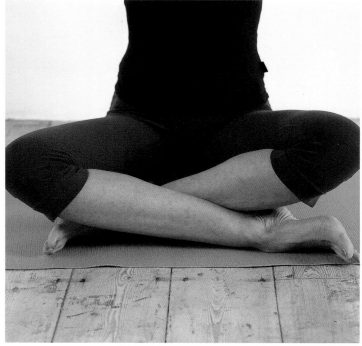

1 Sit on a foam block and cross the legs – place the left foot under the right thigh. Press the fingertips into the floor in order to lift the trunk.

3 Hold for 30–60 seconds. Change the crossover of the legs – so that the other shin-bone is in front – and repeat, extending the spine and then placing the hands on the knees again.

Soften the groin area so that the knees release down towards the floor. Note which shin-bone is in front. Cross at the shins, not the ankles, and ensure the shin-bones cross in line with the centre of the body.

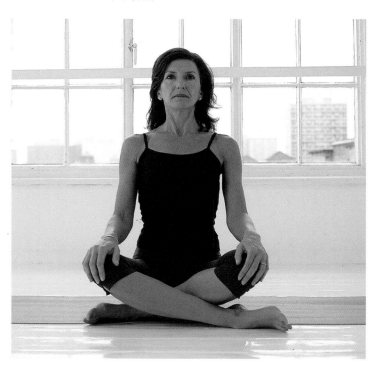

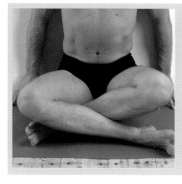

Focus
• Sukhasana can be done with the back against the wall, extending the spine up the wall.
• Broaden the base of the posture by spreading the buttocks to the sides.

2 Extend the spine up, take the shoulders back and open the chest. Maintain the extension of the spine and put the hands on the knees.

Hero Pose
VIRASANA

This pose stretches the tops of the feet, ankles and knees. It helps to relieve leg cramps and is a good remedy for indigestion. It also helps to correct flat feet and reduces discomfort in the legs.

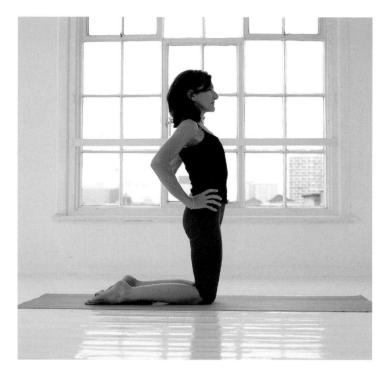

1 Kneel on a blanket or yoga mat with the knees together, the feet hip-width apart and the toes pointing straight back behind you.

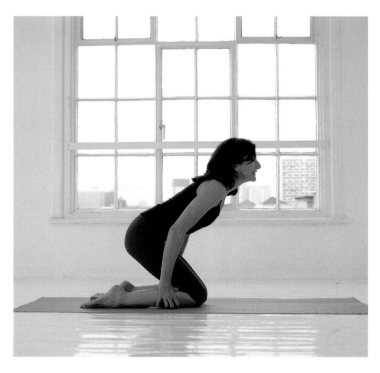

2 Sit between the feet, using the fingers to move the calf muscles away. If you cannot reach the floor comfortably, use a foam block or rolled-up blanket to raise you up.

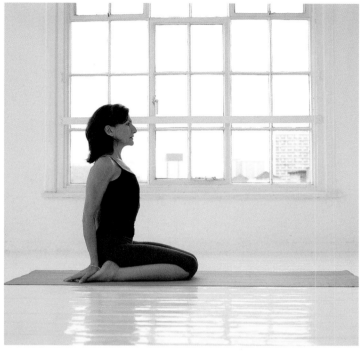

3 Put the palms of the hands on the soles of the feet (fingers pointing towards the toes) and stretch the trunk up. Take the shoulder blades into the body, lift the chest and extend the spine up.

Hold for 1–2 minutes, come out of the pose and straighten the legs.

Modification
• Sit on the edge of a foam block, or two, using as much support as is needed to alleviate knee pain.
• If the tops of the feet are painful, put them on a rolled-up blanket.
• If the knees are uncomfortable, put a rolled-up blanket between the calf and back thigh muscles.

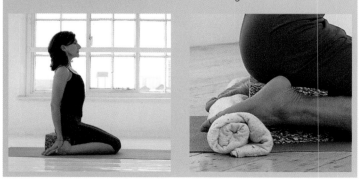

Hero Pose with Extended Arms
VIRASANA WITH PARVATASANA

This pose can also be done sitting in Sukhasana. It creates movement in the shoulder joints and develops the muscles of the chest. The abdominal organs are drawn in and the chest lifts and opens.

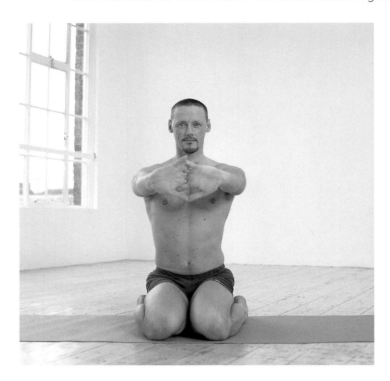

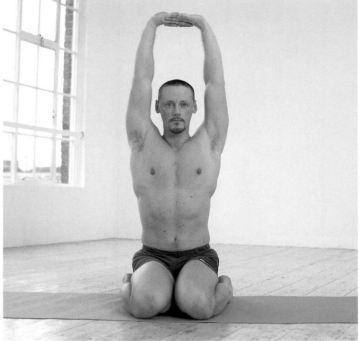

1 Sit in Virasana and interlock the fingers with the right index finger over the left.

Turn the palms away from you, stretch the arms forwards and straighten the elbows.

2 Extend the arms up with the elbows straight. The upper arms are in line with the ears and the palms are facing the ceiling.

Don't overarch in the lower back – extend the trunk and arms strongly upwards. Hold for 30–60 seconds, lower the arms, change the interlock of the fingers (i.e. left index finger over right) and repeat.

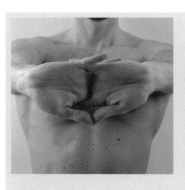
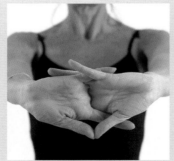

Focus
• Clasp the hands at the root of the fingers and, when extending the arms up, don't allow the fingers to slide apart.
• Change the interlock of the fingers halfway through this pose.

Modification
• If there is difficulty clasping the hands together due to stiffness in the shoulders, then use a strap. Practising this pose will help to relieve the problem.
• If the tops of the feet are painful, put them on a rolled-up blanket.

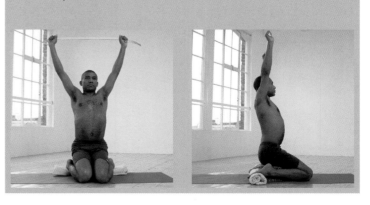

Hero Pose Forward Bend
ADHO MUKHA VIRASANA

This posture helps to soothe and calm the brain, as well as allowing the body to rest. It relieves fatigue and headaches, stretches and tones the spine and relieves back and neck pain.

1 Kneel on a blanket with the big toes together and the knees hip-width apart. Sit on the heels with the buttocks, and if they don't reach the heels, put a folded blanket on the heels.

Once the buttocks are down, extend the trunk forwards and put the forehead on the floor. Stretch both arms and the sides of the trunk forwards, and put the palms on the floor. Don't take the knees too far apart.

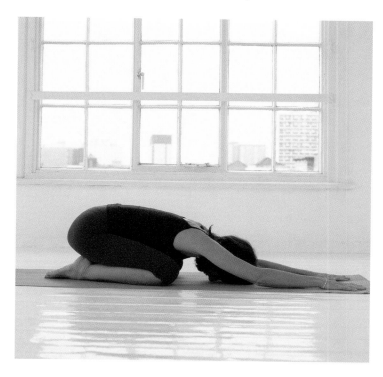

Modification
• The tailbone end of the spine must be supported on the heels. If this cannot be done, put a foam block between the buttocks and the heels.
• If the forehead cannot reach the floor, rest it on a foam block or a folded blanket.

Staff Pose
DANDASANA

This is the basic posture for seated poses and forward bends.
It teaches how to sit up straight and extend the spine up.

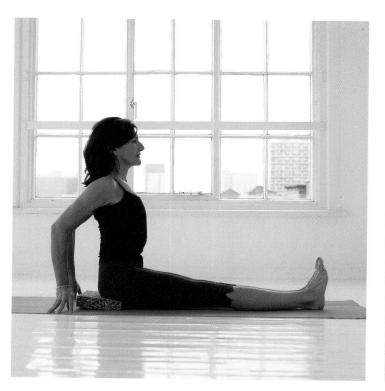

1 Sit on a raise with the legs stretched out in front. Keep the legs and feet together. Tighten the thigh muscles and knees, extend the heels forwards and extend the toes up towards the ceiling. Place the fingertips on the floor behind the hips, press into the floor and extend the trunk up. Don't overarch the lumbar spine. Roll the shoulders back, open the chest. Look straight ahead and relax the eyes. Move the shoulders away from the ears and the shoulder blades towards the front of the body.

Focus
• Balance the head on the spine centrally.
• Open the ribcage.
• Press the backs of the legs into the floor. Extend the inner heels away from the body, keeping feet upright.

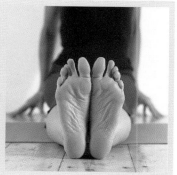

Head of Cow Pose
GOMUKHASANA (ARMS ONLY)

Gomukhasana expands the chest and gives flexibility to the shoulders. As the spine extends strongly upwards, the shoulder joints become less restricted. This pose also makes the wrists more flexible.

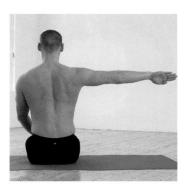 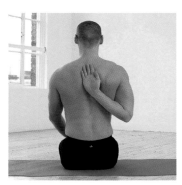

1 Sit in Sukhasana or Virasana and extend the right arm.

2 Bend the right arm behind the back and take the forearm up the back with the palm facing outwards.

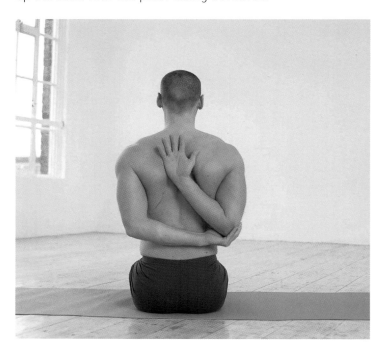

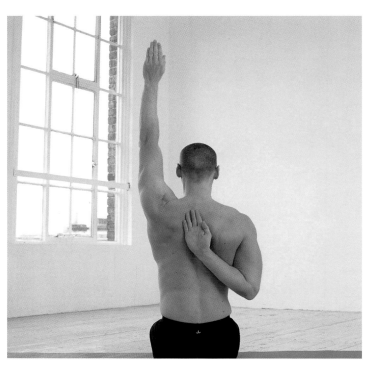

4 Extend the left arm up, turn the palm forwards, bend the elbow, put the palm of the hand below the nape of the neck and clasp the right hand.

3 Use the left hand to bring the right elbow closer to the trunk, so that the right hand moves farther up the back.

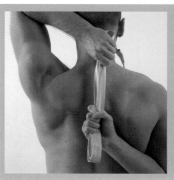

Modification
• Use a strap if the hands cannot grasp one another.
• Keep both sides of the trunk at an equal length and keep the head straight and the eyes level. Don't overarch the lower back.

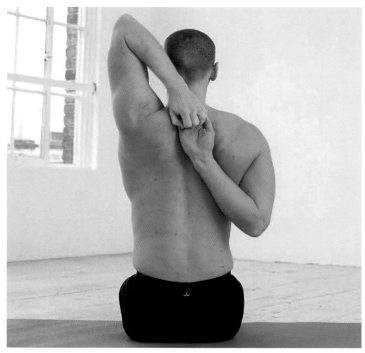

5 Roll the right shoulder back and stretch the left elbow towards the ceiling. Keep the trunk upright and look straight ahead. Hold for 30–60 seconds and repeat on the other side.

Cobbler Pose
BADDHAKONASANA

This pose keeps the knees and hips flexible. It stimulates the pelvis, abdomen and lower back and keeps the kidneys and prostate healthy. It strengthens the bladder and uterus and helps to reduce sciatic pain.

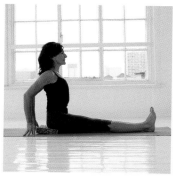 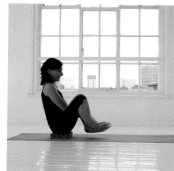

1 Sit in Dandasana on a folded blanket or foam block.

2 Taking the knees out to the side, bend the legs, and use the hands to bring the heels towards the groin.

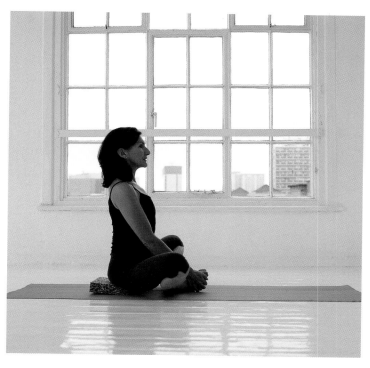

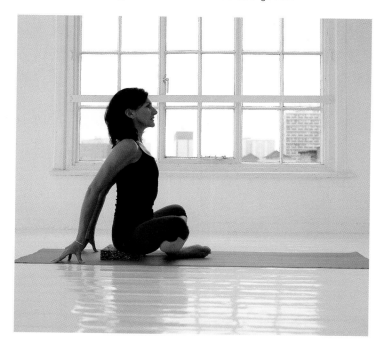

4 Keep the spine lifted, the chest open and hold the ankles, pressing the soles of the feet together.

Roll the shoulders back and down towards the floor, without overarching the lower back.

Hold for 30–60 seconds, release the ankles and come back to Dandasana.

3 With the fingertips on the floor beside the hips, lift up the trunk, take the shoulders back and open the chest.

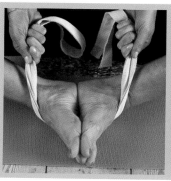

Modification
• If you cannot hold the ankles, use a strap.
• If it is difficult to sit up straight, sit with the back supported against a wall.
• Place a support under the knees to relieve the groin.

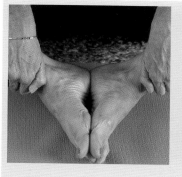 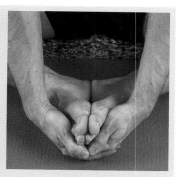

Focus
• Pull the feet in towards the groin as far as you can.
• In the final pose, hold the toes with the hands and lift from the base of the spine.

Seated Angle Pose
UPAVISTAKONASANA

This posture stretches the hamstrings and helps blood circulate in the pelvic region. It strengthens the muscles that support the bladder and uterus, relieves stiffness in the hip joints and alleviates sciatica.

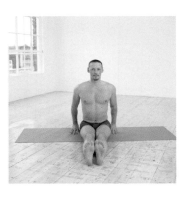 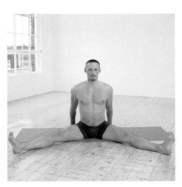

1 Sit in Dandasana on a blanket or mat with no support.

2 Take one leg out to the side, then the other, and widen the distance between the legs. Ensure that the centre of each knee, thigh and foot faces the ceiling. Put the fingertips on the floor behind the hips, press down and extend the spine and trunk upwards.

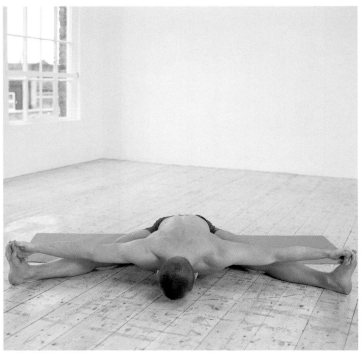

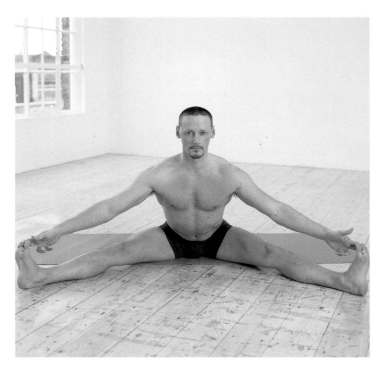

3 Keeping the spine erect, catch the big toes with the first two fingers of each hand and pull on them. Alternatively, put a strap around each foot. Hold the straps as close to the feet as possible.

Extend the spine, keeping the back concave and opening the chest. Look up.

4 Exhale, bend forwards and, keeping the spine stretched, extend the trunk along the floor, trying to get the chest as close to the floor as possible, breathing normally.

Hold for 30–60 seconds and come back to Dandasana.

Modification
- Sit against the wall to support the back.
- Sit on a foam block positioned by the wall for further support.
- Hold the feet with straps if it is difficult to reach.

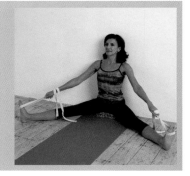

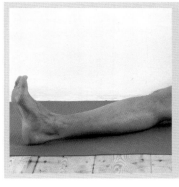

Focus
- Don't allow the feet to roll out. Keep the toes up.
- Extend the inner heels away from the body.
- Press the backs of the legs into the floor and keep the knees facing up.

Boat Pose
PARIPURNA NAVASANA

This pose increases the circulation in the abdomen and tones the abdominal muscles. It improves digestion and relieves lower backache by strengthening the spinal muscles. It also stimulates the thyroid gland.

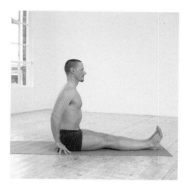
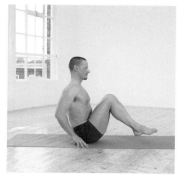

1 Sit in Dandasana on a blanket or mat with no support. Place the hands on the floor beside the hips.

2 Take the trunk slightly back, bend the knees and raise the bent legs, stretching them forwards.

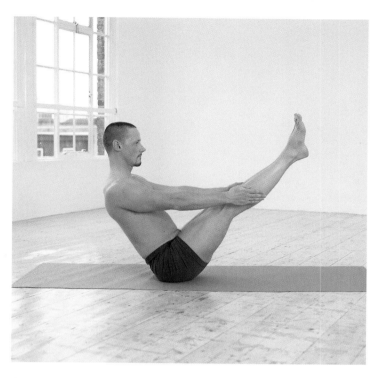

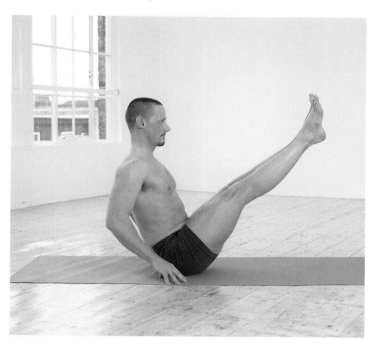

3 Keep both legs very straight (knees and thighs pulled up) and balance on the buttock bones. Raise the feet to 60 degrees, so that they are higher than the head.

4 Stretch both arms forwards, keeping them parallel to the floor with palms facing one another.

Keep stretching the spine and take it into the body so that the trunk doesn't collapse and the chest remains open.

Look straight ahead and make sure there is no tension or strain in the head and neck. There is a tendency to hold the breath in this pose, which causes tension in the eyes, so breathe normally throughout.

Hold for 30–60 seconds, exhale and come back to Dandasana.

Focus
- The abdominal and leg muscles are used to maintain the balance, not the back muscles.
- Don't collapse the lower back – move it into the body and upwards.
- Stretch the backs of the legs strongly.

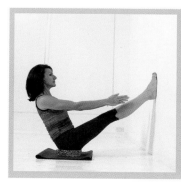

Modification
- If balancing on the buttock bones is difficult, keep the hands on the floor, or put the raised feet against the wall.
- If the back is painful, do the posture with bent knees.

Half Boat Pose
ARDHA NAVASANA

The difference between this pose and Paripurna Navasana is the height to which the legs are lifted. Keeping the legs lower tones the liver, gall bladder and spleen. It also strengthens the spinal muscles.

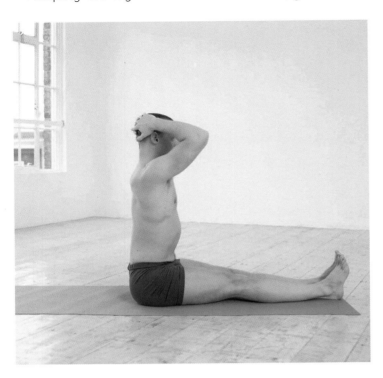

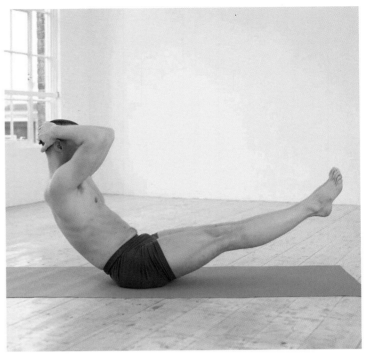

1 Sit in Dandasana on a blanket or mat with no support. Place the hands on the floor beside the hips.

Interlock the fingers and put the hands behind the head just above the neck. Bring the elbows slightly in so that the arms form a semi-circle.

2 Exhale, simultaneously taking the trunk slightly back and raising the legs from the floor to 30 degrees. Keep the knees and thighs pulled up, extend the backs of the legs towards the heels and keep the feet level with the head.

The body rests on the buttock bones and no part of the spine should touch the floor. Look towards the feet.

Breathe normally and keep the eyes soft. Don't strain the neck by pulling the head forwards with the clasped hands – the palms should touch the back of the head and the head should rest lightly on the palms.

Hold for 30–60 seconds, remembering to breathe normally.

Focus
• The difference between Paripurna Navasana and Ardha Navasana is that here the legs are raised to only 30 degrees, not to 60 degrees, and the body is not lowered.
• Interlock the fingers at the back of the head just above the neck.

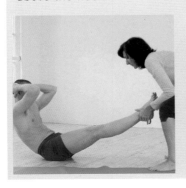

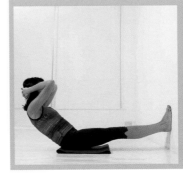

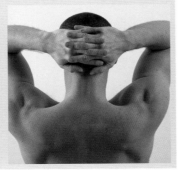

Modification
• If there is a problem with balance, position the raised feet flat against the wall. To hold this position for any length of time requires very strong abdominal muscles, so help may be required.

Head to Knee Pose
JANUSIRSASANA

Janusirsasana stimulates the digestive system, tones the abdominal muscles and brings the brain and heart into a restful state. Forward bends are beneficial for a good night's sleep.

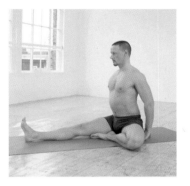
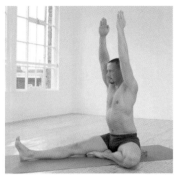

1 Sit in Dandasana on a support, bend the left knee to the side and place the left foot so that the big toe touches the inside of the right thigh.

2 Inhale and extend both arms straight up to the ceiling, moving the shoulder blades into the body. The upper arms are beside the ears. Stretch the spine upwards.

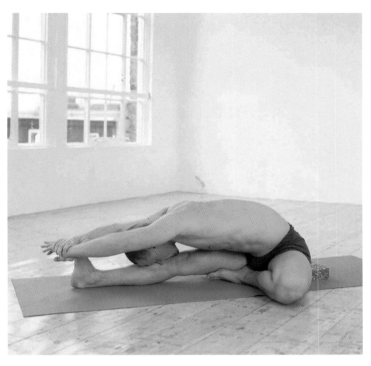

4 Exhale, widen the elbows out to the side, extend the trunk further forwards and take the head down.

Hold for 30–60 seconds, inhale, release the foot, come up and repeat on the other side.

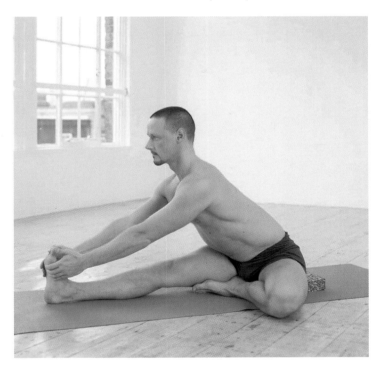

3 Exhale, bend forwards and catch the sides of the right foot with both hands. Make the spine concave and look up. If the lower back aches, do not proceed any further.

Focus
• Keep the right leg straight with the toes pointing up. Press the back of the right leg down on to the floor.

Modification
• If you can't reach the right foot, use a strap around the foot, holding it in a "V" shape with both hands.
• If you are able to catch the foot, hold it around the sides of the foot, not the toes.
• If the lower back is painful, rest the forehead on a stool or bolster.
• Sit on a foam block and support the bent knee on a foam block if it is uncomfortable.

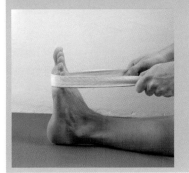
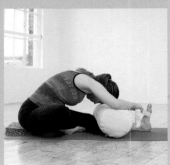

Forward Bend with One Leg Bent Back
TRIANGA MUKHAIKAPADA PASCIMOTTANASANA

This posture improves flexibility of the ankles and knees. It also helps to tone the abdominal muscles and organs.

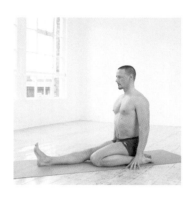 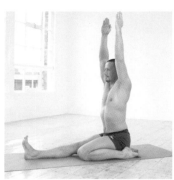

1 Sit in Dandasana on a support. Bend the left leg back and place the foot beside the left hip.

2 Inhale and extend the arms up, palms facing and upper arms beside the ears. Extend the spine and trunk.

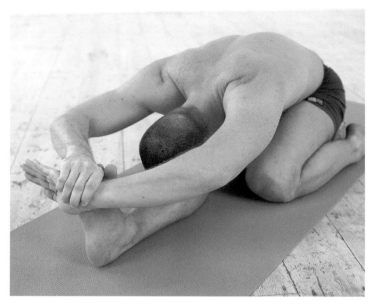

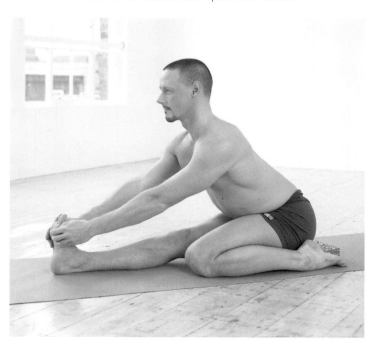

3 Exhale, extend the trunk forwards and clasp the right foot.

4 Inhale, lengthen the spine upwards, make the back concave and look up. Exhale, extend the trunk forwards, elongating the spine and taking the head towards the right leg. Widen the elbows out to the side.

Hold for 1–2 minutes, inhale, release the foot, raise the head and come up. Repeat on the other side.

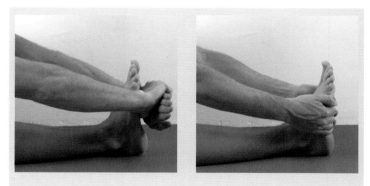

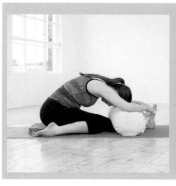

Modification
• An easy version is to rest the head on a bolster or rolled-up blanket.
• It may also help to sit on a raise – a folded blanket or a foam block are both good for this.

Focus
• Try to catch the hands around the foot. If you can't manage this at first, then use a strap, or clutch the foot on either side, but not the toes.
• Press both buttocks down towards the floor. Pull on the foot (or strap) to lengthen the spine and open the chest.
• Move the shoulders away from the ears and relax the neck and head.

Full Forward Bend
PASCIMOTTANASANA

This posture tones and activates the abdominal organs, aids digestion and rejuvenates the spine. As the body is in a horizontal position in forward bend poses, there is less strain on the heart.

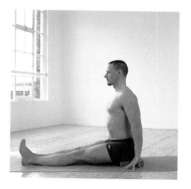
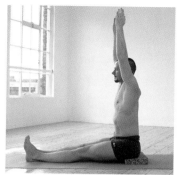

1 Sit in Dandasana on a support.

2 Inhale, extend the arms up (palms facing), keeping the upper arms besides the ears.

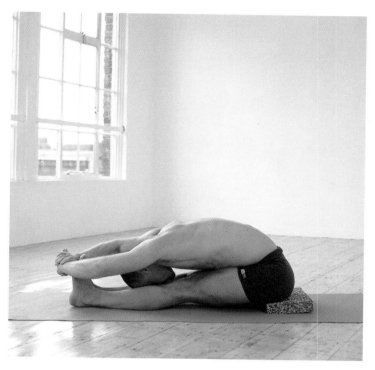

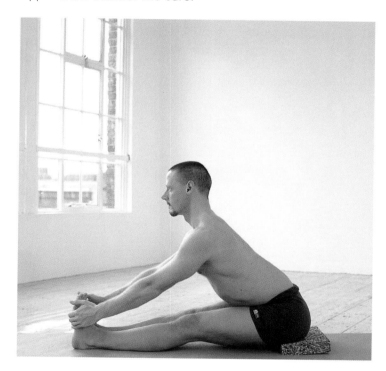

3 Exhale, extend the trunk forwards, clasp the sides of both feet with the hands (or use a strap). Inhale and extend forwards, make the back concave, lift the chest and look up.

4 Exhale, continue extending the spine/trunk forwards over the legs and catch the hands around the foot (or reach further with the strap). Bend the elbows out to the side.

Fully extend the front of the body and the sides of the trunk. Take the head down. If the back aches, rest the head on a bolster or stool. Hold for 30–60 seconds, inhale and come up.

Focus
• Press the backs of the legs down into the floor to extend the spine more.
• Extend the inner heels away, with toes stretching towards the ceiling.
• Pull on the feet or the strap to lengthen the trunk.

Modification
• If the backs of the knees are painful when pressed into the floor, place a rolled-up blanket under the knees.
• If the forehead cannot reach the floor, rest it on a foam block or a folded blanket.
• In cases of extreme stiffness, or pain in the back, rest the head on a stool covered with a blanket.

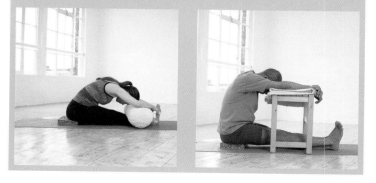

Garland Pose
MALASANA

In this pose the arms hang from the neck like a garland. It relieves lower back pain and reduces stiffness in the knees and ankles. It also activates and nourishes the abdominal organs.

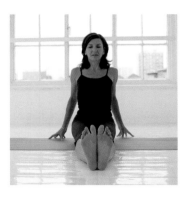
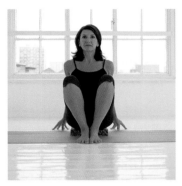

1 Sit in Dandasana on a support.

2 Bend the knees and come up into a squatting position.

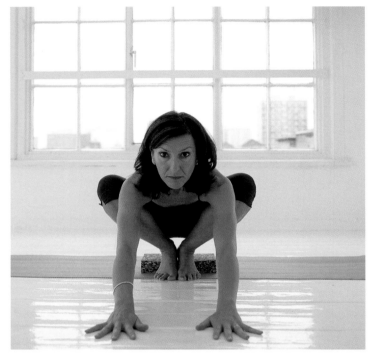

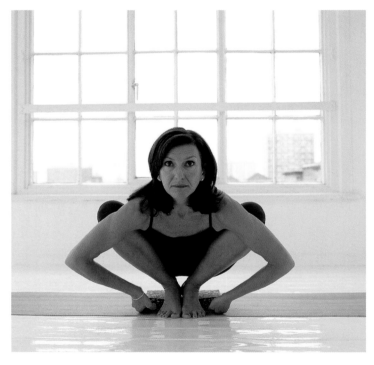

3 Keep the feet together and support the heels by pulling the support forwards underneath the heels. Separate the thighs and knees and extend the trunk forwards between the legs.

Focus
- If the heels come off the support, add another support. The heels must press on to something.
- The inner thighs lightly grip the sides of the trunk.
- Extend the spine and lengthen the side ribs.
- Round the back when taking the head down.

4 Stretch the arms forwards, pressing the palms into the floor, extend the spine towards the head and look up. Wrap the arms around the legs.

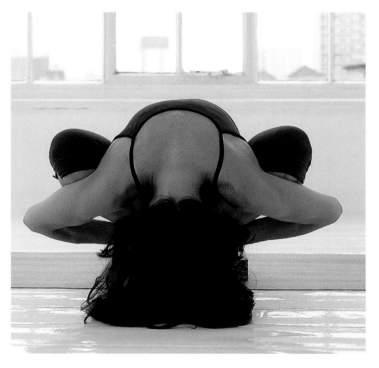

5 Exhale, bend forwards and take the head down towards the floor. Hold the ankles with the hands. Hold for 30–60 seconds and then come up.

Lotus
PADMASANA

Exercise extreme caution when attempting this posture. If the knees are painful, stop immediately and practise Sukhasana as a preparation for Padmasana.

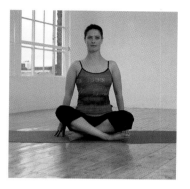 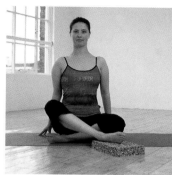

1 Sit in Simple Cross Legs pose (Sukhasana), with the right shin-bone crossed in front.

2 Bring the right foot forwards, supporting it on a foam block if necessary.

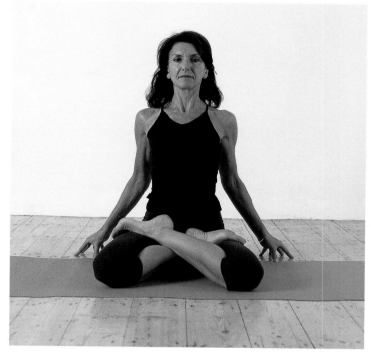

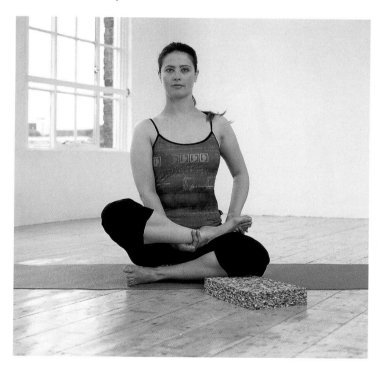

3 Carefully lift the right foot and place it as high up on the left thigh as possible.

Bring the left foot forwards and support it on a block on the other side.

Lift the left foot on to the right thigh. If there is pain in the knees, sit in half-Padmasana, i.e. first leg in Padmasana and second leg in Sukhasana.

4 Press the fingertips into the floor beside the hips to extend the spine up. Continue to lift from the base of the spine upwards through the neck to the top of the head.

Hold for 30–60 seconds. Release the legs, and repeat with the left shin-bone crossed in front of the right.

Many people will find they lack the flexibility in the knees to do this posture at first, but in time suppleness will increase and the posture will become comfortable. Changing the cross of the legs regularly means that they will develop evenly on both sides.

Focus
• When bending the knee, to avoid straining and to create space, use the fingers to draw the top of the calf muscle and the bottom of the back thigh muscle away from the back of the knee.
• For painful knees, place a strap at the back of the knee and pull on it as you take the leg into Padmasana.
• If the right knee doesn't reach the floor, support it on a foam block, then take the left leg into Padmasana.

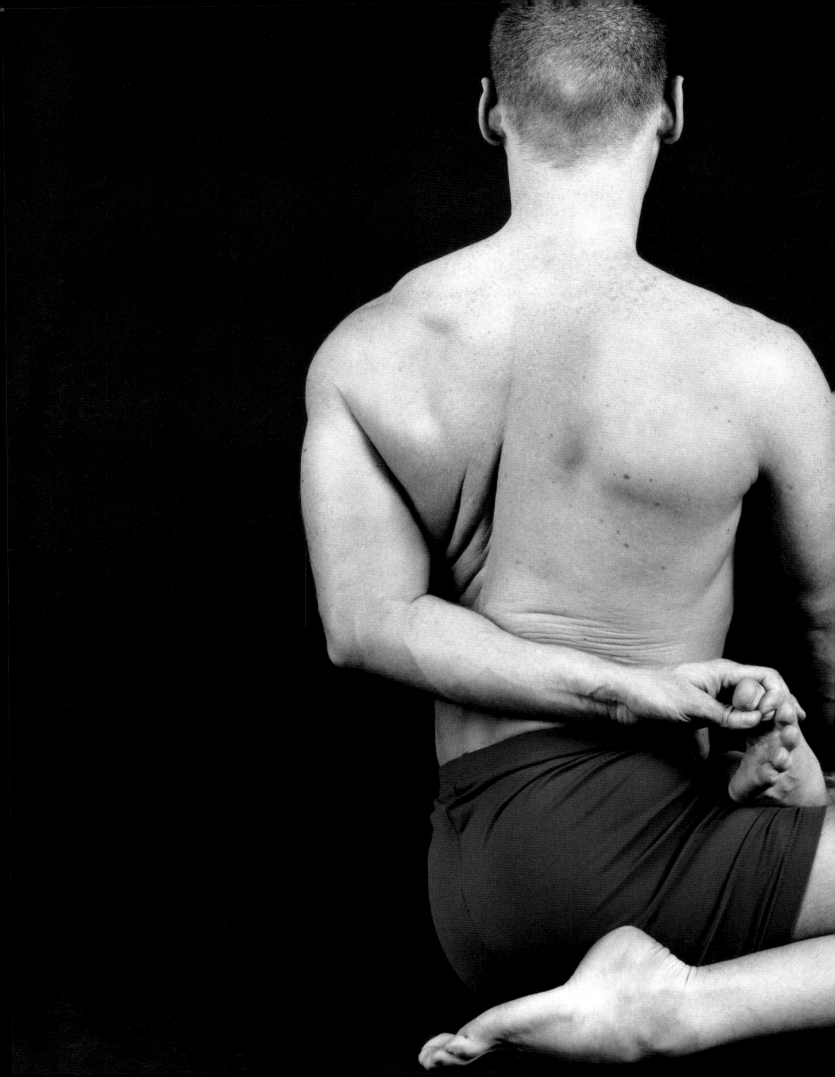

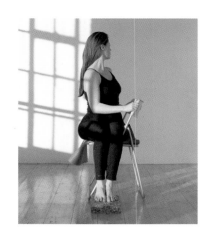

Twists

All lateral extension postures (twists) create flexibility in the spine and shoulders. They activate and nourish the pelvic and abdominal organs, and bring relief to back, hip and groin problems. As the spine becomes more supple, blood flow to the spinal nerves improves, and energy levels are raised. When practising twists, lift the spine first, and then turn the abdomen, chest and finally the head. Moving the shoulder blades into the back will improve the turn.

Standing Twist
STANDING MARICYASANA

This posture reduces stiffness in the neck and shoulders. It improves the alignment of the spine and strengthens the spinal muscles. It also relieves lower back pain and sciatica.

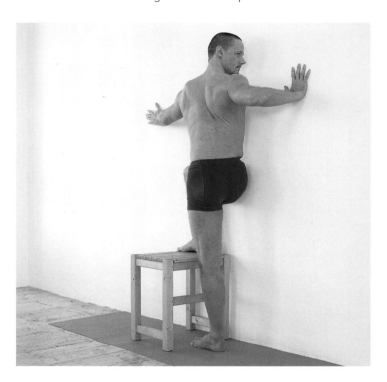

1 Put a stool near the wall. Stand in Tadasana with the wall on your right. Bend the right knee and place the foot on the stool, keeping the right thigh against the wall.

Inhale, stretch the left leg strongly up and keep the toes of this foot facing forwards. Extend the trunk towards the ceiling. Exhale, turn the front body to face the wall, and place the hands on the wall at shoulder level.

Inhale, extend trunk further, exhale, press the hands into the wall to enable the trunk to turn more to the right. Turn as far as you can, look over the right shoulder. Hold for 20–40 seconds, release, and repeat on the other side.

Focus
• Don't allow the front body to lean towards the wall.
• Move the shoulder blades into the body and downwards towards the waist to open the chest.

Easy Pose Twist
SUKHASANA (TWIST)

In this easy, cross-legged twist, use the breath to lift and turn. Relax the shoulders, moving them away from the ears and into the body.

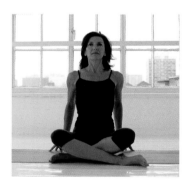

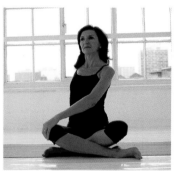

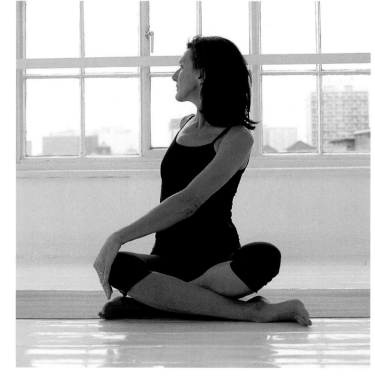

1 Sit in step 1 of Sukhasana, with the fingertips on the floor.

2 Place the palm of the left hand on the outer right thigh. Inhale, press the right fingertips into the floor and extend the spine upwards. Exhale, press the left palm into the thigh and turn towards the right.

3 Look over the right shoulder. Hold for 30–40 seconds, release and repeat to the other side, changing the cross of the legs.

Hero Pose Twist
VIRASANA (TWIST)

This pose strengthens the abdominal muscles and relieves indigestion. Lower backache is eased, the hips become more flexible and the hamstring muscles more supple.

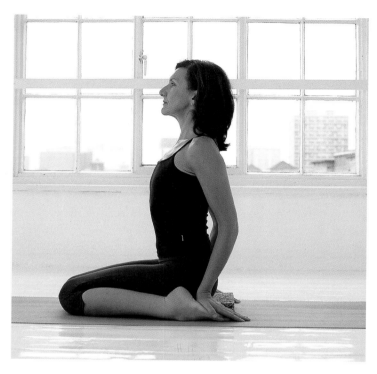

1 Sit in Virasana with the soles of the feet facing the ceiling, and the palms on the feet.

Sit on a foam block or folded blanket if this helps.

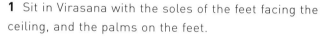

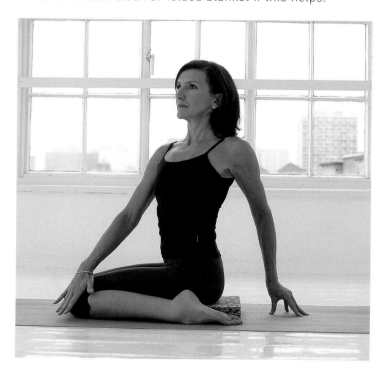

2 Put the left fingertips on the floor/block beside the left hip, and put the right palm on the left thigh.

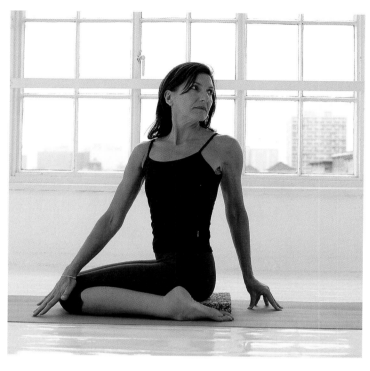

3 Inhale, press the left fingers into the floor and lift the trunk. Exhale, press the right palm into the left thigh and turn to the left. With each exhalation, turn the abdomen, waist, chest and shoulders further to the left and look over the left shoulder.

Hold for 30–60 seconds, release and repeat on the other side.

Focus
• Keep the shoulders relaxed, moving them down, away from the ears and into the body.
• Try to turn a little more with each exhalation.
• Use the breath to lift and turn.

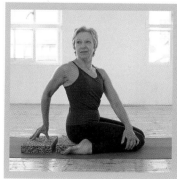

Modification
• Sit on a wooden or foam block and use another block to place the fingertips on, behind the body.
• As with all directional poses, start with the right side and repeat on the left.

Simple Twist Using a Chair
BHARADVAJASANA (CHAIR)

This twist is an easier version of Bharadvajasana I. The chair is used to allow a safe and effective rotation of the trunk. It relieves a stiff back, neck and shoulders, and exercises the abdominal muscles.

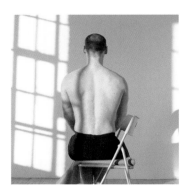 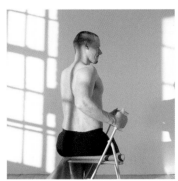

1 Sit on a chair with the right side of the body facing the chair-back. Keep the knees and feet together. Sit up straight and look straight ahead.

2 Inhale, extend the spine up and put the hands on the back of the chair.

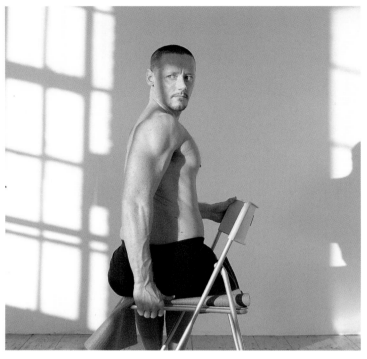

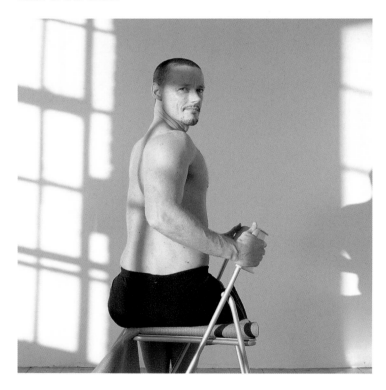

3 Exhale, and turn the trunk to the right, using the hands to help you turn.

Inhale, lift the spine further, take the shoulder blades into the body and open the chest. Rotate the spine further so that the chest is parallel to the back of the chair. Keep the neck free from tension or strain.

4 Exhale, turn the trunk more and look over the right shoulder. Grip the back of the seat for leverage. Hold for 20–30 seconds, exhale, release the hands, face forwards and repeat on the other side.

Focus
• Press the feet firmly into the floor to lift the trunk.
• Press the left buttock down towards the seat of the chair – it wants to lift. Use the inhalation to extend the spine; use the exhalation to turn it.

Modification
• This twist can be made easier by raising the feet, or by placing a block between the knees.

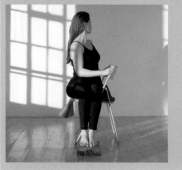 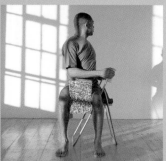

Simple Twist
BHARADVAJASANA I

This twisting posture creates flexibility in the neck and shoulders and relieves lower back pain. It reduces pain in the knees and tones the abdominal organs, particularly the kidneys, liver, spleen and gall bladder.

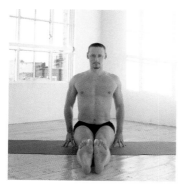

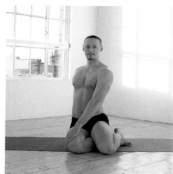

1 Sit in Dandasana on a support.

2 Bend both legs to the left, placing the feet beside the left hip. Put the left foot on top of the arch of the right foot.

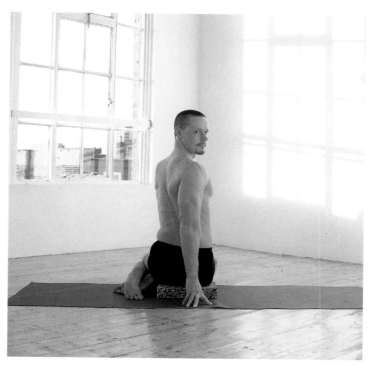

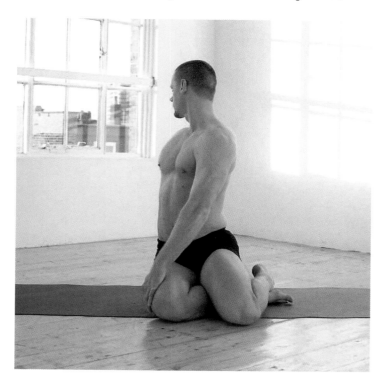

3 Keep the soles of both feet facing the ceiling.

Extend the trunk and spine up. Put the right fingertips beside the right hip and the palm of the left hand on the right knee.

Inhale, press the right fingers into the floor to lift the spine.

Exhale, press the left palm against the right knee to turn the trunk to the right.

4 Repeat, turning the abdomen, waist, chest and shoulders further with each exhalation.

Look over the right shoulder, hold for 30–40 seconds, exhale, release and repeat on the other side.

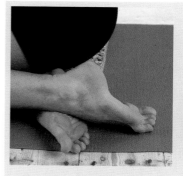

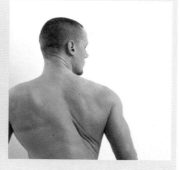

Focus
• Rest the left foot over the instep of the right foot.
• Press the left buttock down towards the floor to get the whole spine turning.
• Use the breath to lift and turn.
• Draw the shoulder blades down and into the body to lift the spine and open the chest.

Catching Arms Behind
MARICYASANA I (TWIST ONLY)

This spinal twist removes stiffness in the shoulders and spine and reduces lower backache. As there is an increased blood flow to the abdominal organs, digestion improves and the organs become toned.

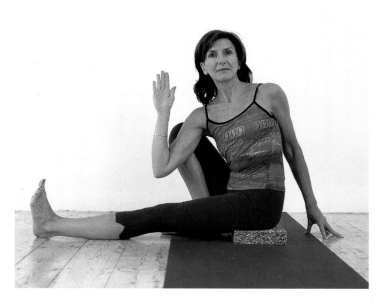

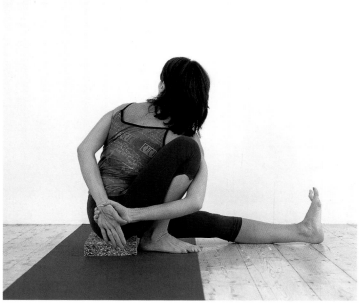

1 Sit in Dandasana on a support. Keep the fingertips pressing into the floor beside the hips. Bend the right leg so that the knee faces the ceiling and the right heel is in line with the right buttock bone, toes pointing forwards.

Extend the left leg along the floor. Turn the trunk to the left and take the right elbow in front of the right knee (fingers pointing to the ceiling). Rotate the trunk more to the left.

2 Press the left fingertips into the floor to lengthen the spine. Wrap the right arm around the right leg and take it behind the body.

Turn the left shoulder slightly back and swing the left arm behind the back, catching hold of it with the right hand. If the hands don't reach, use a strap.

Turn the trunk as far as possible to the left, turn the head and look over the left shoulder. Move the back ribs and shoulder blades into the body to open the chest, and turn more. Extend the front of the body from the pubis to the chin. Hold for 20–30 seconds, then release and repeat on the other side.

Modification
• To ease your body into this posture, use a block under the floor hand and a lift to sit on.
• If you cannot reach your hands behind your back, use a strap. Fold the strap in two and grasp it firmly behind you, pulling the arms around.

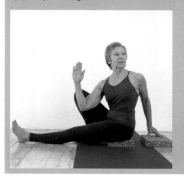

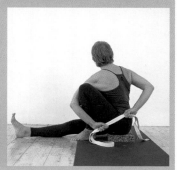

Focus
• Keep the knee of the bent leg facing the ceiling throughout, and the heel close to the body.
• Press the sole of the right foot into the floor to lift the spine as much as possible.
• Move the shoulder blades into the body and down towards the floor to extend and rotate the spine more.
• The full posture, and Maricyasana II, combine a twist with a forward bend suitable for advanced yogis only.

Sitting Twist
MARICYASANA III

This stronger twist increases energy levels. As there is a vigorous rotation, the abdominal organs such as liver, spleen, pancreas, kidneys and intestines are toned and massaged, improving their performance and function.

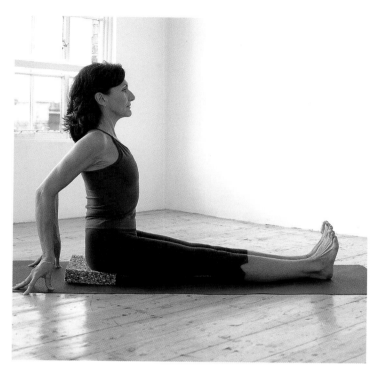

1 Sit in Dandasana on a support. Lift the spine upwards.

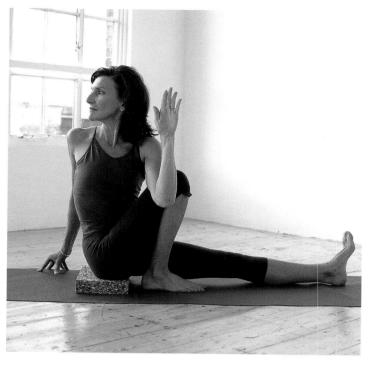

3 Try to get the left armpit closer to the knee. Inhale, press the right fingers into the floor and lift the spine.

Exhale, press the left arm against the knee and the knee against the arm, and turn further to the right.

Repeat the lift and turn. Move the spine into the body, take the shoulder blades into the back and turn further. Look over the right shoulder. Rotate the left side of the ribcage, the left armpit and the left hip towards the right to increase the turn of the spine. Keep the chest lifted and open by moving the shoulders down and the shoulder blades forwards.

Hold for 30–60 seconds, release and repeat on the other side.

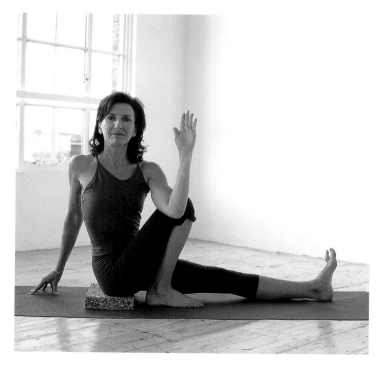

2 Bend the right knee up towards the ceiling, and put the sole of the foot on the floor in line with the right buttock bone. Turn to the right. Put the fingertips of the right hand on the floor/block behind the right hip. Bend the left arm and place the elbow on the outside of the right knee.

Focus
• Press the right foot firmly into the floor, especially the big toes and inner heel, and press the back of the left leg into the floor and stretch it forwards, toes facing up.
• Use the breath to lift and turn.
• Ensure that the bent knee stays facing the ceiling – when placing the bent arm over the knee, don't push it out of alignment.

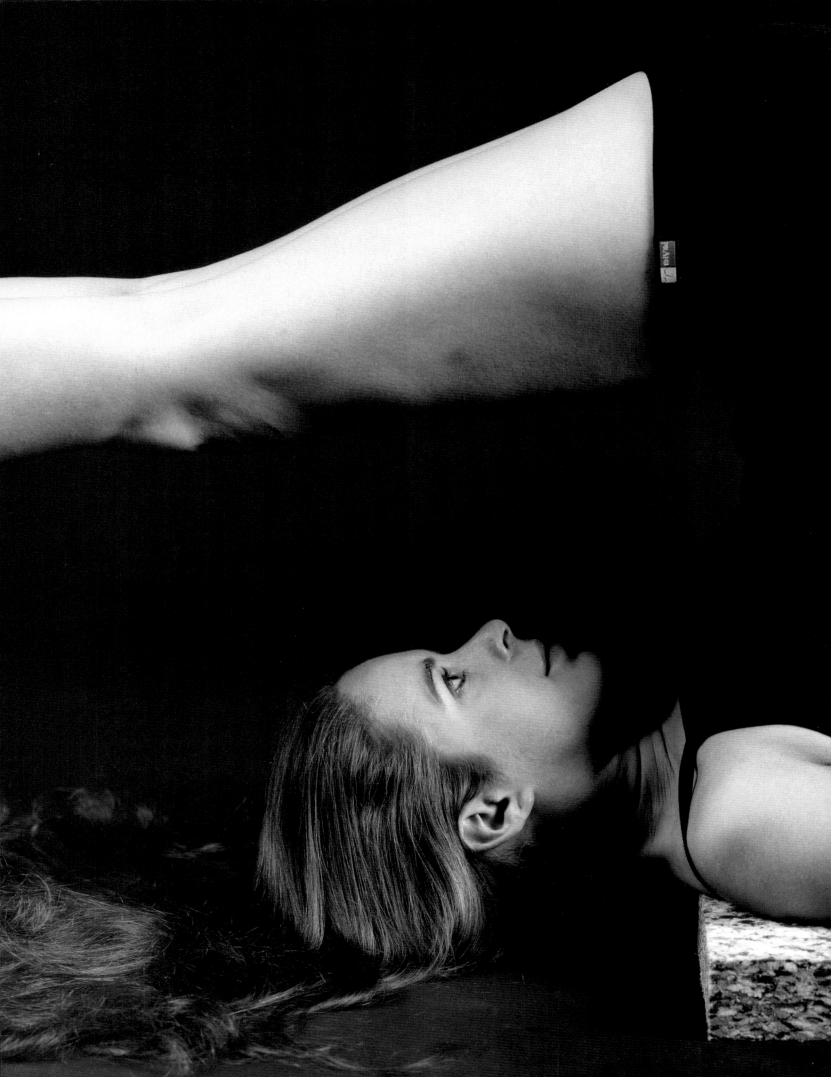

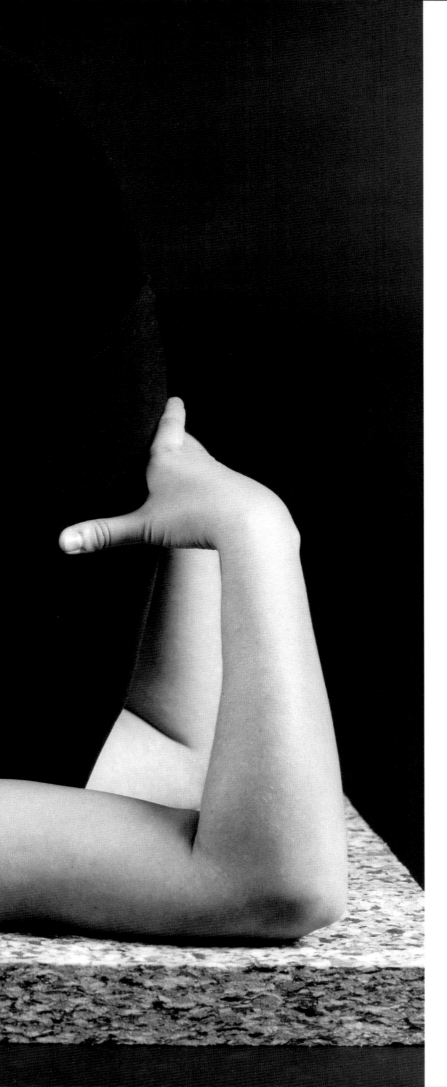

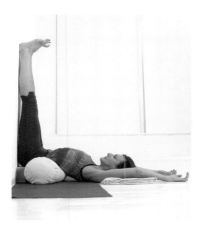

inverted
Asanas

All inverted postures revitalize the entire system of the body. Because the internal organs are inverted, they become energized, and the brain is nourished as blood flow towards it is increased. Since there is no weight on the legs, inversions bring relief to tired, strained legs. Women should not practise any inversions during menstruation as this interferes with the natural flow of blood at this time.

Legs Up the Wall Pose

VIPARITA KARANI

This restorative pose calms the brain, opens the chest and rests the legs. It helps reduce respiratory problems, eases headaches and relieves indigestion and nausea. It is also beneficial for preventing varicose veins.

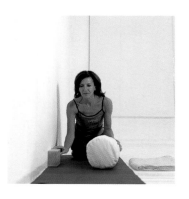
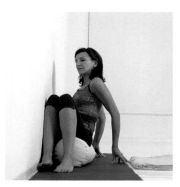

1 Put a wooden block against the wall with a bolster in front and a folded blanket in front of the bolster.

2 Sit on the bolster, sideways to the wall with the hip touching the wall.

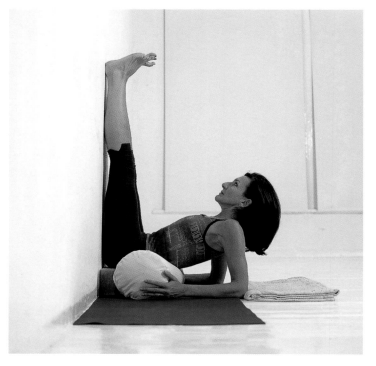

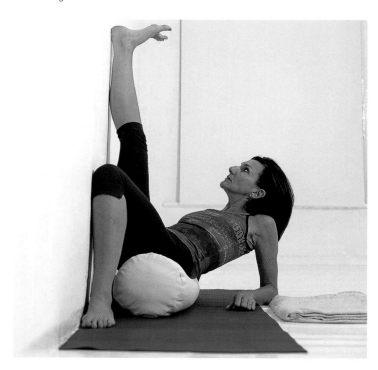

3 Swivel the trunk around, using the hands to balance. Take one leg up the wall, keep the buttocks against the wall and straighten the second leg.

Focus
• Keep the inner edges of the feet together so that the soles of the feet are parallel to the ceiling.
• Keep the abdomen soft and press the shoulders into the floor.

4 Once both legs are up the wall, carefully take the trunk down and lower the shoulders and head on to the floor. Keep the backs of the legs and buttocks against the wall and open the chest.

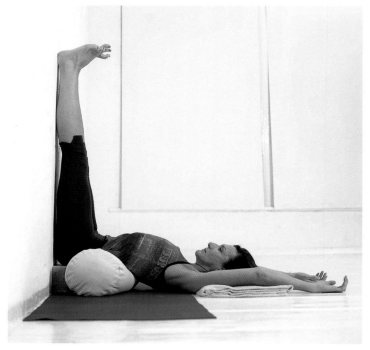

5 Take the arms over the head, breathe evenly and relax. Hold for 5–6 minutes and then come down.

Supported Shoulder Stand
SALAMBA SARVANGASANA

This is known as the queen, or mother, of the postures. It supports the thyroid gland, frees the body of toxins and is beneficial for relieving respiratory problems such as asthma, congestion and sinusitis.

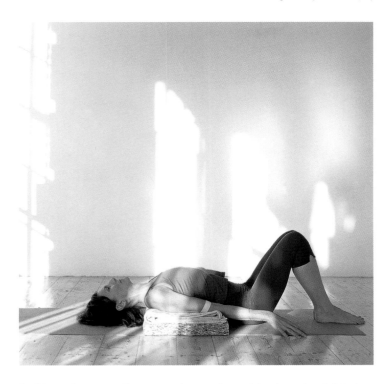

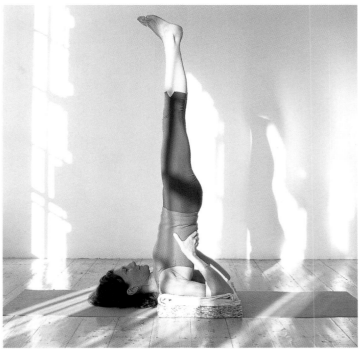

1 Place four small, or one large, foam block and a folded blanket on the mat for comfort. Lie with the shoulders and arms on the support and the head on the floor.

Stretch the arms towards the feet and move the shoulders away from the head.

3 Lift the hips and trunk and immediately support the back with the palms of both hands. Straighten the legs and move the hands up the back towards the shoulder blades to increase the lift of the chest. Bring the chest towards the chin and stretch the whole body straight up. Look towards the chest. Hold for 2–5 minutes.

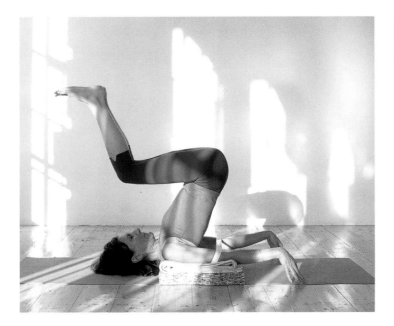

Focus
• Press the hands into the back to move the back ribs towards the front of the chest and to lift the trunk. Press the upper arms into the support.
• If the elbows slip apart, tie a belt around the upper arms (just above the elbows) to keep them shoulder-width.
• Stretch the legs up and keep the soles of the feet parallel to the ceiling – rest the toes on a wall for balance.

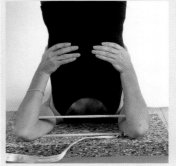

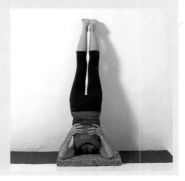

2 Bend the knees towards the chest. Press the fingertips into the floor, and take the knees towards the head.

Supported Shoulder Stand
SALAMBA SARVANGASANA (AGAINST WALL)

This is an easier version of the shoulder stand. If pressure is experienced in the head while in Salamba Sarvangasana, come down immediately and try the pose against the wall or using a chair.

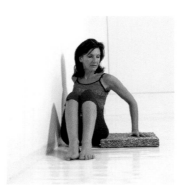

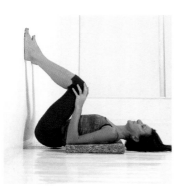

1 Sit as close as possible to the wall and place a foam block just under your left buttock.

2 Lean back, swivel the trunk around and take one leg, and then the second, up the wall. Keep the buttocks against the wall, the shoulders near the edge of the support and the head on the floor.

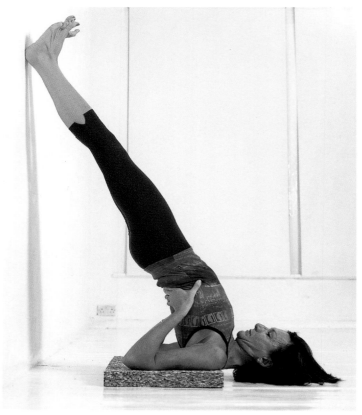

4 Straighten the legs, press the heels firmly into the wall and lift the chest, trunk and hips. Hold for 2–5 minutes, bend the legs and come down.

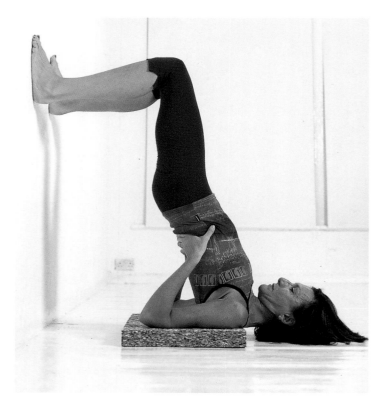

3 Press the feet into the wall and raise the hips and chest. Support the back with the hands and move the elbows towards one another.

Modification
• If you cannot manage Salamba Sarvangasana alone or against a wall, get someone to assist you by holding your legs upright. Begin by resting your feet on their thighs, then allow them to correct your alignment.
• Once you have done the posture with help, you may find it easier to achieve on your own.

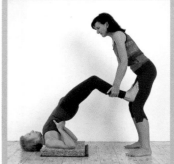

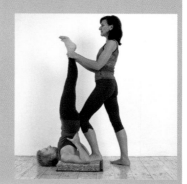

Shoulder Balance in Chair
CHAIR SARVANGASANA

In the classic Salamba Sarvangasana posture, the hands support the back. In this modified version, a chair is used and this allows the pose to be held for longer with minimal strain on the neck and back.

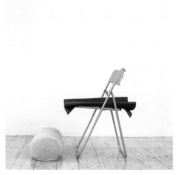

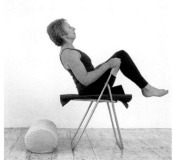

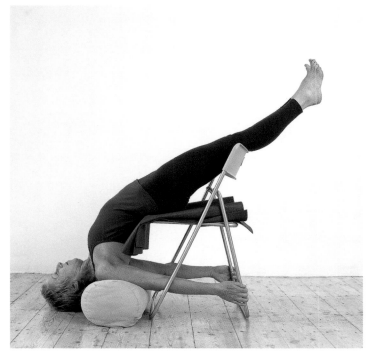

1 Place a bolster on the floor parallel to the front legs of the chair. Fold a mat and put it on the seat of the chair.

2 Sit on the chair and bend the legs over the back of the chair. Hold on to the sides of the chair. Lean the trunk slightly back.

4 Straighten one leg at a time. When both legs are straight, slide the hands further down the back chair legs to increase the stretch of the arms. Move the shoulders away from the ears and the shoulder blades towards the head to open and lift the chest.

Breathe normally and look towards the chest. Hold the pose for up to 5 minutes, keeping the back of the neck soft.

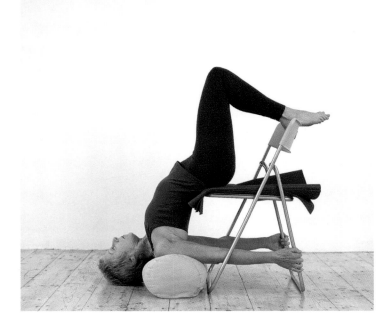

3 Lower the back on to the seat of the chair. Slide the buttocks and back towards the front edge of the chair seat. Carefully rest the shoulders on the bolster and the back of the head on the floor. Hold the back chair legs.

Focus
• As with other inversions, Chair Sarvangasana should not be practised during menstruation.

Coming out of the posture
• Return first one leg, then the other, to step 3. Begin to release the grip of the hands on the chair legs and gently push the chair slightly away.
• Slide the back then buttocks on to the bolster, pushing the chair by the seat. Rest for a moment, roll over to the side, slide off the bolster and come up.

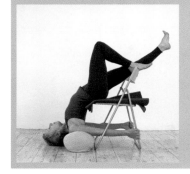

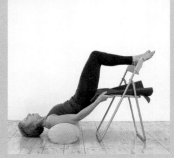

Half Plough Pose
ARDHA HALASANA

This supported version of Halasana reduces the effects of fatigue, anxiety and insomnia, and relieves stress-related headaches. If you have lower back pain, practising Ardha Halasana will not aggravate it.

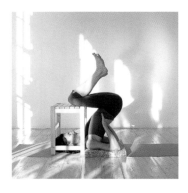
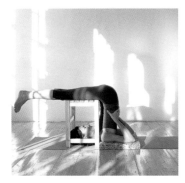

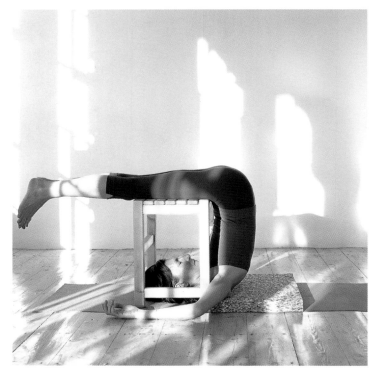

1 Place a chair/stool over the head before going into Salamba Sarvangasana. From this pose, take the legs down on to the stool to support the thighs.

2 Straighten the legs and support the spine with the hands.

3 Take the arms over the head and relax. Hold for 2–5 minutes, bend the knees, slide the thighs off the stool and come down.

Plough Pose
HALASANA

This inversion relaxes the brain. It is beneficial to practise it when you have a cold, and it improves the functioning of the thyroid and parathyroid glands.

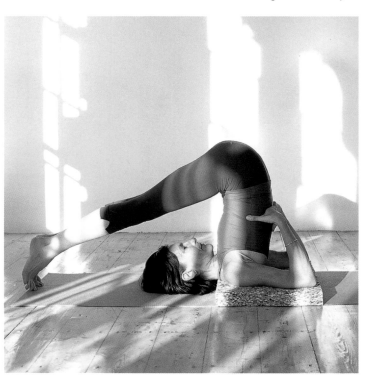

1 Go into Salamba Sarvangasana with the shoulders on a folded blanket or foam support. Take the legs down over the head and put the feet on the floor.

Keep supporting the back with the hands, lift the back and keep the chest open and lifted. Straighten the legs, extending them away from the hips.

Relax the eyes, hold for 2–5 minutes and come down.

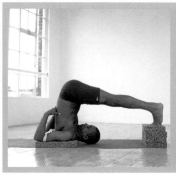

Modification
• If the back hurts, put a support under the toes.
• The tips of the toes press into the floor or bricks. Lift thigh bones towards the ceiling and stretch the heels away from the head.

Shoulder Stand Bridge Pose
SETU BANDHA SARVANGASANA (SUPPORTED)

This pose opens the chest and gives a mild extension to the spine. It calms the brain, reduces depression and relieves headaches. Digestion is improved and the internal organs are strengthened.

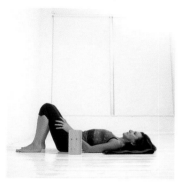
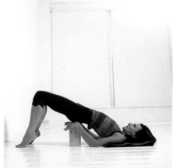

1 Lie on the floor with the knees bent and the toes pointing towards the wall.

2 Keeping the head, neck and shoulders on the floor, press the feet down and lift the hips from the floor. Put a wooden block vertically under the sacrum near the tailbone.

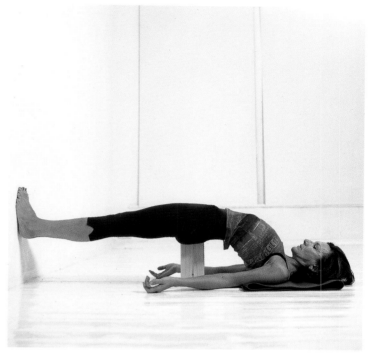

4 Open the chest, and extend the arms towards the feet, which are pressing firmly into the wall. Roll the tops of the shoulders towards the floor and move the shoulder blades towards the front of the body to open the chest.

Hold for 1–2 minutes, then bend the legs, remove the block and come down.

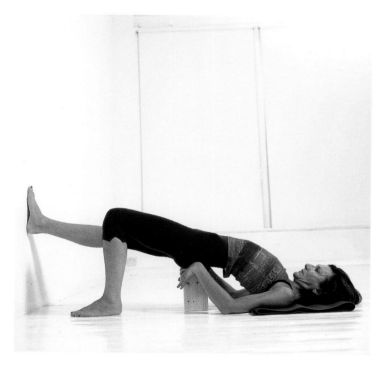

3 Straighten one leg at a time and place the feet on the wall at whatever height is comfortable for the lower back.

Focus
• Maintain a strong stretch on the back of the legs from the buttock bones to the heels.
• There should be no tension in the neck.
• Lift the breastbone towards the chin.

Modification
• If the wooden block is uncomfortable on the sacrum (lower back), use four stacked foam blocks.
• If the lower back hurts, support the feet on wooden blocks or a bolster.

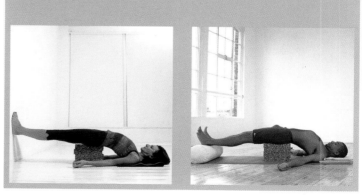

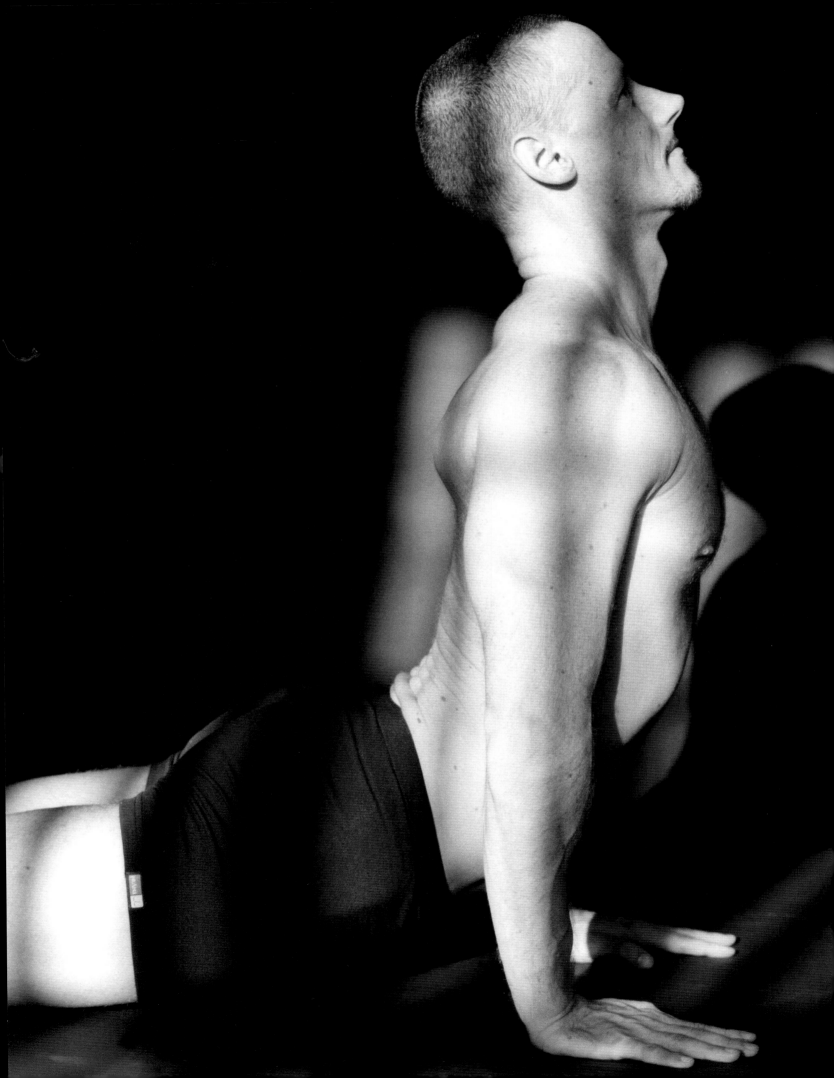

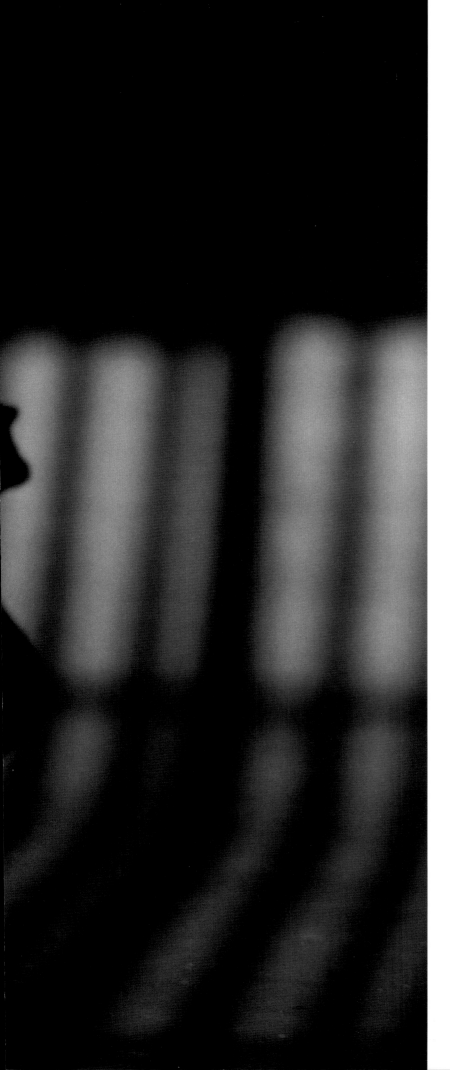

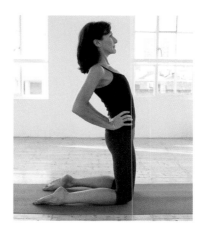

supine and prone
Asanas

There are two types of supine/prone postures: some are restful and are used for recuperation, while others strengthen the back, arms and legs. In all of them, the abdomen is stretched and the spine and hips gain flexibility.

Fish Pose
MATSYASANA (SIMPLE)

Here the muscles of the spine and abdomen are fully stretched. Flexibility in the hips, knees and ankles develops and the chest lifts and opens, so the depth of the breath improves.

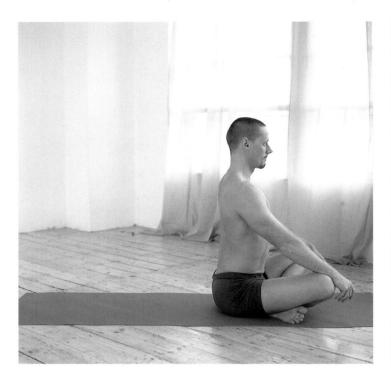

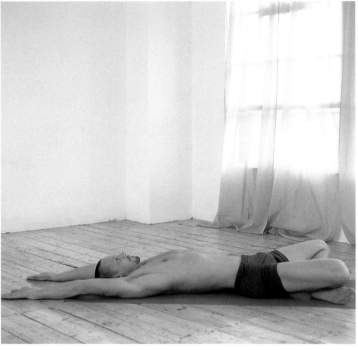

1 Sit in Sukhasana (simple cross legs), crossing the right shin-bone over the left.

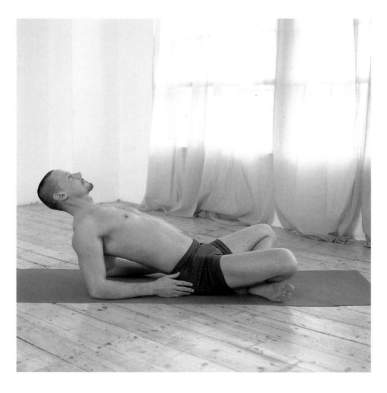

2 Lean back by resting on the elbows and then lie down. Soften the groin to allow the knees to release towards the floor.

3 Take the arms over the head, straighten the elbows and extend the arms strongly back.

Extend the trunk towards the head and the knees away from the head. Keep the lower back long (don't arch it) and move the shoulders away from the floor and towards the ceiling to lift and open the chest.

Hold for 1–2 minutes, come up, change the cross-over of the legs and repeat.

Modification
• If the groin is painful, support each knee with a foam block or bolster.

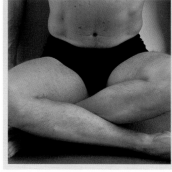

Focus
• Cross the legs evenly at the shins, not at the ankles, and change the cross.
• Don't overarch in the lower back – lengthen it by extending the sacrum towards the feet.

Cross Bolsters

This pose gently stretches the back and soothes the brain. As the back ribs
are supported by the vertical bolster, the chest opens and breathing deepens,
the abdomen extends and the whole body relaxes.

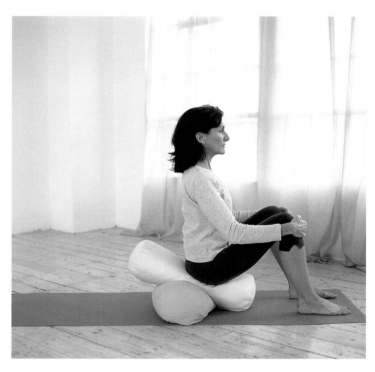

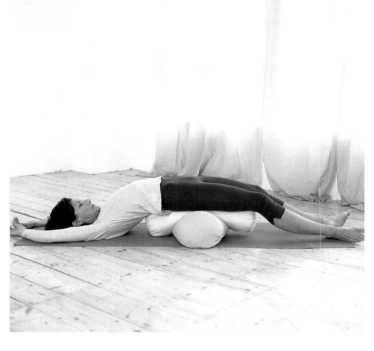

1 Place two bolsters on the floor, the first one horizontal
and the second lengthways on top. Sit on the top bolster
where it crosses over the bottom one, and bend the knees.

3 Extend the legs forwards, take the arms over the head
and relax them.

   Hold for 2–5 minutes, then bend the knees, slide back
towards the head, roll over to the side and get up.

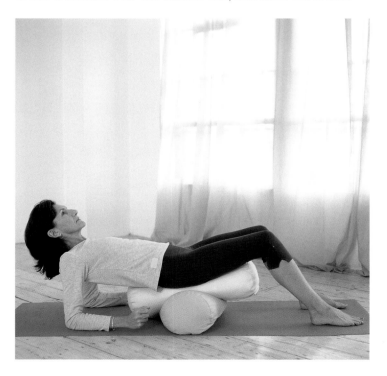

Modification
• The shoulders must rest on the floor. If this is difficult,
put a folded blanket underneath them.
• If the lower back aches, lift the feet and place them on
two or three foam blocks. It may be easier to lie on top
of the bolsters placed separately lengthways.
• To make the posture more relaxing, tie two straps
around the legs, one at the ankles and one across the
middle of the thighs.

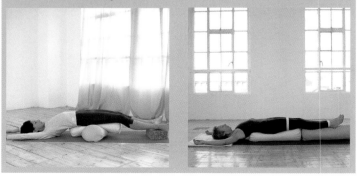

2 Lie back by resting on the elbows, placing the lower back
on the highest part of the top bolster. Lower the shoulders
down on to the floor.

Supine Cobbler Pose
SUPTA BADDHAKONASANA

This recuperative pose is particularly useful for women, especially during menstruation. The strap around the lower back lengthens the spine, and the bolster lifts the chest. This pose also helps sciatica.

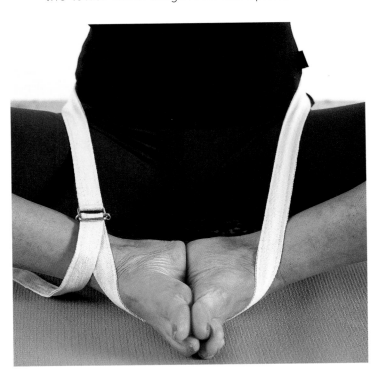

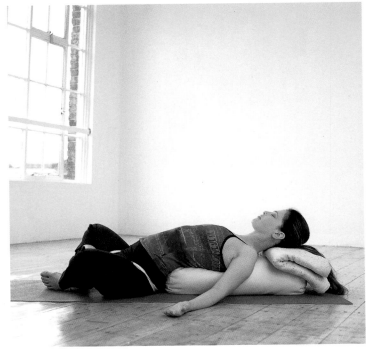

1 Place a bolster lengthways on the floor with a folded blanket at the top end. Sit in front of the bolster with the edge in contact with the lower back. Bend the knees out to the sides, take the soles of the feet together and draw the heels as close to the pubis as possible. Loop the strap across the lower back, over the hips and bind the soles of the feet together at the ankles.

2 Lie back over the bolster, keeping the edge touching the lower back, and support the head and neck with the folded blanket.

Feel the bolster gently moving the spine into the body and the resultant broadening, lifting and opening of the chest. Allow the shoulders to roll down towards the bolster. Keep the face, mouth and throat relaxed.

Take the arms out to the side, keeping the palms facing upwards. Relax them and close the eyes.

Hold for 2–5 minutes, focusing on the breathing, then open the eyes and come up.

Modification
• If the back is aching, put more support on the bolster and under the head.
• If the groin is uncomfortable, support each knee with a foam block or bolster.
• If the back aches in this posture despite the extra support, come out of it and lie over the bolster with the legs crossed as in Sukhasana.

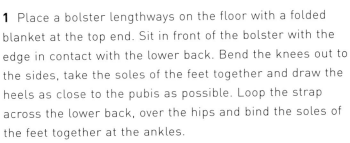

Focus
• Make a circle with a strap and place it over the head. Bring it down to the hips, and hook it over the feet.
• As you lie back, the strap will keep the feet as close to the body as possible.

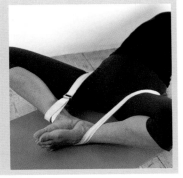

Reclining Hero Pose
SUPTA VIRASANA

This restful posture stretches the abdominal organs and the pelvic region. It also relieves aching legs and is good for digestion. If the back aches despite extra support, lie over the bolster with legs crossed.

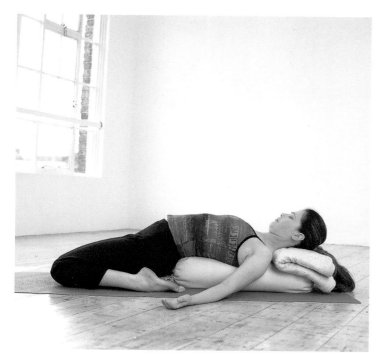

1 Place a bolster lengthways on a mat with a folded blanket at the top end to support the head. Sit in Virasana on a foam block placed against the bolster.

Hold the bolster against the lower back and lie over the bolster, supporting the head and neck on the folded blanket. Take the arms out to the side, palms facing upwards. Hold for 3–5 minutes and come up.

Modification
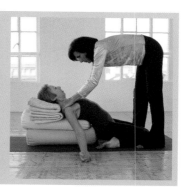
• If the knees or lower back are painful, put another bolster under the first one.
• Keep the shoulders back, the chest open and raised.
• If necessary, place more blankets under the head.

Legs Stretched to 90 Degrees
URDHVA PRASARITA PADASANA

This pose strengthens the lower back and gives relief to tired legs.
The brain stays calm while focusing on the breath.

1 Sit sideways to the wall and move the right hip and buttock as close to the wall as possible. Lean back, swivel the trunk around and take both legs up the wall. The head should be in line with the tailbone.

Lie down and allow the wall to support the legs. Extend both arms over the head, keep the hips down, and stretch the legs up the wall. Hold for 40–60 seconds and come up.

Focus
• Extend the backs of the legs towards the ceiling and press them into the wall.
• Keep the lower back and hips moving towards the floor.
• Take the shoulder blades into the body to open the chest.
• This is considered a supine, relaxing pose, while Viparita Karani raises the hips and back off the floor, and is therefore considered an inverted posture.

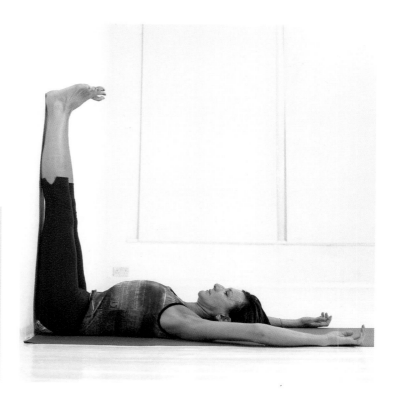

Prone Leg Stretches
SUPTA PADANGUSTHASANA I & II

These postures are good for stretching the hamstrings. They strengthen the knees and hip joints, and help to relieve sciatica. The pelvic area is aligned, removing stiffness from the lower back and easing backache.

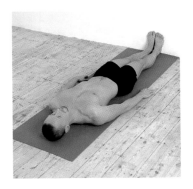
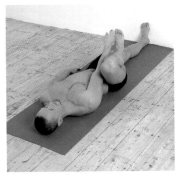

1 Lie down on a mat or blanket, with the soles of both feet touching the wall.

2 Bend the right knee towards the chest, and grab the big toe with the right thumb and forefinger.

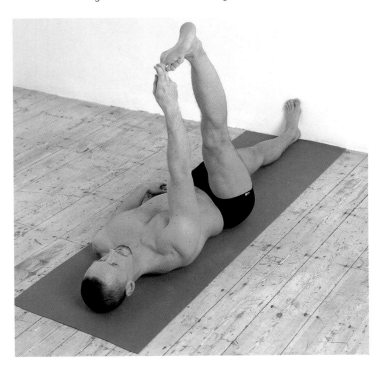

3 Supta Panangusthasana I – Stretch the right leg straight up towards the ceiling while pressing the sole of the left foot more firmly into the wall. Keep the right leg at a 90-degree angle. (If the back is painful, take the leg to a 60-/70-degree angle.)

Lengthen the back of the right leg from the buttock bone to the heel. Press the back of the left leg into, and along, the floor. Pull on the foot to open the chest. Hold for 30–40 seconds, come down and repeat with the left leg.

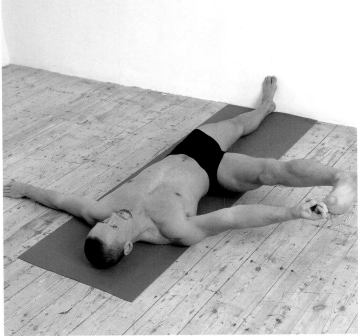

4 Supta Padangusthasana II – following the instructions as before, extend the leg up to 90 degrees and then stretch the right leg and arm sideways to the right. Take the right leg towards the floor without disturbing the alignment of the head, trunk or left leg.

Press the sole of the left foot into the wall and the back of the leg into the floor. If the whole body rolls over towards the right, put a support under the right foot to control the descent of the leg (if using a strap, pull on it with the right hand) and extend the left arm out to the side.

Open the chest. Hold for 30–40 seconds and repeat on the other side.

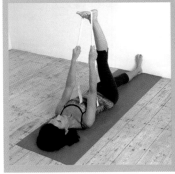

Modification
• Students with tight hamstrings can use a strap around the foot, rather than catching the big toe.
• If difficulty is experienced with the leg to the side, rest the thigh on a bolster.

Dog Pose
ADHO MUKHA SVANASANA

Dog pose is a good all-over stretch. It extends the legs and strengthens the ankles. It also eases stiffness in the neck, shoulders and wrists. Staying longer in this pose removes fatigue and restores energy.

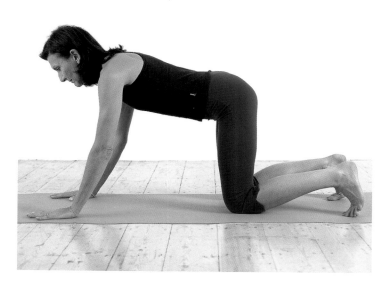

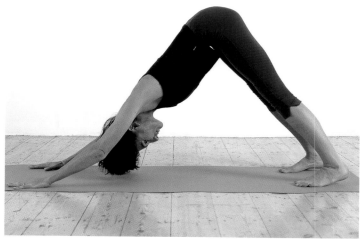

1 Get on to all fours (hands and knees). Place the palms on the floor, hands shoulder-width apart, with the middle fingers pointing forwards. Take the knees hip-width apart and tuck the toes under.

Press the hands firmly into the floor, particularly the thumbs and index fingers. Fully straighten the arms, extending them from the floor towards the shoulders. Move the shoulders away from the ears and the shoulder blades into the body to open the chest.

2 Raise the hips, straighten the legs and extend the heels towards the floor. Press the thighs back. Straighten both elbows, lift the shoulders towards the waist and stretch the trunk up.

Relax the head towards the floor. Keep the arms and legs firm. Push the heels towards the ground.

Hold for 20–30 seconds, bend the knees and come down.

Modification
• For an easier version of this posture, work with the hands or feet supported by a wall.
• Turn the hands out and place the palms on the floor with the index fingers and thumbs against the wall.

• Alternatively, start with the back to the wall, rest the heels up the wall and come into the pose.
• If there is strain in the head or neck, rest the forehead on a bolster for a more restful version of this posture.

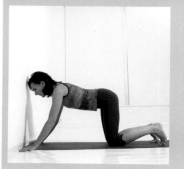

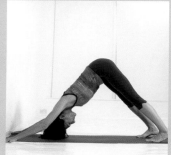

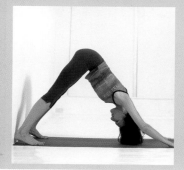

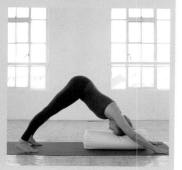

Dog Pose (head up)
URDHVA MUKHA SVANASANA

This pose strengthens the spine, relieves backache and sciatica, and tones the internal organs. It also helps to expand the chest and increase flexibility in the neck and shoulders.

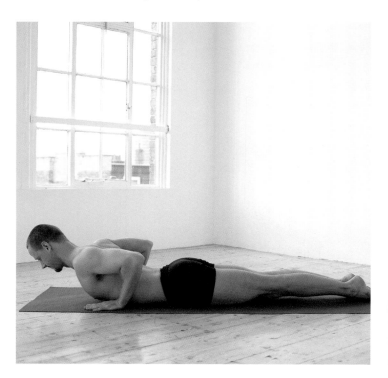

1 Lie face down on the floor and stretch both legs back, pressing the tops of the feet into the floor. (If the lower back hurts, tuck the toes under.) Place the palms on the floor beside the chest and spread the fingers.

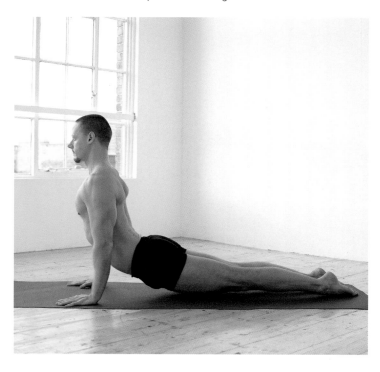

2 Inhale, raise the head and chest, straighten the arms and lock the elbows.

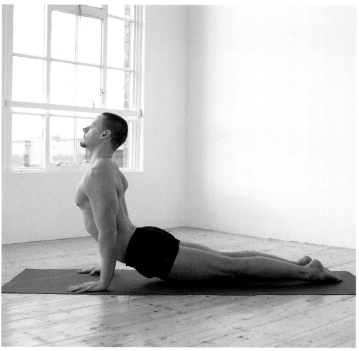

3 Lift the hips, thighs and knees a few centimetres/inches off the floor, bringing the tailbone and sacrum forwards.

Keeping the elbows straight, roll the shoulders back, lift the chest further and curve the trunk back between the arms. Lengthen the back of the neck, take the head back slightly and look up. Stay for 30–40 seconds, breathing evenly.

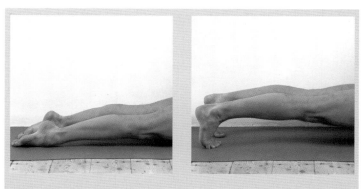

Focus
• Keep the toes pointing backwards, and lift the legs off the floor. If difficulty is experienced lifting the legs off the floor, tuck the toes under and then lift up.
• To lift the trunk and chest more, put each hand on a wooden block.

Locust Pose
SALABHASANA I

Salabhasana strengthens the back and improves flexibility in the spinal muscles. The abdominal muscles become stronger, improving digestion. Stiffness is reduced in the neck and shoulders.

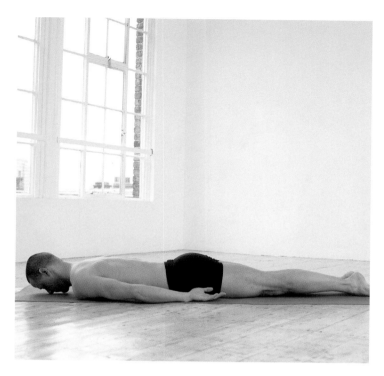

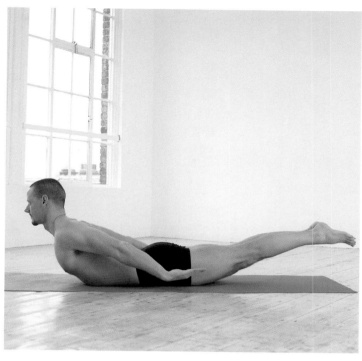

1 Lie face down on the floor with the arms beside the trunk, feet together, knees straight and the toes stretching back. Turn the palms up. Stretch the arms and raise them so the hands are parallel to the floor. Press the sacrum down and raise the head, chest and legs as high as they will go without causing any back pain.

2 Extend the trunk forwards, the legs and arms back and lift the chest.

Balance on the lower abdomen, look straight ahead and breathe normally. Hold the pose for 20–30 seconds and then release and lower the chest, head and legs.

Focus

• In everyday life we are continually bending forwards, but have little reason to bend backwards. Back bends help to extend the heart muscles, stretch the front side of the lungs and maintain flexibility in the respiratory muscles, thereby increasing lung capacity. They are also useful for nourishing and toning the abdominal organs and stimulating the adrenal glands.

• Back bends have not been featured here, as they are advanced postures that should be carried out only under the supervision of an experienced and qualified teacher. For a preliminary back bend try Ustrasana, over the page, in the moderated version at first.

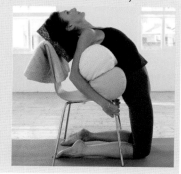

Modification

• Don't raise the arms and legs too high, as this will cause pain in the lower back.
• Stretch the shoulders back, keeping the arms parallel.
• Keep the legs together and the knees straight.
• If it is difficult to do the pose with the feet together, place a foam block between the feet, press the inner edges of the feet into the block and lift the legs.
• In order to open the chest more, and increase the extension in the arms, put a wooden block on the palm of each hand. Imagine the blocks are heavy weights, and without actually lifting the hands any higher, push the palms into the blocks as if trying to lift them.

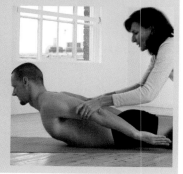

Camel Pose
USTRASANA

Although neither supine nor prone, this posture is preparation for more advanced back bends. It strengthens the spinal muscles and enables you to understand the curvature of the spine.

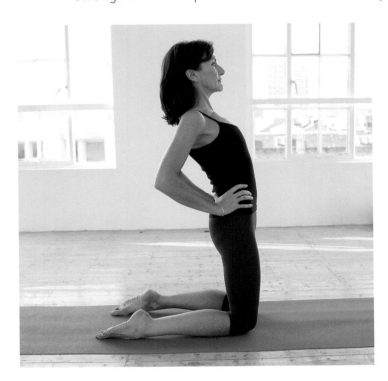

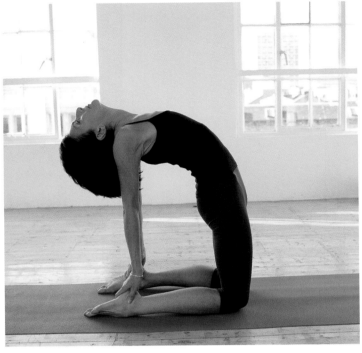

1 Kneel with the knees and feet hip-width apart. Press the shin-bones and tops of the feet firmly into the floor. Place the hands on the waist, and lengthen the trunk upwards.

3 Keep the neck long and take the head back. Look behind you. Keep lifting and opening the chest.

Hold for 15–20 seconds, inhale, raise the head, release the hands and lift the trunk.

Focus
• Move the back ribs and shoulder blades more deeply into the back to open the chest more.
• Straighten the arms and hold the heels more firmly to activate the shoulders.
• Finish this pose by leaning forwards to extend the spine in the opposite direction.
• Keep the thighs perpendicular to the floor.

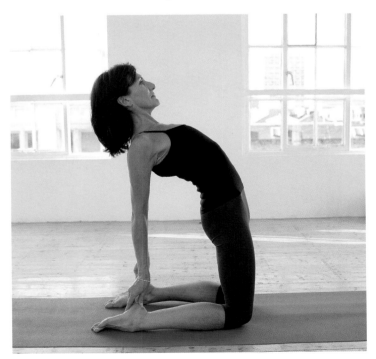

2 Exhale, keep the chest lifting and curve the spine back, moving the spine deeply into the body. Extend the arms towards the heels and hold the heels with the hands.

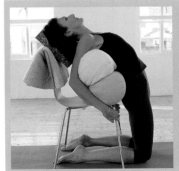

Modification
• Students who cannot reach their heels can arch over bolsters propped on a chair, or place a rolled-up blanket under the tops of their feet so the heels are easier to reach.

Corpse Pose
SAVASANA

After performing the asanas, this relaxation pose helps to release tension in the muscles, settle the breathing and calm the mind. Energy flows into and through the body, recharging it and removing stress.

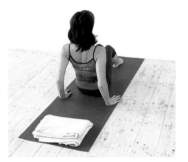
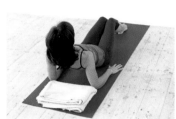

1 Sit in the centre of the mat with the knees bent and the feet on the floor. Put a folded blanket at the head end of the mat.

2 Lower the trunk down, rest on the elbows and check the body alignment, then carefully lower the trunk on to the floor. Place the centre of the back of the head on the support.

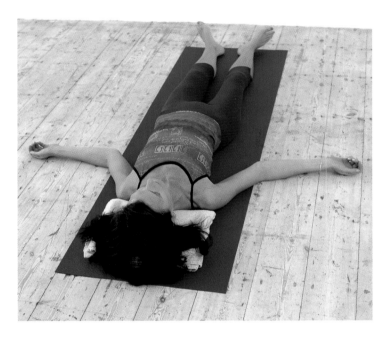

4 Stretch the arms out to each side, slightly away from the sides of the trunk, and turn the palms so that the knuckles of the little fingers are on the floor as much as the knuckles of the index fingers. Shut the eyes by lowering the upper eyelids towards the lower eyelids.

Relax the eyes and facial features and allow the body to sink into the floor. Breathe evenly and focus on the breath in order to keep the brain calm and passive. Don't go to sleep.

Hold for 5–10 minutes, then slowly open the eyes, bend the knees, roll over to the side and slowly come up.

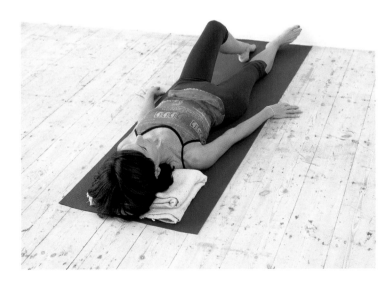

3 Straighten one leg at a time and, when straight, keep the legs and feet together.

Release the tension in the legs and allow the feet to drop out to the side.

Focus
• Let your body go and surrender to the floor.
• Relax the fingers and palms of the hands.
• Keep the head straight, with the bridge of the nose facing the ceiling.
• Relax the thigh muscles and let the legs roll away from one another.
• Draw the organs of perception (eyes, ears and tongue) inwards so that the mind and body become one and inner silence is experienced.

Breathing
UJJAYI PRANAYAMA

In Pranayama the brain becomes quiet which allows the nervous system to function more effectively.
It generates a store of energy in the body, while strengthening and increasing the capacity of the lungs.

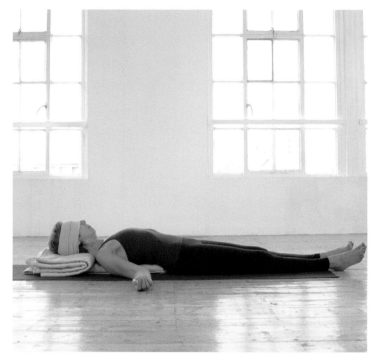

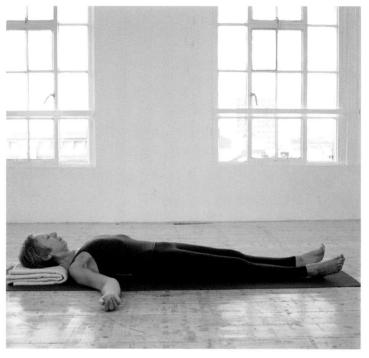

1 Normal Inhalation/Extended Exhalation

Lie in Savasana on a bolster or blanket, with another folded blanket under the head. Cover the eyes with a bandage. Spend a few minutes becoming aware of your normal breathing. Exhale, relax the abdomen. Inhale normally.

Exhale slowly, quietly and smoothly, lengthening the breath without straining. Inhale normally again. Exhale slowly, deeply and smoothly.

If breathlessness or fatigue is experienced in between cycles, take a few normal breaths before proceeding. Continue in this manner for 5 minutes. Return to normal breathing to allow the lungs to recover.

Focus
- Beginners should master the postures and gain control over the body before attempting Pranayama.
- Keep the face, eyes, mouth and throat relaxed.
- Keep the chest and ribcage lifted throughout.
- Keep the shoulders moving away from the ears.
- Keep the abdomen soft in inhalation and exhalation.
- Soften the palms of the hands and relax the fingers.
- If the mind is racing, an eye bandage will aid calmness.

2 Extended Inhalation/Normal Exhalation

Exhale, completely emptying air from the lungs.

Take a slow, soft inhalation, filling the lungs from the bottom to the top.

Don't strain or jerk the chest, breathe smoothly and lengthen the breath calmly.

Exhale normally. Inhale once more, slowly drawing the breath into the lungs.

Exhale normally.

Repeat these two cycles for about 5 minutes, then return to normal breathing. Once you've returned to normal breathing, check that there is no tension in the shoulders, throat, mouth or hands.

Exercise caution when practising Pranayama – incorrect practice may strain the lungs and diaphragm.

These two cycles can be practised separately or together and should be done for a few months before proceeding to breathing with extended inhalation and extended exhalation.

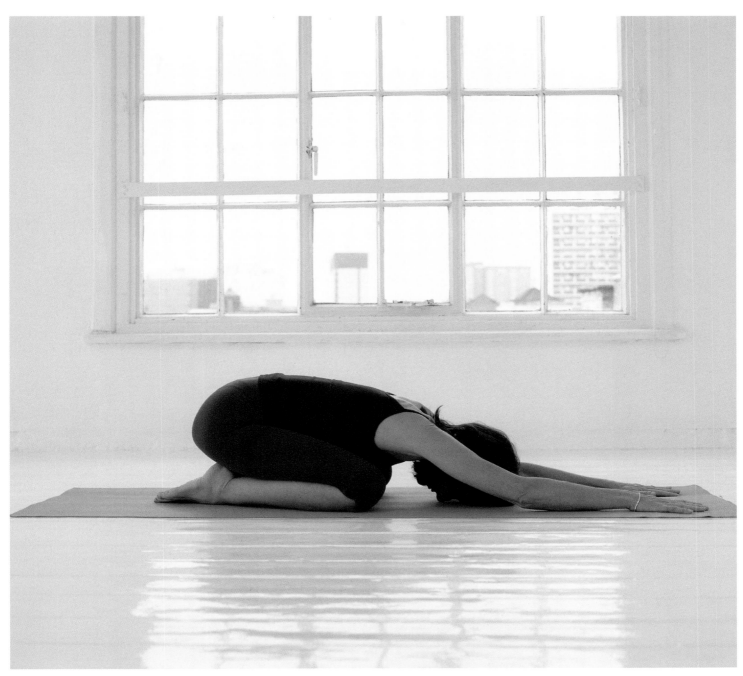

3 Extended Inhalation/Extended Exhalation
Exhale, completely emptying the lungs of air. Inhale slowly and smoothly, lengthening the breath.

Maintain the lift of the chest, and exhale slowly and deeply without straining the throat.

Control the flow of breath so that the body doesn't shudder or strain. Take a few normal breaths.

Repeat for about 5 minutes. Return to normal breathing.

To end the above cycles, bend the knees, roll over to the side and remove the bolster. Lie flat, with the head still supported, in Savasana for 5 minutes, keeping the brain quiet and releasing the body to the floor. Slowly open the eyes, turn to one side, stay for a moment, then turn to the other side. Come up and sit in Adho Mukha Virasana before getting up.

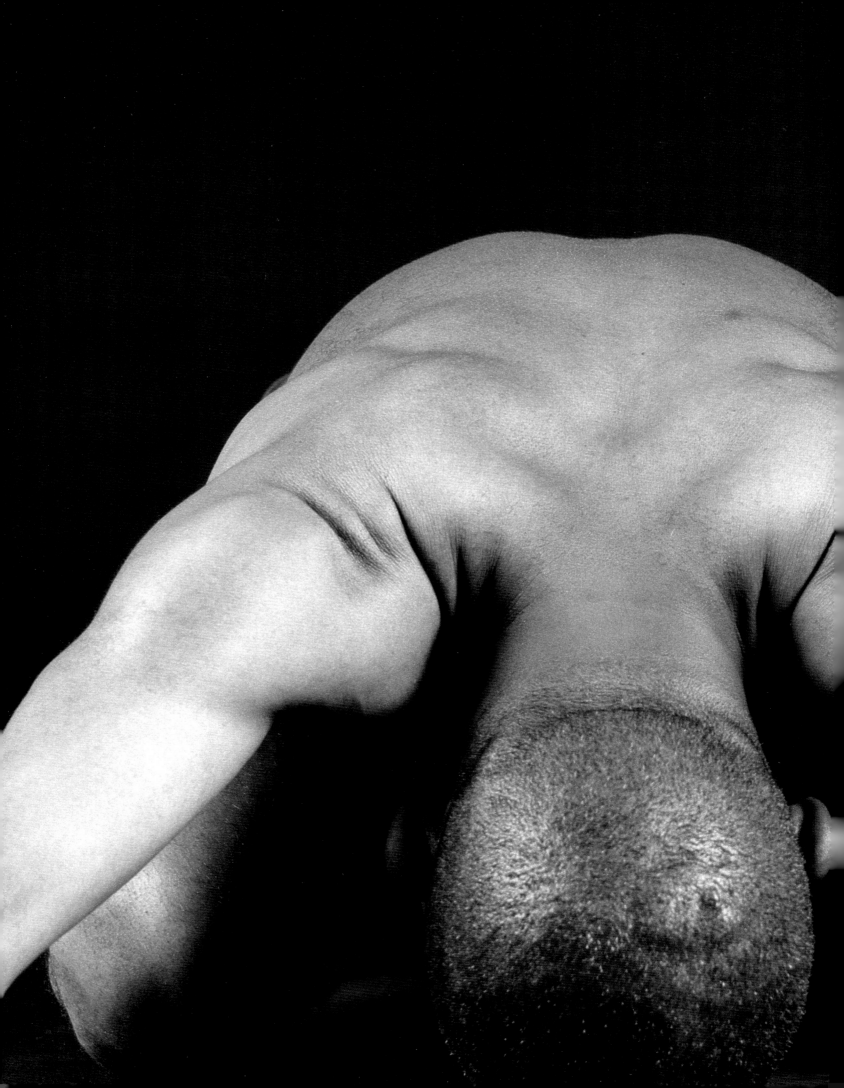

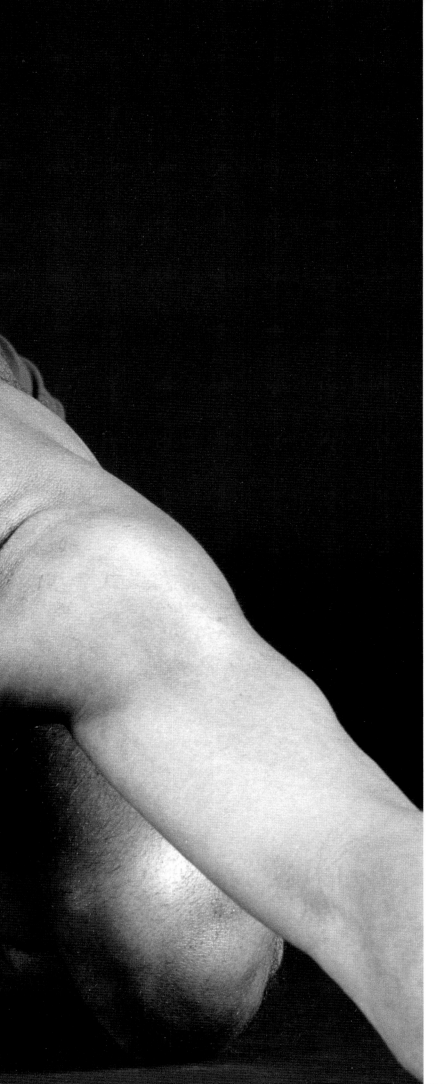

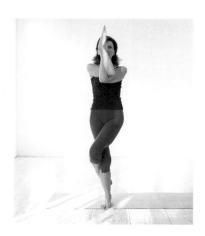

routine
Practice

The sage Patanjali states in Yoga Sutra 11.47: "Perfection in an asana is achieved when the effort to perform it becomes effortless, and the infinite being within is reached."

Practising postures in a set order increases their effectiveness as well as the student's understanding of each posture. The subtleties and details of the poses and their effect on the mind and body become more obvious as one's practice becomes more established.

Routines and Sequences

The practice of postures has a beneficial impact on the entire body. The postures tone the muscles, tissues, ligaments, joints and nerves, as well as maintaining and improving the health and functioning of all the body systems. It is important to keep practising until you become familiar with, and comfortable in, the postures. When this happens, the full benefits are felt. This is why routines should be practised as often as possible.

Classification of postures

Broadly speaking, standing postures are dynamic and exhilarating. They refresh both body and mind by removing tension, aches and pains. The standing postures form the basis of all other postures, and, through them, practitioners become familiar with various parts of their bodies, their muscles and joints, and use their intelligence to bring action and awareness to these parts. Most routines begin with standing postures in order to waken the physical body – the arms, legs and spine – and stimulate the brain by connecting movements to specific areas of the body. They also build stamina and strength as well as determination.

The seated postures are introduced after standing postures to rest and remove strain from the legs. Seated forward bends are calming. They remove fatigue, soothe the nerves and calm the mind. In standing postures the brain is stimulated; in seated postures an agitated, fluctuating mind becomes passive.

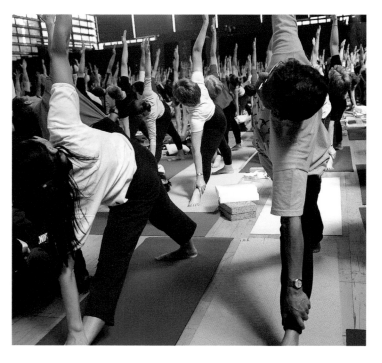

Twisting postures extend and rotate the spine. These postures are good for relieving backache and stiffness in the neck and shoulders. The internal organs are stimulated as the trunk turns, and this improves digestion.

Inverted postures energize the entire system. They relieve strain in the legs, activate and nourish the inner organs, stimulate the brain and improve the respiratory, circulatory and nervous systems. Standing, seated and twisting postures prepare the body and mind for inversions. Women should not practise inversions while menstruating.

Supine, prone, or lying-down postures are also known as abdominal postures, and a routine should never begin with these. Standing postures tone the stomach muscles so they can be used correctly, and inverted postures protect the organs so they are not damaged when doing abdominal postures, so these should be done before attempting abdominal postures.

Savasana (relaxation) should be done for 5–10 minutes (depending on time) at the end of each routine.

Suggested practice plan

The following routines are suggested to enable students to practise systematically and progressively. It is more beneficial to practise for a shorter time each day than a longer session once or twice a week. Attend a regular yoga group with a qualified teacher, as they can make sure you are progressing at the correct pace.

Each routine can be practised daily, starting with Sequence 1 on the first day and progressing to Sequence 5 by the end of the week. Repeat the first 5 sequences over a 2–3 week period to consolidate the postures, then continue with the Sequences 6–10. Ultimately, discrimination should be used with regard to the length of time and which postures to

left Try to get to an organized class, led by a qualified teacher, at least once or twice a week, and supplement this by practising at home every day, and you will feel the difference very quickly.

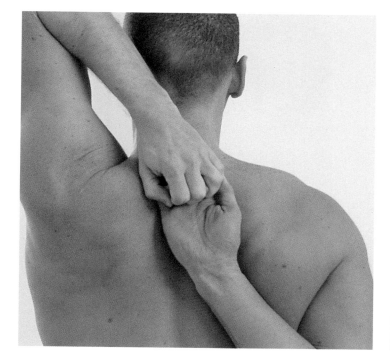

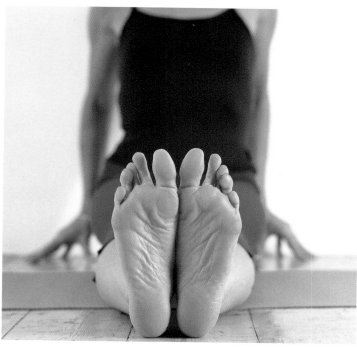

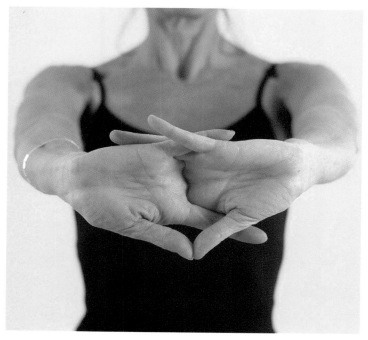

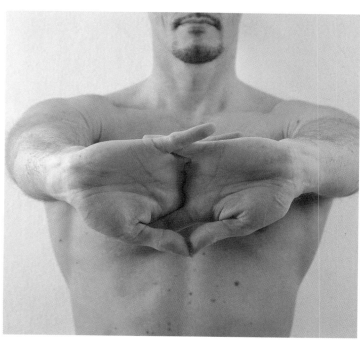

above Time and patience are required to understand the subtleties and technical requirements of the postures.

practise, the aim being to have a physical and spiritual rhythm to your practice. Confidence is gained by working at an even pace, learning about the postures and their effects on the body, and then proceeding with knowledge and understanding on to the next routine. Move on to the next set of routines only when you feel able to do so.

As you progress in your practice, flexibility and stamina improve and the postures can be held for longer periods of time. The effects of the postures are not instant, and timing is dependent on energy, intelligence and awareness. However, if time doesn't permit it, you can tailor your practice to suit the circumstances.

Sequence 1 – Simple Standing Postures

In this first sequence, the shapes of the postures should be studied and worked on. Then, as these become more familiar, detailed instructions should be incorporated to make the postures more correct and to feel the effects. Think about keeping the spine long in all postures. If fatigue or exhaustion is felt, do supported Uttanasa I to recover.

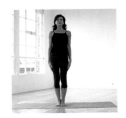

1 **Tadasana**

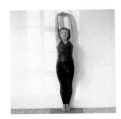

2 **Tadasana** with hands in Parvatasana

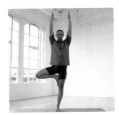

3 **Vrksasana**

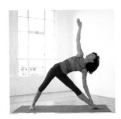

4 **Utthita Trikonasana**

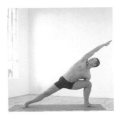

5 **Utthita Parsvakonasana**

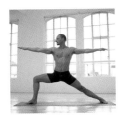

6 **Virabhadrasana II**

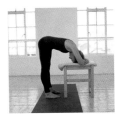

7 **Uttanasana I** (s)

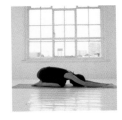

8 **Adho Mukha Virasana**

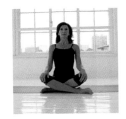

9 **Sukhasana**

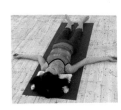

10 **Savasana**

Focus
• Where the moderated posture is used it is marked (s) for supported or (w) if the wall is used.

Sequence 2 – Simple Seated Postures

In this group of seated postures, one supine pose (Adho Mukha Svanasana) and two inverted postures (Setu Bandha Sarvangasana and Viparita Karani) have been introduced, but inversions should not be done if you are menstruating. It is advisable to sit on a support in the seated postures, as this helps to lift and extend the spine. The lower back should not be arched forwards, but lengthened upwards towards the head. In Virasana, ensure that the support under the buttocks is high enough so that there is no pain in the knees. If any discomfort is felt in the lower back in Setu Bandha Sarvangasana, raise the feet higher so as to remove strain from the lumbar region.

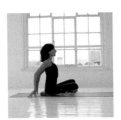

1 **Sukhasana**

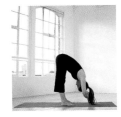

2 **Uttanasana I**

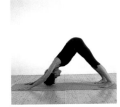

3 **Adho Mukha Svanasana**

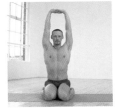

4 **Sukhasana**

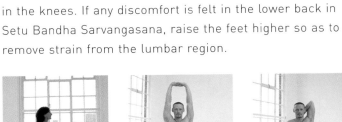

5 **Virasana with Parvatasana**

6 **Gomukhasana**

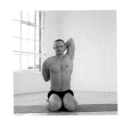

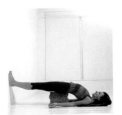

7 **Setu Bandha Sarvangasana**

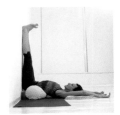

8 **Viparita Karani**

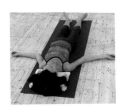

9 **Savasana**

Focus
• Each routine can be practised daily, starting with Sequence 1 on the first day and progressing to Sequence 5 by the end of the week. Then repeat over a 2–3 week period before progressing to sequences 6–10.

Sequence 3 – Consolidation of Simple Standing Postures

Parsvottanasana has been introduced here, in which the back foot is turned in much more than in the other standing postures. Ensure that both hips are level and facing in the same direction. Use wooden blocks to support each hand in this posture, and lengthen and extend the spine upwards. Begin to increase the timings in these postures.

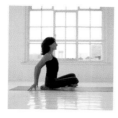
1 **Sukhasana**

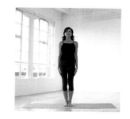
2 **Tadasana**

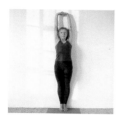
3 **Tadasana** (Parvat.)

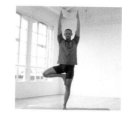
4 **Vrksasana**

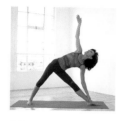
5 **Utthita Trikonasana**

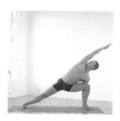
6 **Utthita Parsvakon.**

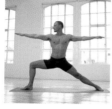
7 **Virabhadrasana II**

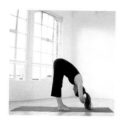
8 **Parsvottanasana** (s)

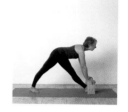
9 **Uttanasana I**

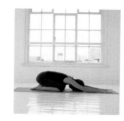
10 **Adho Mukha Vir.**

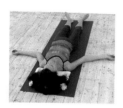
11 **Savasana**

Sequence 4 – Introduction of Salamba Sarvangasana and Ardha Halasana

Virabhadrasana I is brought into this routine as a slightly more challenging standing posture. It is very important to have the back leg well turned in and both hips turned to their maximum in this pose. The back leg in all standing postures is strong and stable – this leg is the "brain" of the posture. If Salamba Sarvangasana is uncomfortable, just lie with the legs up against the wall. Do not do Salamba Sarvangasana or Ardha Halasana if you are menstruating.

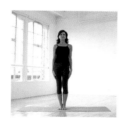
1 **Tadasana**

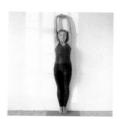
2 **Tadasana** (Parvat.)

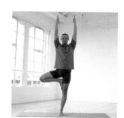
3 **Vrksasana**

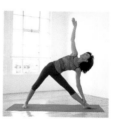
4 **Utthita Trikonasana**

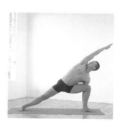
5 **Utthita Parsvakon.**

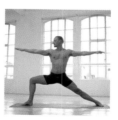
6 **Virabhadrasana II**

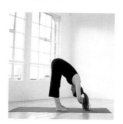
7 **Uttanasana I**

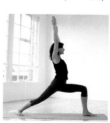
8 **Virabhadrasana I**

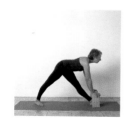
9 **Parsvottanasana** (s)

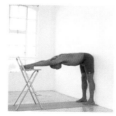
10 **Uttanasana I** (s)

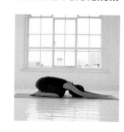
11 **Adho Mukha Vir.**

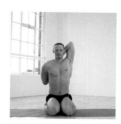
12 **Gomukhasana**

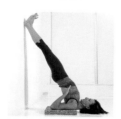
13 **Salamba Sarv.** (w)

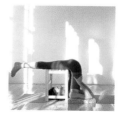
14 **Ardha Halasana**

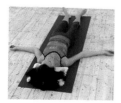
15 **Savasana**

Sequence 5 – Quiet, Calming Practice

This routine focuses on postures with the head supported and the chest lifted. If you are feeling tired or out of sorts, this quietening practice will help. Try to hold the postures for as long as possible in order to experience their calming effects. Keep the face relaxed throughout and the breathing normal, but be aware of the change of depth and rhythm of the breath as you relax. In Adho Mukha Svanasana, keep the spine ascending to the ceiling even though the head is down. Move the shoulders towards the front of the chest in order to broaden and create space in the chest cavity.

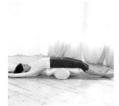

1 **Cross Bolsters**

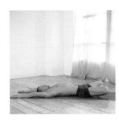

2 **Matsyasana**

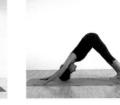

3 **Uttanasana I**

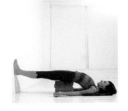

4 **Adho Mukha Svanasana**

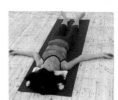

5 **Setu Bandha Sarvangasana**

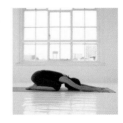

6 **Savasana**

Sequence 6 – Hamstring-stretching Poses

In these standing postures, pay attention to the feet by ensuring the soles of the feet make maximum contact with the floor. Stretch all five toes of each foot into and along the floor, and extend the legs strongly up from the ankles to the hips. In Utthita Hasta Padangusthasana (I & II), ensure the front of the trunk is lengthening up towards the ceiling, and the sides extending. In Prasarita Padottanasana, extend and lengthen the spine forwards before taking the head towards the floor. Pay attention to the feet in this posture. If they roll on to the little toe side, extreme discomfort will be felt on the side of the shin-bones, so ensure that all four corners of the feet are pressing equally into the floor.

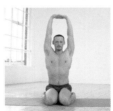

1 **Virasana with Parvatasana**

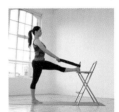

2 **Utthita Hasta Padangusthasana I** (s)

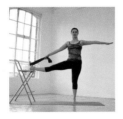

3 **Utthita Hasta Padangusthasana II** (s)

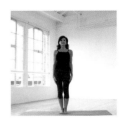

4 **Tadasana**

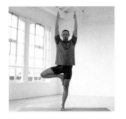

5 **Vrksasana**

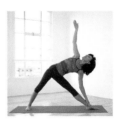

6 **Utthita Trikon.**

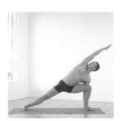

7 **Utthita Parsvakon.**

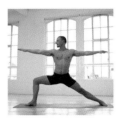

8 **Virabhadrasana II**

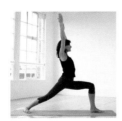

9 **Virabhadrasana I**

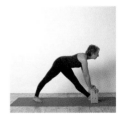

10 **Parsvottan.** (s)

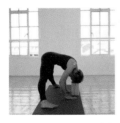

11 **Prasarita Pad.** (s)

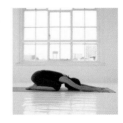

12 **Adho Mukha Vir.**

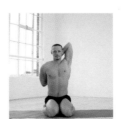

13 **Gomukhasana**

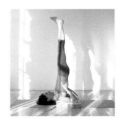

14 **Salamba Sarvang.**

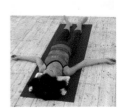

15 **Ardha Halasana**

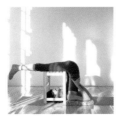

16 **Savasana**

Focus

• Repeat the Sequences 1–5 over a 2–3 week period to consolidate the postures, then continue with Sequences 6–10. Ultimately your discrimination should be used with regard to the length of time and which postures to practice.

Sequence 7 – Sitting Postures with Simple Twists

In the twisting postures, the spine must first be extended and lengthened, and then turned. Move the whole trunk around when you turn, keep the shoulders moving away from the ears, and turn your head without tensing the neck. In Virasana with Parvatasana, ensure that the shoulders move away from the ears so the neck can lengthen and extend.

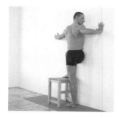

1 Standing Maricyasana

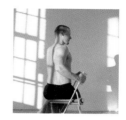

2 Bharadvajasana chair

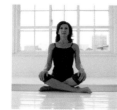

3 Sukhasana

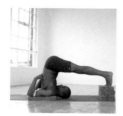

4 Virasana with Parvatasana

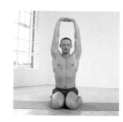

5 Gomukhasana

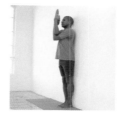

6 Garudasana (s)

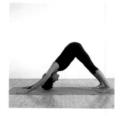

7 Adho Mukha Svan.

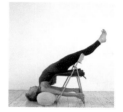

8 Chair Sarvang.

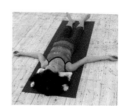

9 Halasana

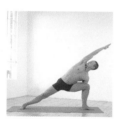

10 Savasana

Focus
• Halasana is introduced without a stool for support. If the back aches or the neck becomes painful, use a support (Ardha Halasana) until the discomfort goes away.

Sequence 8 – Introduction of Utkatasana and Garudasana

When the arms are extended, ensure that they stretch from the tops of the shoulders to the tips of the fingers, and keep the palms of the hands broad. Virabhadrasana I can be attempted, but if this causes backache, put the hands on the hips. Garudasana may be done standing in Tadasana, but gradually work towards doing the full posture.

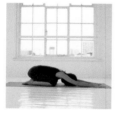

1 Adho Mukha Vir

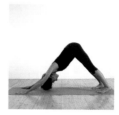

2 Adho Mukha Svan.

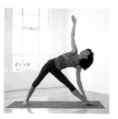

3 Tadasana

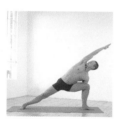

4 Utthita Trikon.

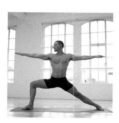

5 Utthita Parsvakon.

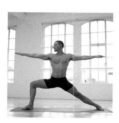

6 Virabhadrasana II

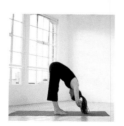

7 Uttanasana I

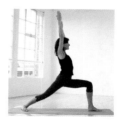

8 Virabhadrasana I

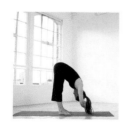

9 Uttanasana I

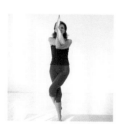

10 Parsvottanasana

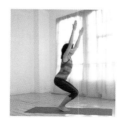

11 Garudasana

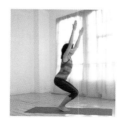

12 Utkatasana

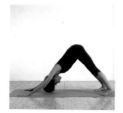

13 Adho Mukha Svan.

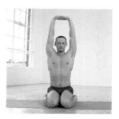

14 Virasana/Parvat.

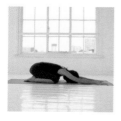

15 Adho Mukha Vir.

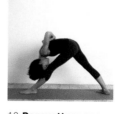

16 Chair Sarvang.

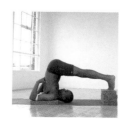

17 Halasana (s)

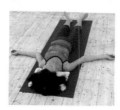

18 Savasana

Sequence 9 – Relaxation Practice

Ensure that the chest is lifted and open in these postures. The brain should remain passive, with the mind quietly focusing on the breath, throughout the poses. These postures can be held for 3–5 minutes to gain maximum benefit. If the muscles of the groin are painful in Supta Baddhakonasana, place foam blocks under each thigh to lessen the stretch. If the back and/or knees hurt in Supta Virasana, add as much support as is needed to relieve the discomfort. To eliminate visual distractions, close your eyes and keep them still, focusing on the breath.

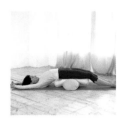 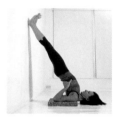 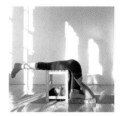 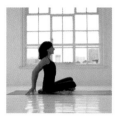 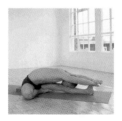 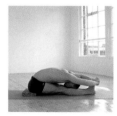

1 **Cross Bolsters**   2 **Matsyasana**   3 **Supta Baddhkonasana**   4 **Supta Virasana**   5 **Adho Mukha Virasana**   6 **Adho Mukha Svanasana**

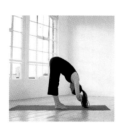 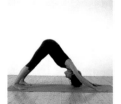 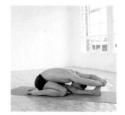

7 **Salamba Sarv.** (w)   8 **Ardha Halasana**   9 **Sukhasana**

Focus
• Practise Sequences 6–10 by repeating them over several weeks and learn to increase timings before proceeding to the next five.

Sequence 10 – Introduction to Seated Forward Bends

Sit on a support for these seated postures to help lift the spine. The forward bends are done with a concave back, an action achieved by lifting and opening the chest, moving the shoulders away from the ears and moving the shoulder blades towards the front of the body. If the back hurts, hold a strap caught around the foot, so the angle between the trunk and the leg lessens and the backache is relieved. Keep the arms straight when holding the strap. In Urdhva Prasarita Padasana, the entire backs of both legs (from buttock bones to heels) should be against the wall.

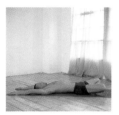 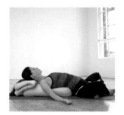 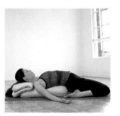 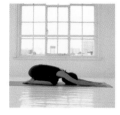 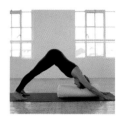 (row one)

1 **Uttanasana I**   2 **Adho Mukha Svanasana**   3 **Dandasana**   4 **Janusirsasana**   5 **Trianga Mukha. Pascimottanasana**   6 **Pascimottanasana**

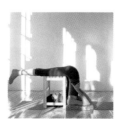 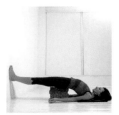 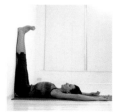 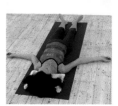

7 **Ardha Halasana**   8 **Setu Bandha Sarvangasana**   9 **Urdhva Prasarita Padasana**   10 **Savasana**

Sequence 11 – Standing Poses Held for Longer

This sequence consolidates the standing postures and should be done with more awareness and attention to detail. If discomfort is experienced, try to locate it, think about what has caused it and, by understanding the technique of the pose, try to remove it. Try to hold each posture for a little longer than you have done previously.

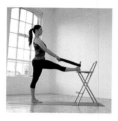

1 Utthita Hasta Padangusthasana I (s)

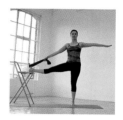

2 Utthita Hasta Padangusthasana II (s)

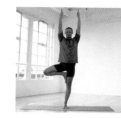

3 Tadasana

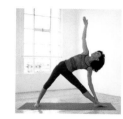

4 Vrksasana

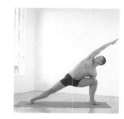

5 Utthita Trikonasana

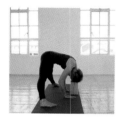

6 Utthita Parsvakonasana

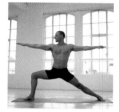

7 Virabhadrasana II

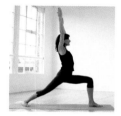

8 Virabhadrasana I

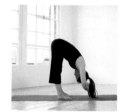

9 Uttanasana I

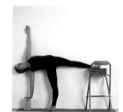

10 Ardha Chandr. (s)

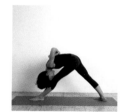

11 Parsvottanasana

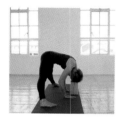

12 Prasarita Pad. (s)

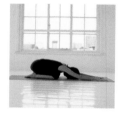

13 Adho Mukha Vir.

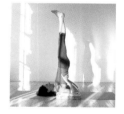

14 Salamba Sarvang.

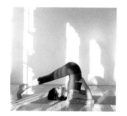

15 Halasana

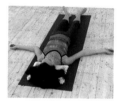

16 Savasana

Focus
• This sequence should take longer than the others so far, as the timing of each posture is increased.

Sequence 12 – Increased Timings in Seated Forward Bends with Concave Back

Doing the forward bends with a concave back improves the elasticity of the spine and helps to open the chest. The whole trunk must be lengthened. When looking up, be careful not to compress the back of the neck.

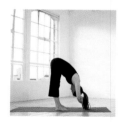

1 Uttanasana I

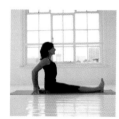

2 Adho Mukha Svanasana

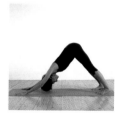

3 Dandasana

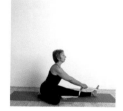

4 Paripurna Navasana (s)

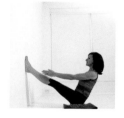

5 Janusirsasana (s)

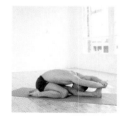

6 Trianga Mukha. Pascimottanasana

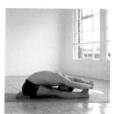

7 Pascimottanasana

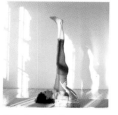

8 Salamba Sarvang.

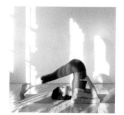

9 Halasana

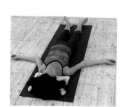

10 Savasana

Focus
• In Paripurna Navasana, lift the trunk upwards. If the lower back becomes painful, do the posture with the fingertips on the floor.

Sequence 13 – Basic Standing Postures and Introducing Seated Postures

Try to practise the standing postures with less strain and more composure. By now the technicalities of the poses should be physically ingrained, so try to just "be" in the posture and allow the psychological effects to emerge.

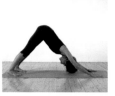
1 **Adho Mukha Svan.**

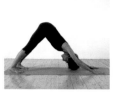
2 **Uttanasana I**

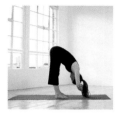
3 **Tadasana**

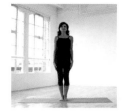
4 **Utthita Trikonasana**

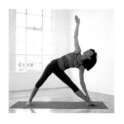
5 **Utthita Parsvakon.**

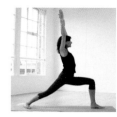
6 **Virabhadrasana I**

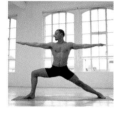
7 **Virabhadrasana II**

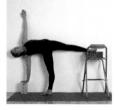
8 **Ardha Chandr.** (s)

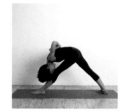
9 **Parsvottansana**

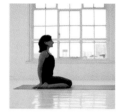
10 **Virasana**

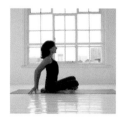
11 **Sukhasana**

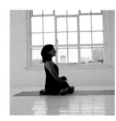
12 **Baddhakonasana**

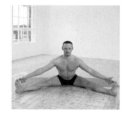
13 **Upavistakonasana**

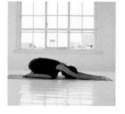
14 **Adho Mukha Vir.**

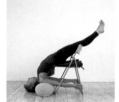
15 **Chair Sarvang.**

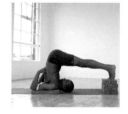
16 **Halasana** (s)

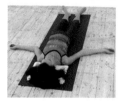
17 **Savasana**

Sequence 14 – Twists and Seated Forward Bends

After doing the first two twists, which allow the spine to extend and rotate, the forward bends become easier. In this sequence, full forward bend poses are done, where the trunk is extended and, if possible, the foot of this leg is caught with the hands. If you cannot reach the foot or the lower back is painful, catch a strap around the foot.

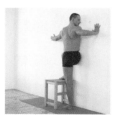
1 **Standing Maricyasana**

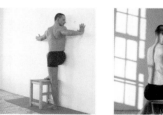
2 **Bharadvajasana (chair)**

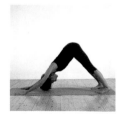
3 **Adho Mukha Svanasana**

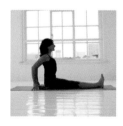
4 **Dandasana**

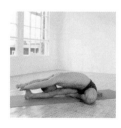
5 **Janusirasana**

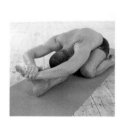
6 **Trianga Mukha. Pascimottanasana**

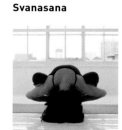
7 **Maricyasana I**

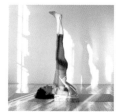
8 **Pascimottanasana**

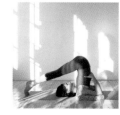
9 **Malasana**

10 **Salamba Sarvang.**

11 **Halasana**

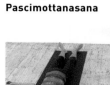
12 **Savasana**

Sequence 15 – Relaxing and Recuperative Postures

This sequence should not be rushed and the postures can be safely held for up to 5 minutes. The chest should be lifted and open, the eyes soft and closed, the facial features relaxed and the brain calm and focused on the breathing. Do not fall asleep, just relax and breathe. The back should feel comfortable in all the poses, so use support if necessary.

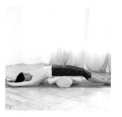

1 **Cross Bolsters**

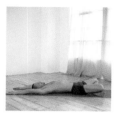

2 **Matsyasana**

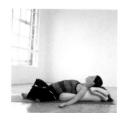

3 **Supta Baddhakon.**

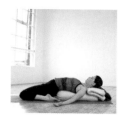

4 **Supta Virasana**

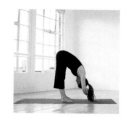

5 **Uttanasana I**

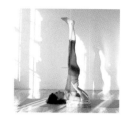

6 **Salamba Sarvangasana**

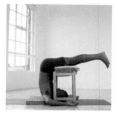

7 **Ardha Halasana** (s)

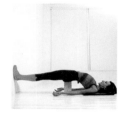

8 **Setu Bandha Sarv.**

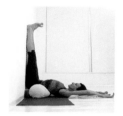

9 **Vipariti Karani**

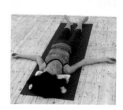

10 **Savasana**

Focus
• Consolidate these postures, going back to the ones you find more difficult and practising them again until they feel easier.

Sequence 16 – Standing Postures and Standing Forward Bends

This routine can take up to two hours to complete. If fatigue is experienced, do Uttanasana I in between to rest the brain and allow the body to recover. Increase timings in the postures, especially Salamba Sarvangasana and Halasana.

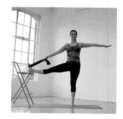

1 **Utthita Hasta Pad. I & II** (s)

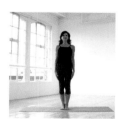

2 **Tadasana**

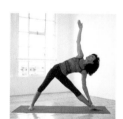

3 **Utthita Trikonasana**

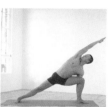

4 **Utthita Parsvakonasana**

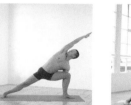

5 **Virabhadrasana I**

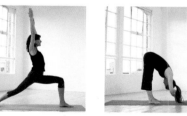

6 **Uttanasana I**

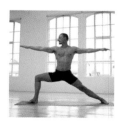

7 **Virabhadrasana II**

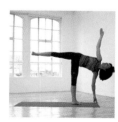

8 **Ardha Chandrasana**

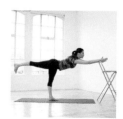

9 **Virabhadrasana III** (s)

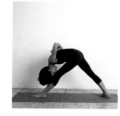

10 **Parsvottanasana**

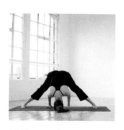

11 **Prasarita Padattonasana**

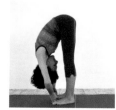

12 **Padangusthasana**

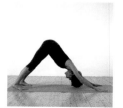

13 **Adho Mukha Svan.**

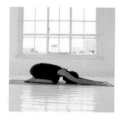

14 **Adho Mukha Vir.**

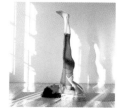

15 **Salamba Sarvang.**

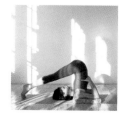

16 **Halasana**

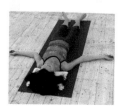

17 **Savasana**

102

Sequence 17 – Stronger Forward Bends and Floor Twists

Lift, open and broaden the chest in all these seated poses. Sit on a support to help with the lift of the spine. While practising the twists, make sure the spine is extended and lengthened before twisting. Both buttock bones should remain on the support in the twists. Increase the timing of the forward bends and keep the brain passive.

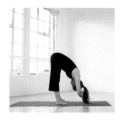 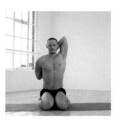 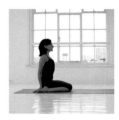 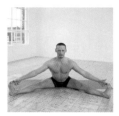 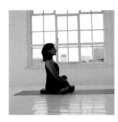 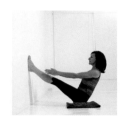

1 **Uttanasana I**   2 **Virasana**   3 **Gomukhasana**   4 **Baddhakonasana**   5 **Upavistakonasana**   6 **Paripurna Nav.** (s)

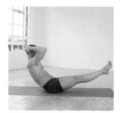 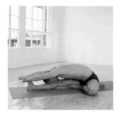 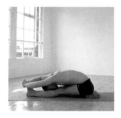 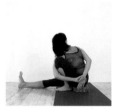 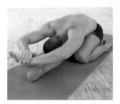 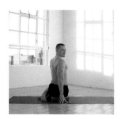

7 **Ardha Navasana**   8 **Janusirsasana**   9 **Trianga Mukha.**   10 **Maricyasana I**   11 **Pascimottanasana**   12 **Bharadvajasana I**

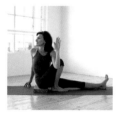 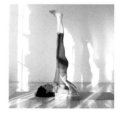 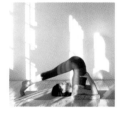 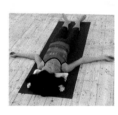

13 **Maricyasana III**   14 **Salamba Sarvang.**   15 **Halasana**   16 **Savasana**

Focus
• In Paripurna Navasana and Ardha Navasana, try to straighten the legs. If the back hurts, practise these postures with bent knees.

Sequence 18 – Progressively More Difficult Postures

At this stage of practice, your stamina, endurance and flexibility should have improved, so this sequence of postures should be challenging but manageable. Practise Virabhadrasana III with only the hands supported, and fully extend the back (lifted) leg away from the head while the arms stretch strongly towards the fingertips.

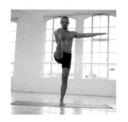 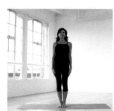 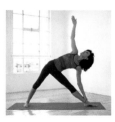 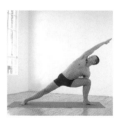 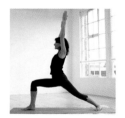 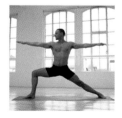

1 **Utt. Hasta Pad. I & II**   2 **Tadasana**   3 **Utthita Trikonasana**   4 **Utthita Parsvakon.**   5 **Virabhadrasana I**   6 **Virabhadrasana II**

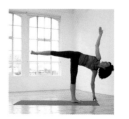 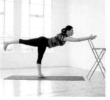 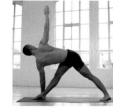 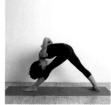 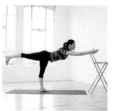 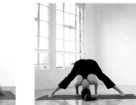 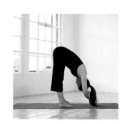

7 **Ardha Chandrasana**   8 **Virabhadrasana III** (s)   9 **Parivrtta Trikonasana**   10 **Parsvottanasana**   11 **Prasarita Padottanasana**   12 **Uttanasana I**   13 **Savasana**

Sequence 19 – Relaxation

In this relaxation routine, forward bends are practised with the head supported. Once the head touches the support, the brain should become calm and passive, allowing you to focus on the breath. Do not strain or create tension while practising supported forward bends, just allow the body to take on the shape of the posture and let go.

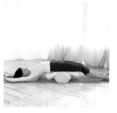
1 **Cross Bolsters**

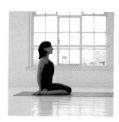
2 **Virasana**

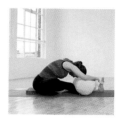
3 **Janusirsasana**

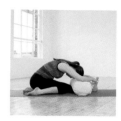
4 **Trianga Mukha.**

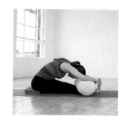
5 **Pascimottanasana**

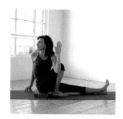
6 **Maricyasana III**

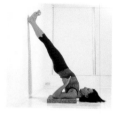
7 **Salamba Sarv.** (w)

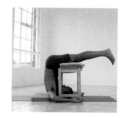
8 **Ardha Halasana** (s)

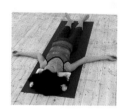
9 **Savasana**

Focus
• If the sequences are becoming too challenging, go back to Sequence 1. There is no race to get through all the sequences as quickly as possible. It is more sensible to work slowly, methodically and intelligently than to rush ahead and lay yourself open to pain and injury.

Sequence 20 – Prone Poses and Basic Standing Poses

Urdhva Mukha Svanasana is one of the preparatory postures for backbend work. In this posture the centre of the tops of the feet should be on the floor, the inner legs should lift up towards the ceiling, and the elbows and knees should be locked. If difficulty is experienced with lifting the body off the floor, use blocks under the hands and tuck the toes under.

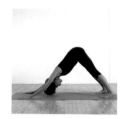
1 **Adho Mukha Svan.**

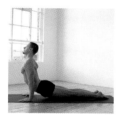
2 **Urdhva Mukha Sv.**

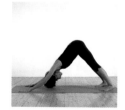
3 **Adho Mukha Svan.**

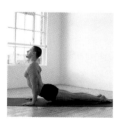
4 **Urdhva Mukha Sv.**

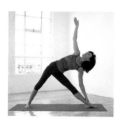
5 **Utthita Trikonasana**

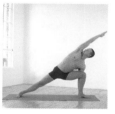
6 **Utthita Parsvakon.**

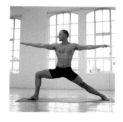
7 **Virabhadrasana II**

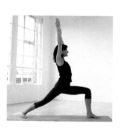
8 **Virabhadrasana I**

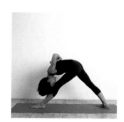
9 **Parsvottanasana**

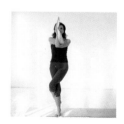
10 **Vrksasana**

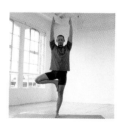
11 **Garudasana**

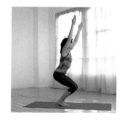
12 **Utkatasana**

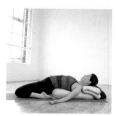
13 **Supta Virasana**

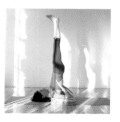
14 **Salamba Sarvang.**

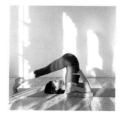
15 **Halasana**

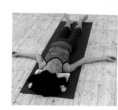
16 **Savasana**

Focus
• As a result of opening the chest and extending the spine upwards, the standing postures require less effort and are improved.

Sequence 21 – Seated Postures and Knee Work

Practising Padmasana incorrectly may result in severe knee problems, so never force the knee. Practise Sukhasana a few times prior to Padmasana in order to "lubricate" the hip and knee joints, and then practise Padmasana with one leg in Sukhasana – be patient, consolidate your practice and, with courage and determination, you will achieve your goal.

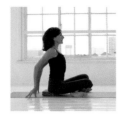

1 **Sukhasana**

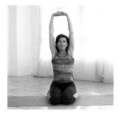

2 **Virasana with Parv.**

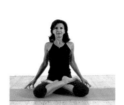

3 **Padmasana**

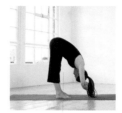

4 **Dandasana**

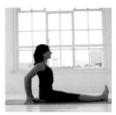

5 **Uttanasana I**

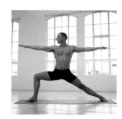

6 **Virabhadrasana II**

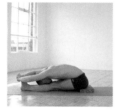

7 **Pascimottanasana**

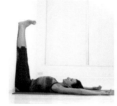

8 **Urdhva Pras. Pad.**

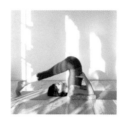

9 **Salamba Sarvang.**

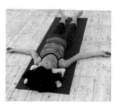

10 **Halasana**

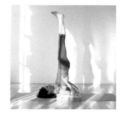

11 **Savasana**

Sequence 22 – Standing, Reverse Standing and Seated Posures

This group of mixed postures requires stamina, strength and flexibility and should be practised with care. Rest in Uttanasana I between the standing postures if necessary. You should set aside at least two hours to do this practice, doing the directional postures twice on each side, and at the end of the sequence practise Savasana for 10 minutes.

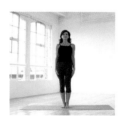

1 **Tadasana**

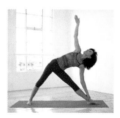

2 **Utthita Trikonasana**

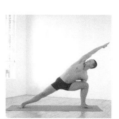

3 **Utthita Parsvakon.**

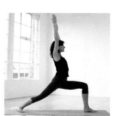

4 **Virabhadrasana I**

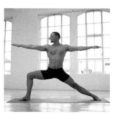

5 **Virabhadrasana II**

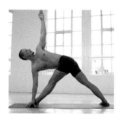

6 **Parivrtta Trikon.**

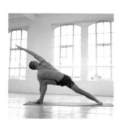

7 **Parivrtta Pars.**

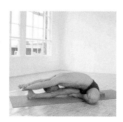

8 **Parsvottanasana**

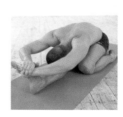

9 **Janusirsasana**

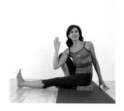

10 **Trianga Mukha.**

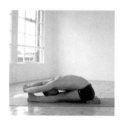

11 **Maricyasana I**

12 **Pascimottanasana**

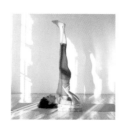

13 **Salamba Sarvang.**

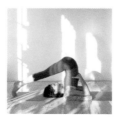

14 **Halasana**

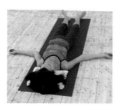

15 **Savasana**

Sequence 23 – Relaxation and Pranayama (Breathing)

Increase the timings in this group in order to open the chest more and deepen relaxation. Never strain the lungs or become agitated in Pranayama – both inhalation and exhalation must be smooth, calm and flowing. The quality of your Pranayama is more important than the quantity. If you feel uncomfortable and tense, return to normal breathing.

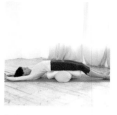
1 **Cross Bolsters**

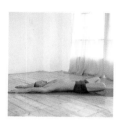
2 **Matsyasana**

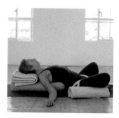
a3 **Supta Baddha.** (s)

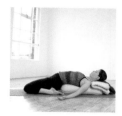
4 **Supta Virasana**

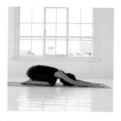
5 **Adho Mukha Vir.**

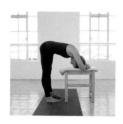
6 **Uttanasana I** (s)

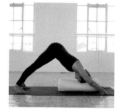
7 **Adho Mukha Svanasana** (s)

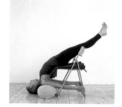
8 **Chair Sarvangasana**

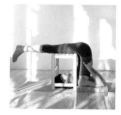
9 **Ardha Halasana**

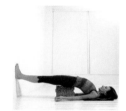
10 **Setu Bandha Sarvangasana**

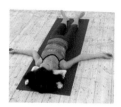
11 **Savasana**

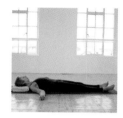
12 **Pranayama**

Sequence 24 – Standing Postures to Consolidate your Practice

In this sequence, focus on fully stretching the backs of both legs. Spend time in Tadasana, analysing and correcting the posture from the feet to the head. Repeat each standing posture twice using the "information" acquired from Tadasana to deepen your understanding and execution of the poses. Extend timings in Salamba Sarvangasana and Halasana.

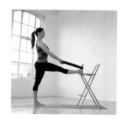
1 **Utt. Hasta Pad. I** (s)

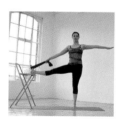
2 **Utt. Hasta Pad. II** (s)

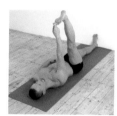
3 **Supta Pad. I**

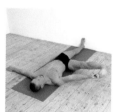
4 **Supta Pad. II**

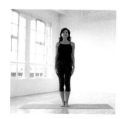
5 **Tadasana**

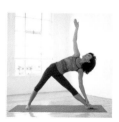
6 **Utthita Trikonasana**

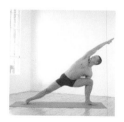
7 **Utthita Parsvakon.**

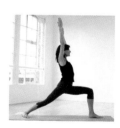
8 **Virabhadrasana I**

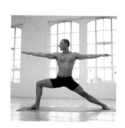
9 **Virabhadrasana II**

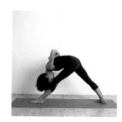
10 **Ardha Chandr.**

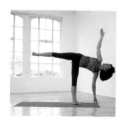
11 **Parvottanasana**

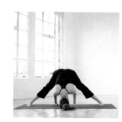
12 **Prasarita Pad.**

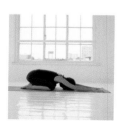
13 **Adho Mukha Vir.**

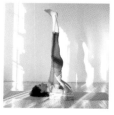
14 **Salamba Sarvang.**

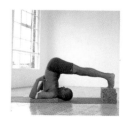
15 **Halasana** (s)

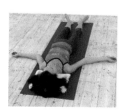
16 **Savasana**

Sequence 25 – Seated Postures

Practise Adho Mukha Svanasana and Urdhva Mukha Svanasana three times, opening the chest and lengthening the spine progressively. In Urdhva Mukha Svanasana, look up without compressing the back of the neck and keep the head in a comfortable position. In Dandasana, Paripurna Navasana, Ardha Navasana and Pascimottanasana, fully stretch and lengthen the backs of the legs and keep the thighs and knees pressing towards the floor. In Baddhakonasana – and Upavistakonasana, keep the front of the body extending from pubis to chin and move the shoulder blades towards the front of the trunk to lift and open the chest. Twist further and breathe more deeply in Bharadvajasana I.

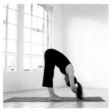 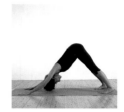 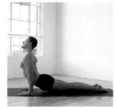 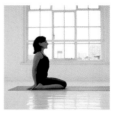 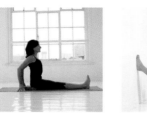 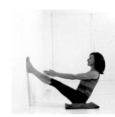

1 **Uttanasana I**   2 **Adho Mukha Svan.**   3 **Urdhva Mukha Svan.**   4 **Virasana**   5 **Dandasana**   6 **Paripurna Nav.** (s)

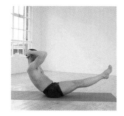 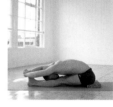 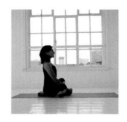 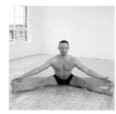 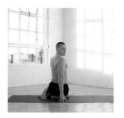 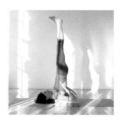

7 **Ardha Navasana**   8 **Pascimottanasana**   9 **Baddhakonasana**   10 **Upavistakonasana**   11 **Bharadvajasana I**   11 **Salamba Sarvang.**

Sequence 26 – Standing and Prone Postures

After the standing poses in this routine, Adho Mukha Svanasana is followed by Urdhva Mukha Svanasana,which prepares the spine for Salabhasana. In the latter two poses, the pubis and sacrum move towards the floor to avoid a painful pinching sensation in the lower back. Salabhasana should be practised with the legs together, though if the back is painful, you should separate them slightly. Extend both legs strongly towards the heels, keeping the soles of the feet long and broad. Lengthen the arms from the shoulders and stretch back towards the fingertips, keeping the palms broad and facing the ceiling. Lift and open the chest as much as possible and look straight ahead, keeping the eyes soft. After Salabhasana, practise Urdhva Mukha and Adho Mukha Svanasana quietly to release the spine gently. Ensure that the back is comfortable in Ardha Halasana. If it is sore in Savasana, rest the legs on a stool.

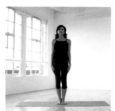 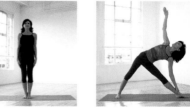 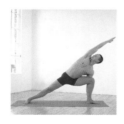 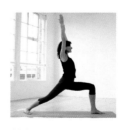 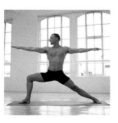 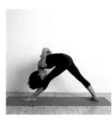

1 **Tadasana**   2 **Utthita Trikonasana**   3 **Utthita Parsvakon.**   4 **Virabhadrasana I**   5 **Virabhadrasana II**   6 **Parsvottanasana**

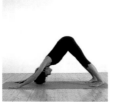 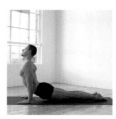 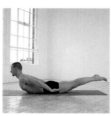 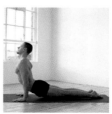 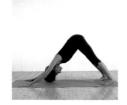 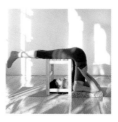

7 **Adho Mukha Svanasana**   8 **Urdhva Mukha Svanasana**   9 **Salabhasana**   10 **Urdhva Mukha Svanasana**   11 **Adho Mukha Svanasana**   12 **Ardha Halasana**
13 **Savasana**

Sequence 27 – Relaxation

Try to let go while practising these poses. When in each posture, settle the body and focus on the breath. If the body becomes restless, the brain will follow. Once the head is resting on the support in the forward bends, soften the abdomen, relax the shoulders and back, keep the face, mouth and throat passive, and unite the breath with the mind and the mind with the breath. Extend the Pranayama practice without causing strain or tension.

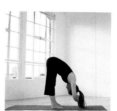

1 **Uttanasana I**

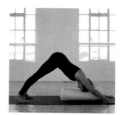

2 **Adho Mukha Svanasana** (s)

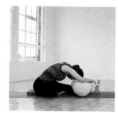

3 **Janusirsasana** (s)

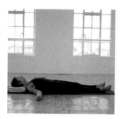

4 **Pascimottanasana** (s)

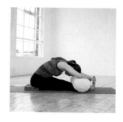

5 **Salamba Sarvangasana** (w)

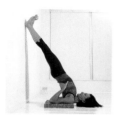

6 **Ardha Halasana**

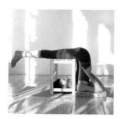

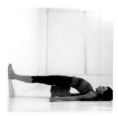

7 **Setu Bandha Sarvangasana**

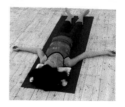

8 **Savasana**

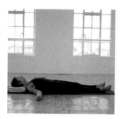

9 **Pranayama**

Surya Namaskara – Sun Salutation

In this short routine the postures are linked together in a flowing movement. It can be practised only when the individual postures have been learnt and understood, which may be after completing the previous 27 sequences. The cycle of postures can be repeated 4–12 times, depending on the time available and the energy of the practitioner.

Surya Namaskara involves quick postures and movement, with each pose held for a few breaths only. Regular practice improves mobility, alertness, agility and speed, while developing willpower and physical strength. The brain becomes active and refreshed.

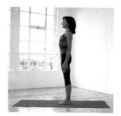

1 **Tadasana**

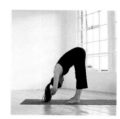

2 Exhale, extend into **Uttanasana I**

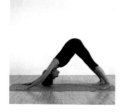

3 Step back into **Adho Mukha Svanasana**

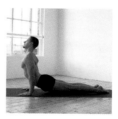

4 Inhale, roll forward into **Urdhva Mukha Svanasana**

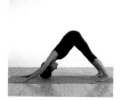

5 Exhale, come back to **Adho Mukha Svanasana**

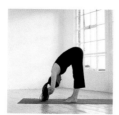

6 On the next exhale jump forwards into **Uttanasana I**

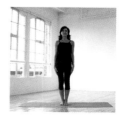

7 Exhale, release the arms and come back into **Tadasana**

Focus
• People with hea rt problems and women who are menstruating should not practise this routine.
• Breathe normally for 3–4 breaths before jumping or stepping into the next posture.

• Synchronize the inhalation and exhalation as you move from one position to another.
• Repeat the routine 4–12 times.
• After completion, rest in Uttanasana I to recover.

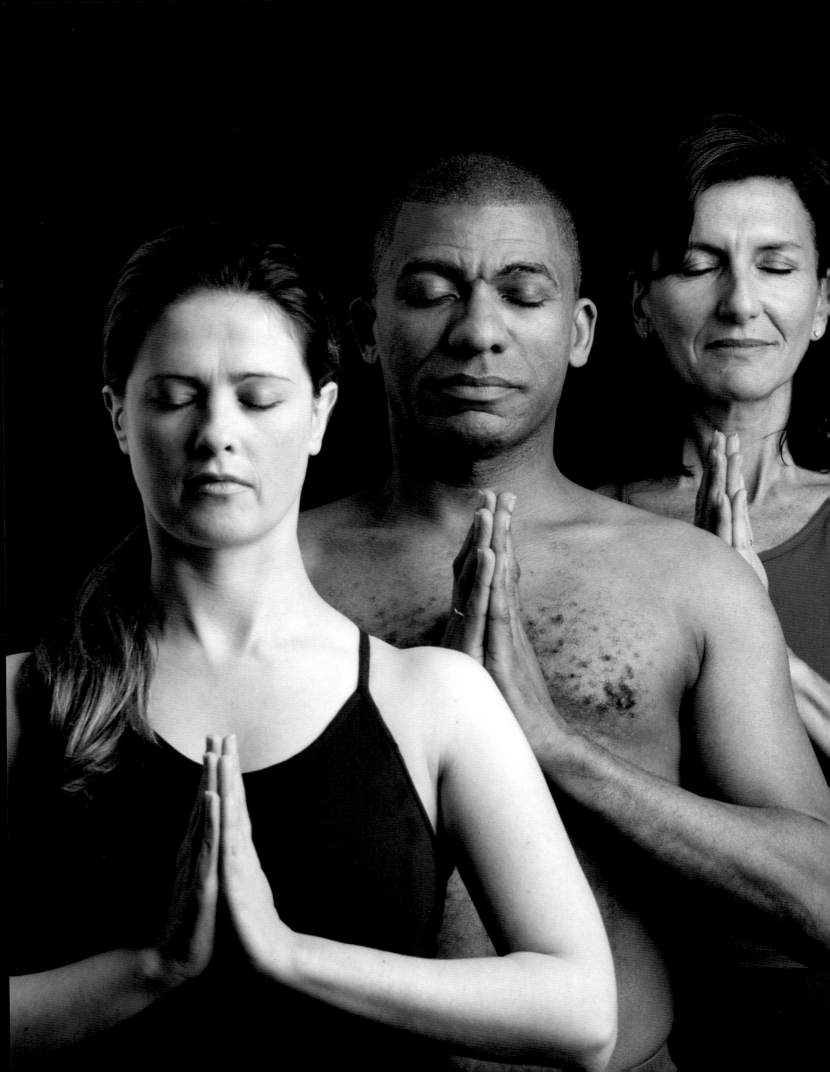

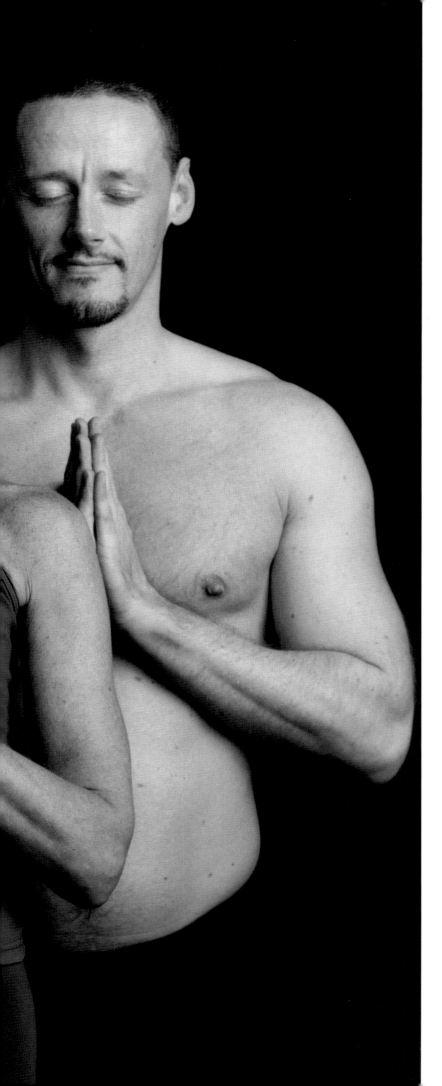

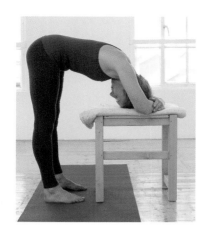

yoga Therapy

"Yoga's system of healing is based on the premise that the body should be allowed to function as naturally as possible. Practising the recommended asanas will first rejuvenate the body, and then tackle the causes of the ailment."

B.K.S. Iyengar

Therapeutic Yoga

Yoga can help to improve and heal parts of the body that are injured, traumatized or neglected. Movement of the body in asanas stimulates injured joints, muscles or organs by increasing the flow of blood to these parts. The practice of yoga also increases the pain threshold. This chapter on therapeutic yoga is based on the sequencing of selected postures to treat specific minor ailments. The postures are adapted by using props and are therefore accessible to all students, regardless of their complaints or the condition of their bodies.

Healing with yoga

When the body is tired and lethargic as a result of minor illness or injury, your regular yoga practice need not be discontinued. Even if you feel unable to follow your sequence of postures in the normal way, practising with props helps to improve the posture and maintain balance, and allows you to stretch fully while experiencing a state of relaxation during practice. This feeling of peace and tranquillity is the beginning of the healing process.

In some cases, the practice of yoga will not result in a complete cure, but in most cases it will alleviate some of the suffering and discomfort associated with the condition, and boost confidence and morale. Practising the asanas with dedication and patience calms the brain and soothes the nerves. This feeling of relaxation reduces the anxiety

that is created by the pain, which in itself helps to reduce the actual pain and improve your pain threshold.

Working through a sequence of postures using the necessary supports can effect remarkable changes in both your physical and mental state, At the end of your practice you are likely to feel more flexible and fluid, with greater mobility, a lessening of pain and a renewed sense of serenity and peace.

This section of the book offers programmes for a range of minor ailments and common problems. It does not include sequences aimed at alleviating any serious medical conditions, as these should be done only under the guidance and supervision of a suitably qualified Iyengar teacher. The student of yoga will readily understand the tremendous need to include yoga in their daily life, and the suggestions that follow show how it can be used effectively with conventional medicine, or alone, to improve or alleviate many common disorders.

The postures for everyday ailments are shown on the following pages. The props and supports used are explained in detail, but you may also find it useful to refer back to the original descriptions of the postures and the various modifications suggested there.

Commonsense should prevail when you are practising these adapted postures, and the poses should be held for only as long as is comfortable. When following a sequence for a specific condition, it is best to continue with this programme until some relief is obtained. If difficulty is experienced with a programme, it is advisable to consult an experienced teacher.

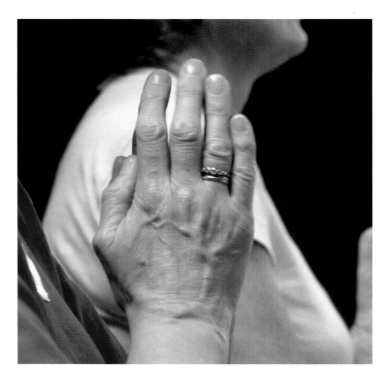

left Iyengar Yoga is a gentle and supportive system of exercise that can help to fend off illness and keep the body supple, whatever the age of the practitioner.

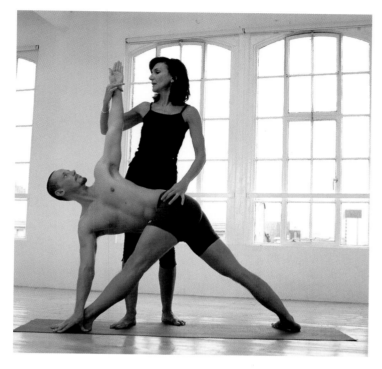

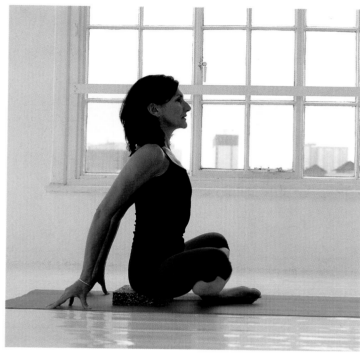

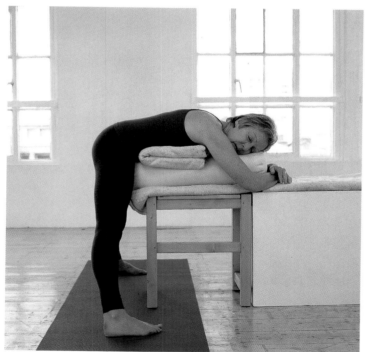

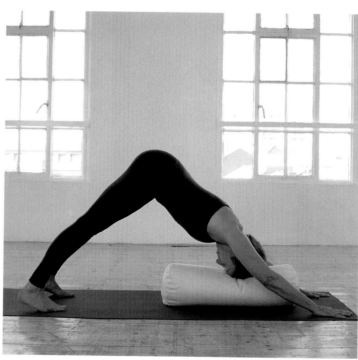

above Clockwise: correcting the alignment of the trunk in Parivrtta Trikonasana; sitting in Baddhakonasana, lifting the chest; supported Adho Mukha Svanasana, with the head resting on a bolster; supported Prasarita Padottanasana – a quiet, passive posture that allows the brain to stay calm. These postures are all potentially therapeutic when used in conjunction with an appropriate routine.

Mental Fatigue and Exhaustion

Stress and physical exertion contribute to fatigue and exhaustion, and if this is not checked it can develop into chronic fatigue syndrome. The pace of daily life has an impact on the body and the emotions.

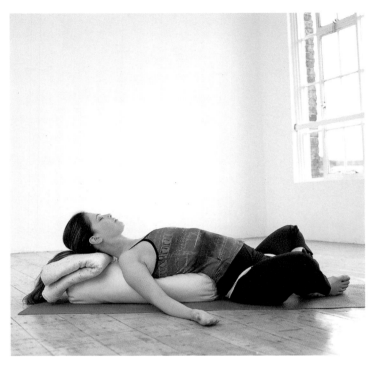

1 Supta Baddhakonasana using a bolster and folded blanket to support the head and neck and a strap to keep the feet close to the body.

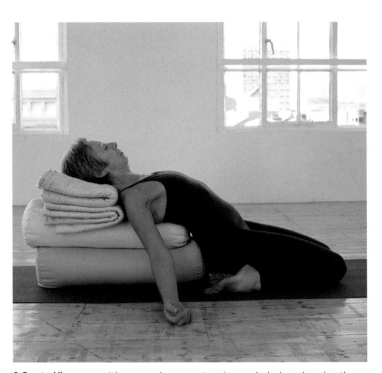

2 Supta Virasana with as much support as is needed placed under the spine, neck and head to allow the back and knees to release. Keep the chest open and up, and the shoulders relaxed and back.

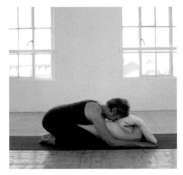
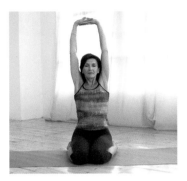

3 Virasana with Parvatasana extending the palms towards the ceiling.
4 Adho Mukha Virasana with the head and trunk supported on a bolster and/or blanket.

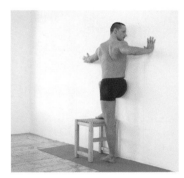
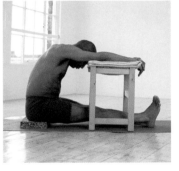

5 Pascimottanasana with the forehead supported on a stool to avoid straining the back.
6 Standing Maricyasana using the wall and the stool for support.

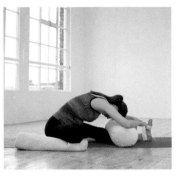
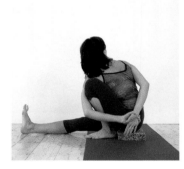

7 Janusirsasana with the head, elbows and knee supported on bolsters, and using a strap.
8 Maricyasana I sitting on a support to aid the lift of the spine, and turning the chest.

Focus

• In yoga, strong emotions are linked to hormonal imbalances, which leave one vulnerable to infections and illness. This sequence works on stimulating and nourishing the internal organs and the nervous system to pacify and calm the nerves, body and mind.

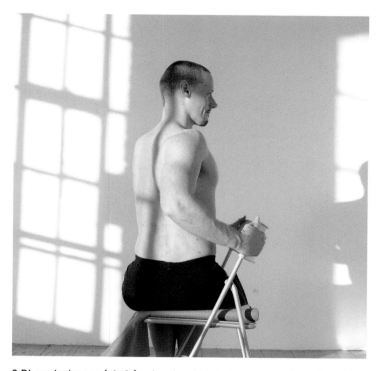

9 Bharadvajasana (chair) using the chair to increase the turn. Keep the feet on the floor, parallel to one another, to stabilize the hips. Turn from the waist, moving a little more with each exhalation.

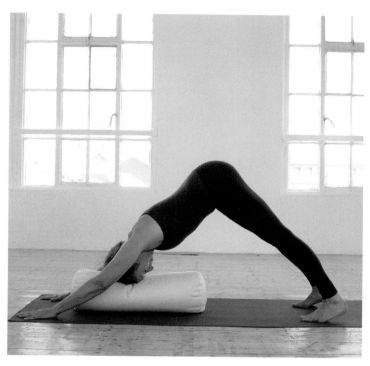

11 Adho Mukha Svanasana with the head supported on a bolster to calm the brain.

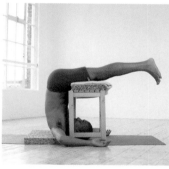

12 Ardha Halasana with the legs supported on foam blocks on a stool, and the brain quiet.

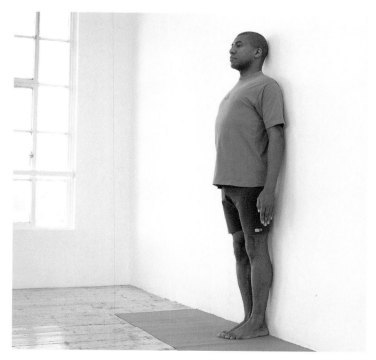

10 Tadasana standing against a wall. Use the wall to aid balance, keeping the feet parallel and together and the heels against the wall. Lift the chest, keeping the face and eyes soft.

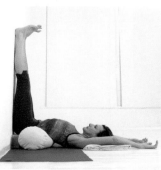

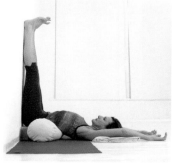

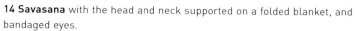

13 Viparita Karani using a wooden block and a bolster to support the lower back and hips.
14 Savasana with the head and neck supported on a folded blanket, and bandaged eyes.

Headache/Migraine

A headache may be a result of tension in the neck muscles and scalp after a stressful event, or due to fatigue and lack of rest. In the case of migraine, an intense throbbing pain in the head may be accompanied by nausea and vomiting.

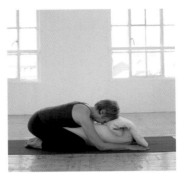 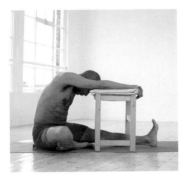

1 Adho Mukha Virasana with the head and trunk supported on a bolster and blanket.
2 Janusirsasana with the forehead and arms supported on a stool.

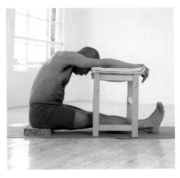 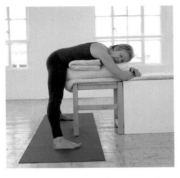

3 Pascimottanasana with the forehead and arms supported on a stool.
4 Prasarita Padottanasana with the head, trunk and arms supported on a stool and blankets.

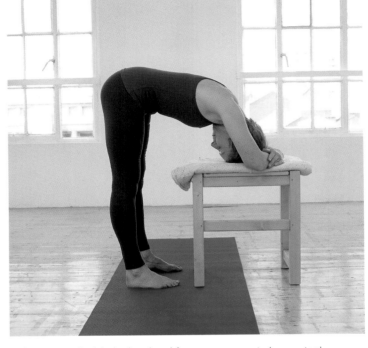

6 Uttanasana I with the head and forearms supported on a stool softened with a blanket. This posture, with the head lowered, allows more blood to flow to the area, helping to relieve any discomfort.

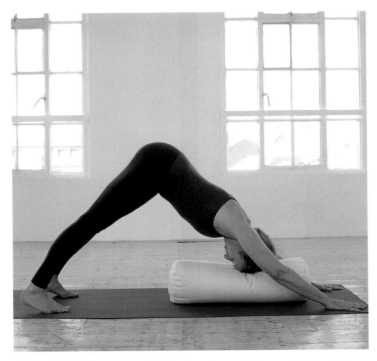

5 Adho Mukha Svanasana with the head supported on a bolster, or a pile of blankets, in order to keep the brain calm.

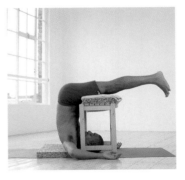 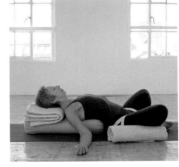

7 Ardha Halasana with the legs supported on a stool, the height adjusted with foam blocks.
8 Supta Baddhakonasana with a strap around legs, bolster under spine, and head supported.

Focus
• These postures for relieving headaches and migraines increase blood flow to the brain and restore the stability of the nervous system. While doing the postures, be aware of lengthening the muscles of the neck and try to keep the brain as quiet as possible.

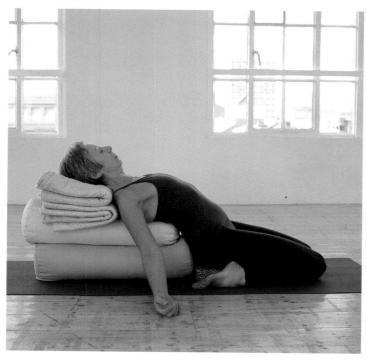

9 Supta Virasana with the spine, neck and head supported on two bolsters and two folded blankets.

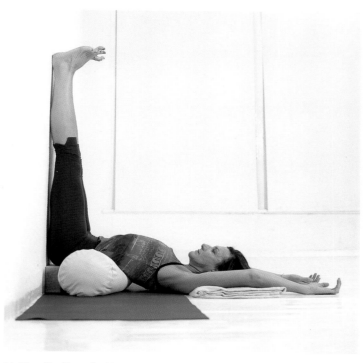

11 Viparita Karani with the backs of the legs against the wall and the body lying over a bolster and wooden block. Use a blanket for comfort under the head, arms extended over the head, palms facing upwards.

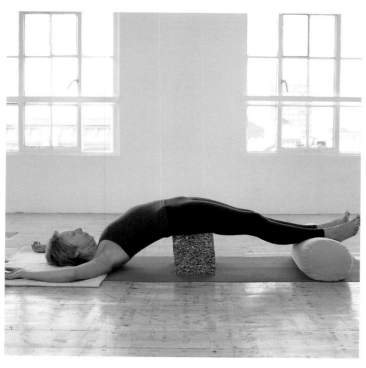

10 Setu Bandha Sarvangasana using foam blocks to support the sacrum and a bolster to support the feet, arms extended over the head, palms facing upwards.

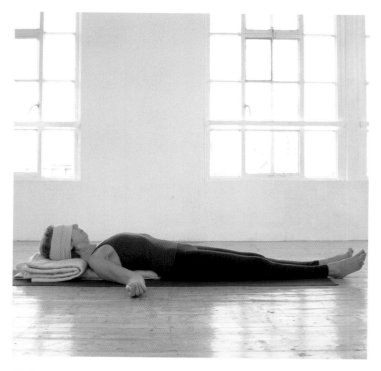

12 Savasana with the neck and head supported on a folded blanket. A bandage firmly tied around the head and/or eyes is very soothing and calming when experiencing headache.

Stress/Anxiety

These postures work on tense muscles and encourage blood to circulate. This stabilizes the heart rate and blood pressure. Shallow, fast breathing becomes deeper, slower and more rhythmical, which results in a higher intake of oxygen, and this helps to remove stress.

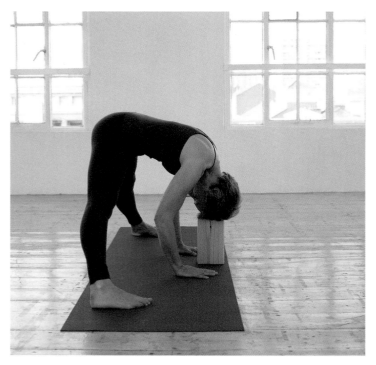

1 Uttanasana I with the head supported on a blanket and stool. When one part of the body is strained and tense, circulation to that body part is decreased – increasing it again will help to calm the mind and body.

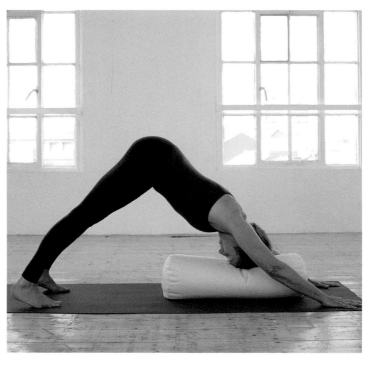

3 Adho Mukha Svanasana with the head supported on a bolster to keep the mind quiet.

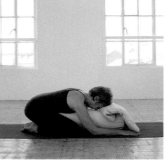

4 Adho Mukha Virasana with a bolster and blanket supporting the trunk and head.
5 Janusirsasana with the head and arms supported on a bolster and a strap around the foot. If necessary, you may also use a bolster to support the bent knee.

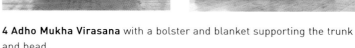

2 Prasarita Padottanasana with the head supported on a wooden block. If the hands don't reach the floor, use foam blocks under the palms to raise the level of support. It may be necessary to use more blocks under the head as well.

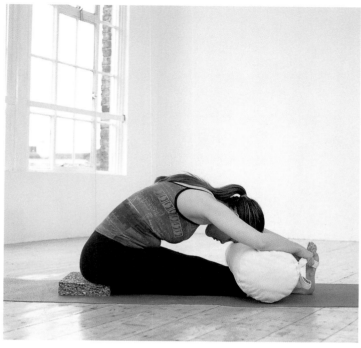

6 Pascimottanasana with the head and forearms supported on a bolster and using a strap around the foot. Keep the eyes closed and the mind still and quiet.

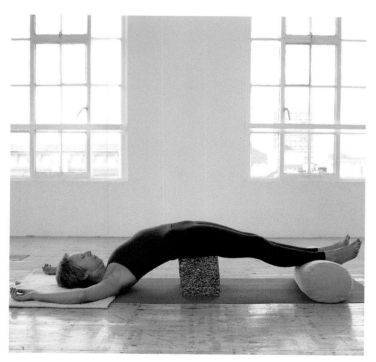

7 Setu Bandha Sarvangasana with four foam blocks under the sacrum, feet resting on a bolster and head and shoulders supported on a folded blanket – arms over head, palms facing the ceiling.

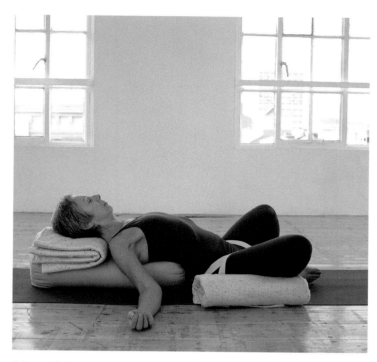

8 Supta Baddhakonasana with bolsters and blankets supporting the spine and head, and a strap around the legs and feet. The thighs are supported with rolled-up blankets.

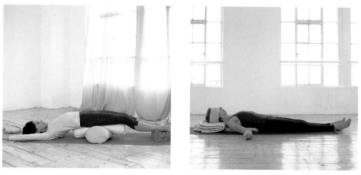

9 Cross Bolsters with the feet resting on blocks. This gentle arch opens the chest.

10 Savasana with a folded blanket supporting the head and neck, and with the eyes covered.

Focus

• Postures here are done with a support under the head. This allows the brain to become quiet and calm. Breathe normally throughout and focus the mind on the breath. Keep the face, mouth and throat relaxed.

• In order to deal with stress and anxiety, both the mind and body must be treated. Tension associated with stress is stored mainly in the muscles, diaphragm and nervous system and if these areas are relaxed, stress is reduced.

Insomnia

The physiological symptoms of insomnia – raised or lowered blood pressure and exhaustion – can be dealt with by doing these postures with the face, mouth, throat and stomach soft and relaxed, in order to keep the mind and brain quiet.

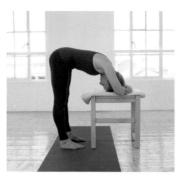
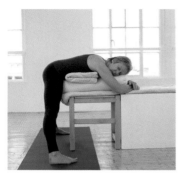

1 Uttanasana I with the head and arms supported on a stool.
2 Prasarita Padottanasana with trunk, arms and head supported.

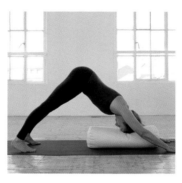
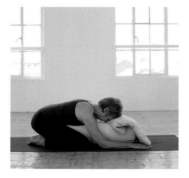

3 Adho Mukha Svanasana with the head supported on a bolster.
4 Adho Mukha Virasana with the forehead and trunk supported.

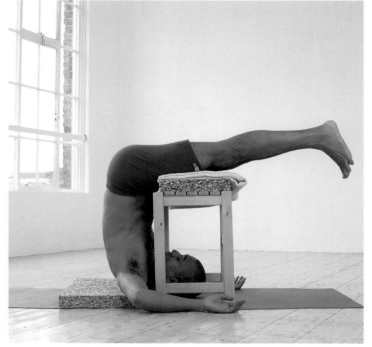

9 Ardha Halasana with a stool and foam blocks for support.

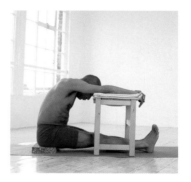
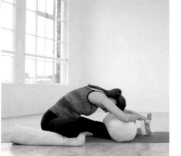

5 Pascimottanasana with the forehead and arms supported.
6 Janusirsasana with the forehead and arms supported, using a strap.

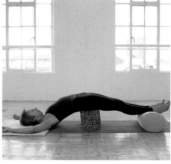
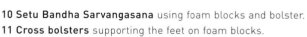

10 Setu Bandha Sarvangasana using foam blocks and bolster.
11 Cross bolsters supporting the feet on foam blocks.

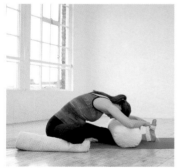

7 Supta Baddhakonasana using a strap and bolster support.
8 Chair Sarvangasana shoulder stand using a chair and bolster.

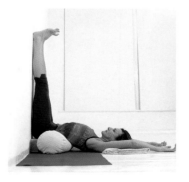
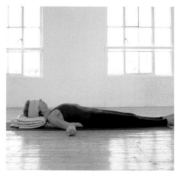

12 Viparita Karani legs against wall, support under lower back.
13 Savasana head and neck supported, eyes bandaged.

Depression

While performing the postures, there needs to be a balance between the mind, body, emotions, and soul. Since the head is supported in these postures, the mind becomes calm and the heart is energized, bringing about courage and a healthier mental state.

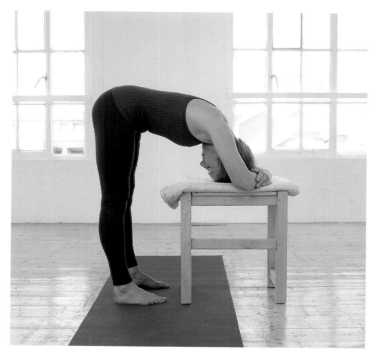

1 Uttanasana I with the head and forearms supported on a stool. This position encourages an increased flow of blood to the head, which helps to calm the mind.

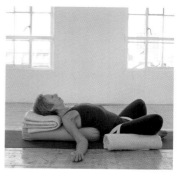

6 Supta Baddhakonasana with a strap and supports.
7 Supta Virasana with several bolsters for support.

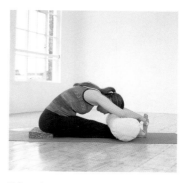

8 Pascimottanasana with the head and arms supported on a bolster.
9 Janusirsasana with forehead and arms supported, using a strap.

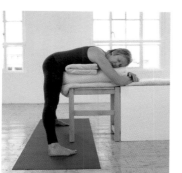

2 Prasarita Padottanasana with trunk, head and arms supported.
3 Adho Mukha Svanasana with the head supported on a bolster.

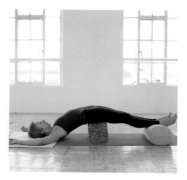

10 Setu Bandha Sarvangasana with supports under sacrum/feet.
11 Cross Bolsters This gentle arch helps breathing.

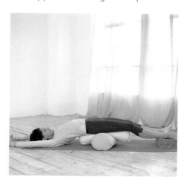

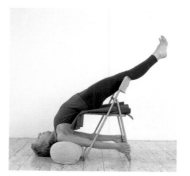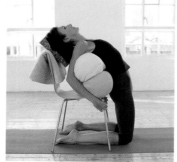

4 Chair Sarvangasana using a bolster for the shoulders.
5 Ustrasana with a chair and bolsters supporting the spine.

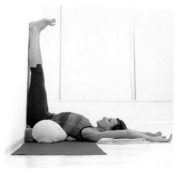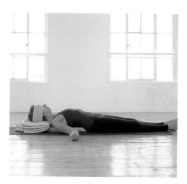

12 Viparita Karani with legs up the wall and a bolster for support.
13 Savasana using support and with the eyes covered.

Colds

In some of the postures listed below, the head is down, which helps to drain the nasal passages and sinuses. In others, the chest is supported and lifted to facilitate easier breathing.

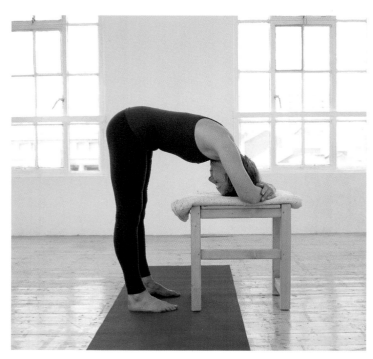

1 Uttanasana I with the head and forearms supported on a stool softened with a blanket. Broadening the chest in this posture will facilitate easier breathing.

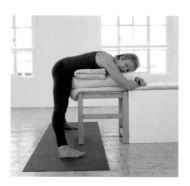 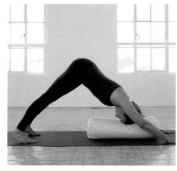

2 Prasarita Padottanasana with the arms and trunk supported on a stool, bolster and blankets.
3 Adho Mukha Svanasana with the head supported on a bolster.

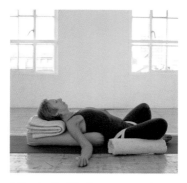 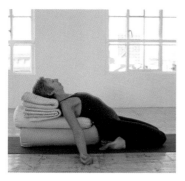

4 Supta Baddhakonasana using a strap and bolster support.
5 Supta Virasana with bolsters and blankets supporting the spine.

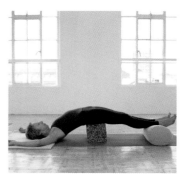 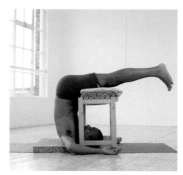

6 Setu Bandha Sarvangasana with foam blocks supporting the sacrum.
7 Ardha Halasana with thighs supported on a stool and shoulders on a foam block.

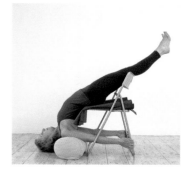 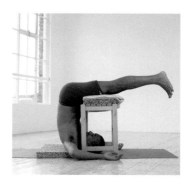

8 Chair Sarvangasana with the shoulders and neck supported on a bolster.
9 Ardha Halasana with the thighs supported on a stool and the shoulders on a foam block.

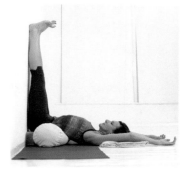

10 Viparita Karani with the legs against the wall and the lower back raised with block and bolster.

Focus
• In the sequences for colds and asthma, attention should be paid to opening and broadening the chest while in the postures. Breathing should be normal and the brain passive. Regular practice of these routines will build up the strength of the respiratory system.

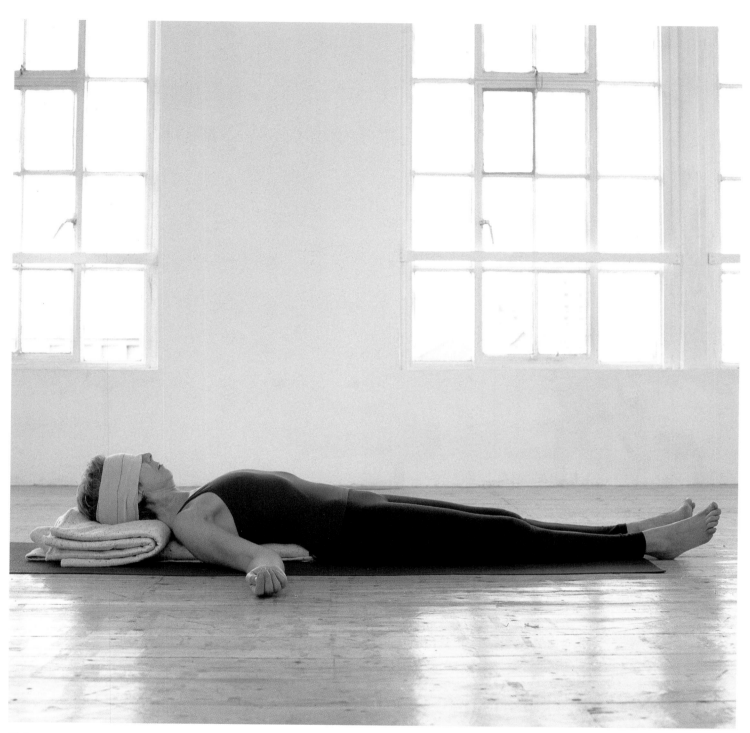

11 Savasana with the head supported and eyes covered. Arms out with
palms facing upwards. Allow the body to let go completely in this posture.
Sink towards the floor. Focus on the breath.

Asthma

These postures facilitate dilation of the air passages in order to make exhalation easier during an attack. They also help to prevent constriction of these passages, thus reducing the number and intensity of further attacks.

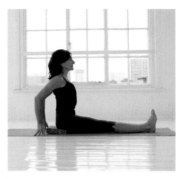 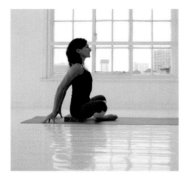

1 Dandasana with the inner edges of the feet together and the backs of the legs pressing into the floor.

2 Baddhakonasana with the soles of the feet pressed together, sitting up, lifting and opening the chest.

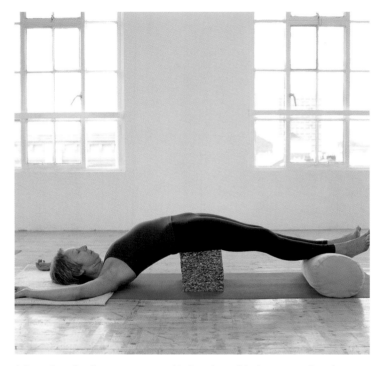

6 Setu Bandha Sarvangasana with four foam blocks supporting the sacrum and a bolster to support the feet.

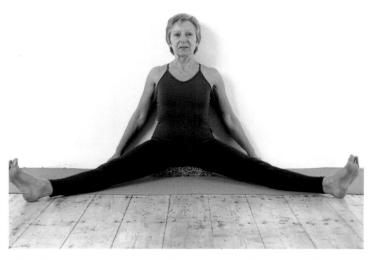

3 Upavistakonasana sitting on a foam block for lift, and using the wall to support the back.

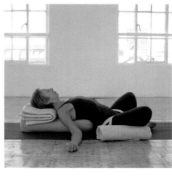 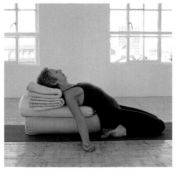

4 Supta Baddhakonasana with the head, neck and spine supported by bolsters and blankets.

5 Supta Virasana supporting the spine with several bolsters and blankets.

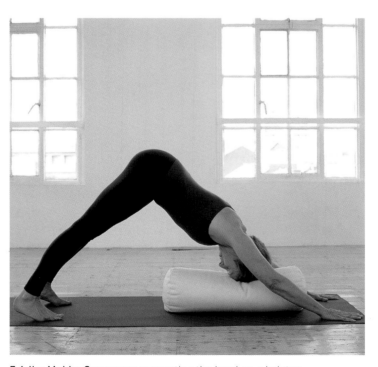

7 Adho Mukha Svanasana supporting the head on a bolster.

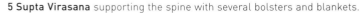

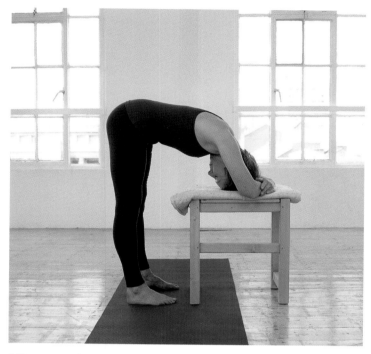

8 Uttanasana I with the head and arms supported on a stool softened with a blanket.

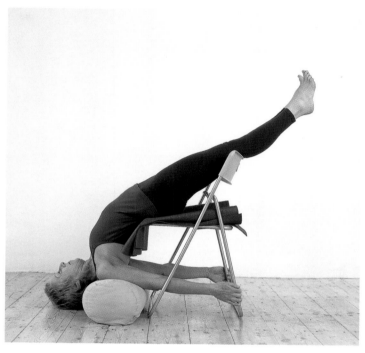

13 Chair Sarvangasana using a chair to support the spine and a bolster for the neck and shoulders. Stretch the arms through the chair and pull on the legs to open the chest, keeping the shoulders back.

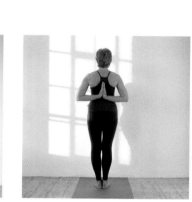

9 Tadasana with the hands in Parvatasana, using the wall to support the body.
10 Tadasana with the hands in Namaste, opening the chest.

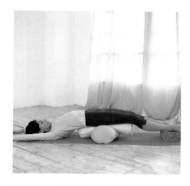
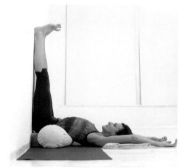

14 Cross Bolsters with two bolsters crossing to help lift and broaden the chest.
15 Viparita Karani with the legs against the wall and support for the back.

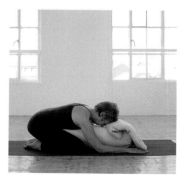
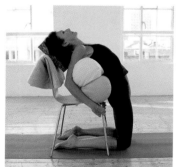

11 Adho Mukha Virasana with the trunk and head supported.
12 Ustrasana using a support for the spine as it arches back.

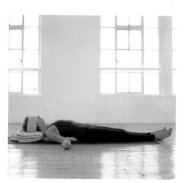

16 Savasana using support for the head and with the eyes covered.

Indigestion

Digestion problems occur as a result of the sluggish movement of food through the stomach and the intestines. In these postures there is increased blood flow to the abdominal organs, which improves the functions of the digestive system.

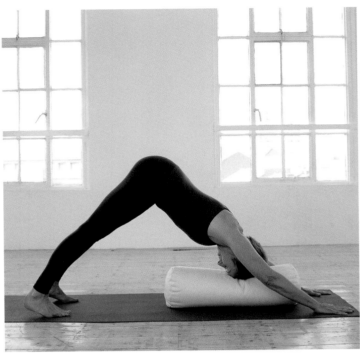

1 Adho Mukha Svanasana with the head supported on a bolster. This posture can also be done with the heels resting on a wall for balance.

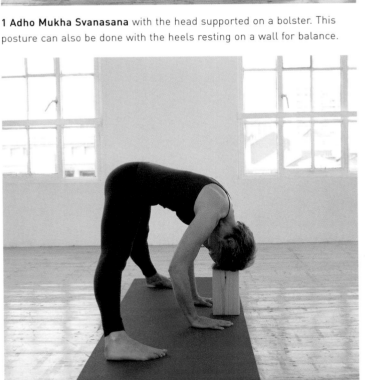

2 Prasarita Padottanasana with the legs apart and with the head supported on a wooden block or several foam blocks.

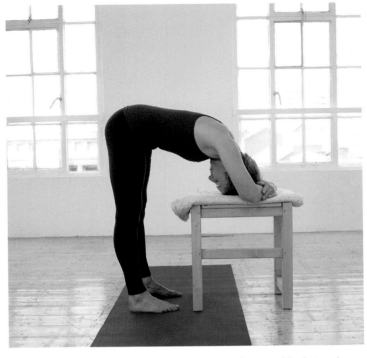

3 Uttanasana I with the head and forearms resting on a blanket and stool. If you do not have a Halasana stool, use a chair and blocks.

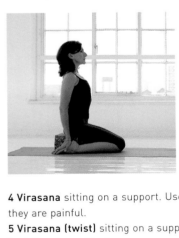

4 Virasana sitting on a support. Use a rolled-up blanket under the feet if they are painful.
5 Virasana (twist) sitting on a support, turning the trunk, resting the back hand on a block.

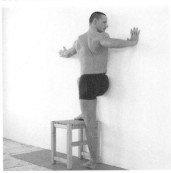

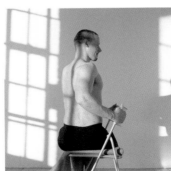

6 Standing Maricyasana using the wall and stool as support.
7 Bharadvajasana (chair) using the back of the chair to turn.

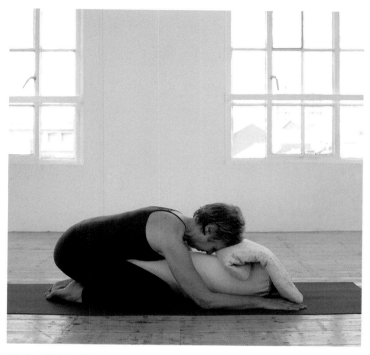

8 Adho Mukha Virasana with the head and trunk supported on a bolster and folded blanket.

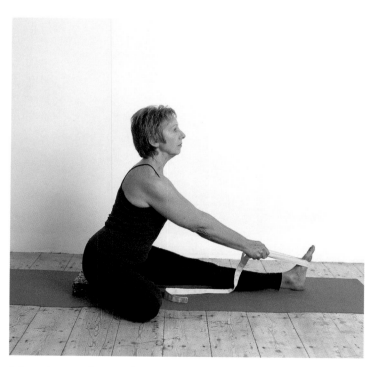

9 Janusirasana (concave) using a strap around the foot and keeping the back concave. Hold the strap in a "V" shape, one end in each hand.

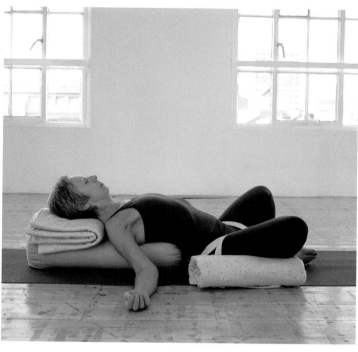

10 Supta Baddhakonasana with bolsters and blankets supporting the spine, head and knees, and a strap around the legs and feet.

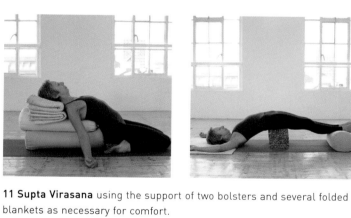

11 Supta Virasana using the support of two bolsters and several folded blankets as necessary for comfort.
12 Setu Bandha Sarvangasana supported sacrum and raised feet.

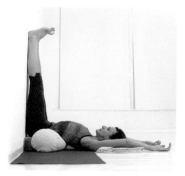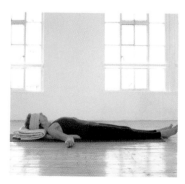

13 Viparita Karani with the legs against the wall, bolster and block supporting the lower back.
14 Savasana with the head supported by blankets and the eyes covered.

Constipation

In these postures the abdominal organs are compressed and massaged and this improves their digestive, absorptive and excretory functions. In the inverted poses, there is a positive displacement of the abdominal organs, which helps to relieve stress and strain.

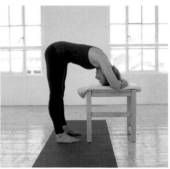 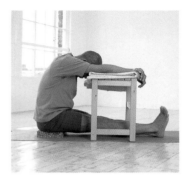 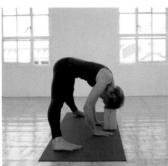 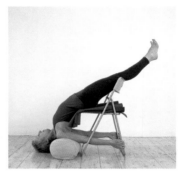

1 Uttanasana I with head and forearms supported on a stool.
2 Prasarita Padottanasana with the head supported on a wooden block.

9 Pascimottanasana supporting the head on a stool.
10 Chair Sarvangasana using a bolster to support the shoulders.

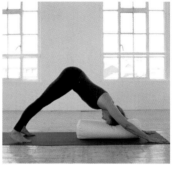 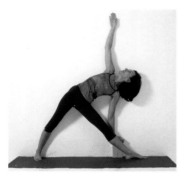 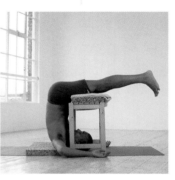 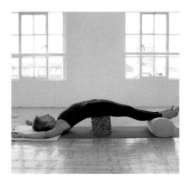

3 Adho Mukha Svanasana with a bolster to support the head.
4 Utthita Trikonasana against the wall, using a block to support the hand.

11 Ardha Halasana using a stool and blocks to support the thighs and a block for the shoulders.
12 Setu Bandha Sarvangasana supporting the sacrum, and feet.

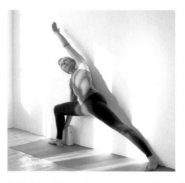 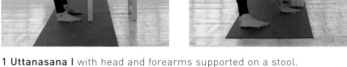 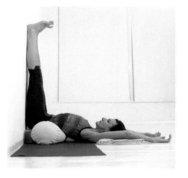 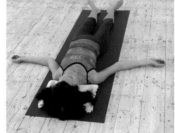

5 Utthita Parsvakonasana against the wall, using a wooden block.
6 Ardha Chandrasana against a wall supporting the leg with a stool.

13 Viparita Karani with the legs against the wall and a block and bolster to support the lower back.
14 Savasana with a blanket supporting the head and neck. Palms are open and up.

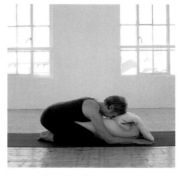 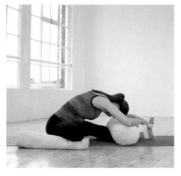

7 Adho Mukha Virasana supporting the head with a bolster and blanket.
8 Janusirsasana supporting the head and knee with bolsters and strap.

Diarrhoea

This condition is often accompanied by abdominal pain or fever. In the postures below, the abdomen should remain soft and the brain passive and calm. A combination of restful and stretching postures will aid comfort.

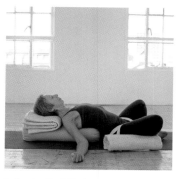

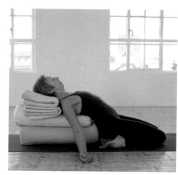

1 Supta Baddhakonasana with a strap around the feet and legs, and support for the spine and legs.
2 Supta Virasana supporting the back and body on bolsters and blankets.

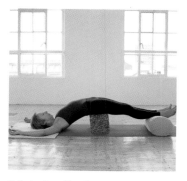

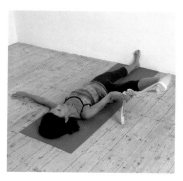

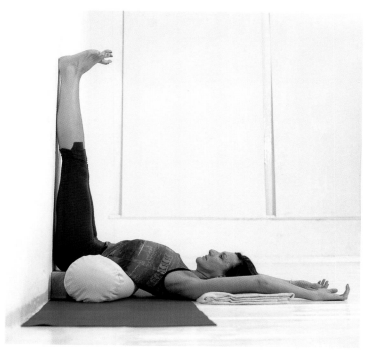

6 Viparita Karani with the backs of the legs against the wall and a bolster and wooden block supporting the lower back. Use a folded blanket to support the head and shoulders.

3 Setu Bandha Sarvangasana supporting the sacrum with foam blocks.
4 Supta Padangustasana II using a strap around the foot, and pressing the other foot to the wall.

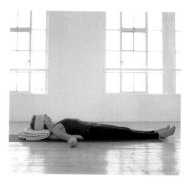

7 Savasana with the head and neck on a folded blanket, and the eyes loosely covered. Keep the whole body relaxed, allow the feet to drop and the arms to be loose, with the palms facing the ceiling.

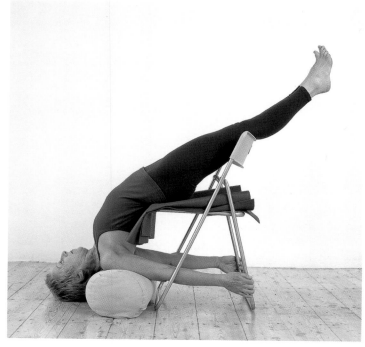

5 Chair Sarvangasana using a bolster to support the shoulders and neck. Inversions will help to relieve any stress on the bowels and abdomen.

Focus
• These sequences to aid digestion include standing postures that stimulate, as well as twists and forward bends that "squeeze" and massage the abdominal organs. While performing these postures, ensure that the abdomen is not restricted or cramped.

Backache

The following five sequences offer poses that will strengthen bones, stretch muscles and help to free and release the affected areas. Flexibility and mobility improve with sustained practice, and pain and discomfort diminish.

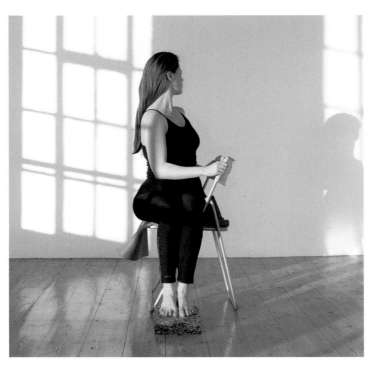

1 Bharadvajasana (chair) with hands on chair back to help rotate the spine safely. Try to turn a little more on each exhalation, turning from the waist. Use a block under the feet if they don't touch the floor easily.

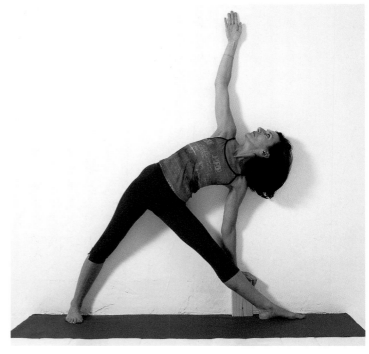

3 Utthita Trikonasana against the wall for balance, using a wooden block to support the hand.

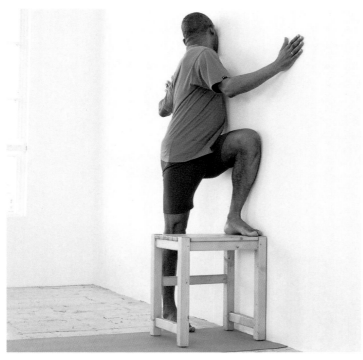

2 Standing Maricyasana using a stool to support the foot of the bent leg and the wall to support the hands in order to turn the trunk.

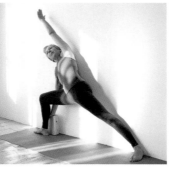

4 Utthita Parsvakonasana against the wall, using a wooden block to support the hand.
5 Ardha Chandrasana against a wall, using a stool for the foot.

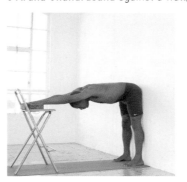

6 Uttanasana I against a wall, with the arms supported on a stool.

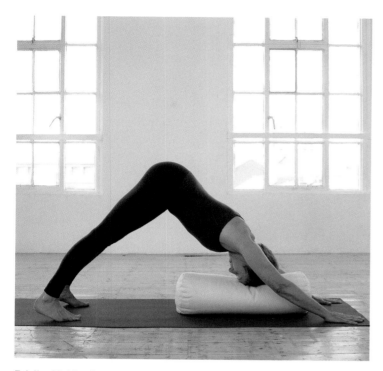

7 Adho Mukha Svanasana with the head supported on a bolster.

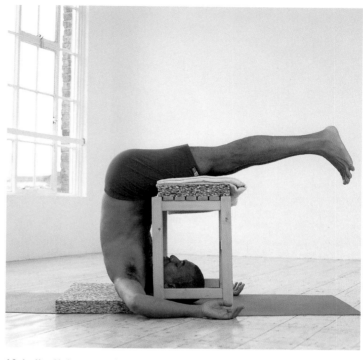

10 Ardha Halasana using a stool and blocks to support the thighs.

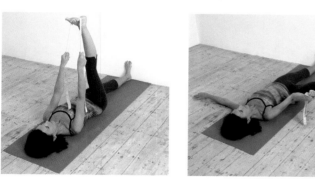

8 Supta Padangustasana I with a strap around the foot and the other foot against the wall.

9 Supta Padangustasana II using a strap around the foot, the leg going out to the side.

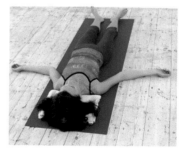
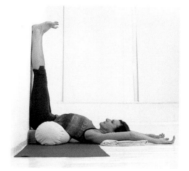

11 Viparita Karani with the legs against the wall and a block and bolster to support the lower back.

12 Savasana with a blanket supporting the head and neck. Palms are open and up.

Focus

• Back problems are caused by a number of factors – stiffness in the lower back muscles, weak abdominal muscles, muscle strain, arthritis, slipped discs or inflammation of muscles and tendons.

• The spine is made up of 32 vertebrae, which work in unison. Weakness and strength is transmitted from one vertebra to another. If one of the vertebrae is overworked it weakens itself, and the other bones – and the muscles and ligaments – have to take the strain until they too begin to weaken.

• When doing postures for backache, the spine must always be lifted, particularly in the lower back. Never hold the breath – breathe normally in the postures, and keep the neck and facial muscles relaxed.

Sciatica

This condition is due to inflammation and compression of the sciatic nerve. The postures in this sequence help to strengthen the leg muscles, increase flexibility in the hips and improve circulation in the legs.

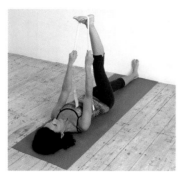
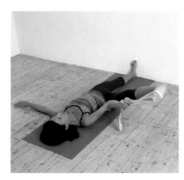

1 Supta Padangustasana I with a strap around the foot and the other foot against the wall.
2 Supta Padangustasana II using a strap, the leg going out to the side.

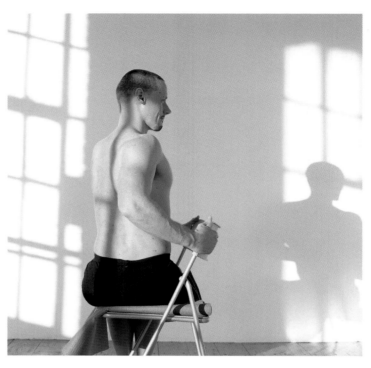

6 Bharadvajasana (chair) with the feet parallel on the floor and using the hands on the chair to increase the turn.

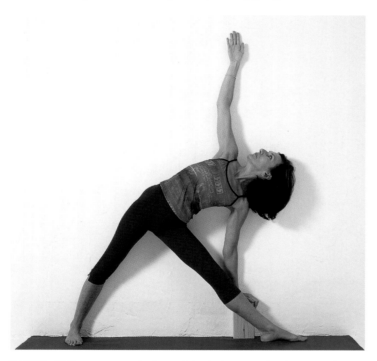

3 Utthita Trikonasana against a wall for balance, and using a wooden block to support the hand.

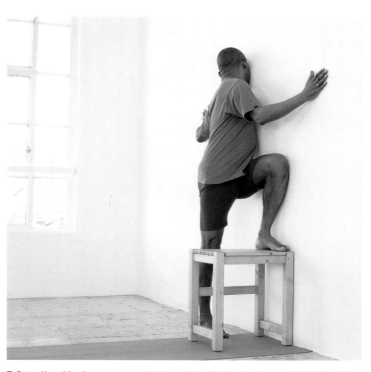

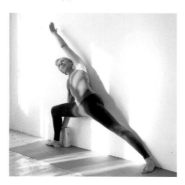
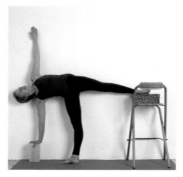

4 Utthita Parsvakonasana against a wall, using support for the hand.
5 Ardha Chandrasana against a wall, using a foam block on a stool to support the extended leg.

7 Standing Maricyasana against a wall, with the foot on a stool. Push the hands into the wall to turn.

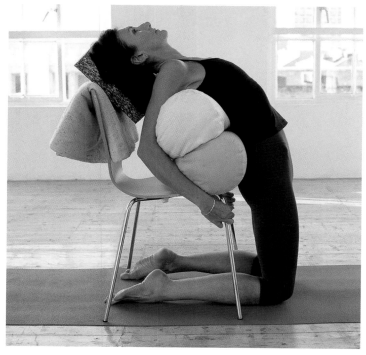

8 Ustrasana using a chair and bolsters to support the arch of the spine. Lean back, allowing the head and neck to relax backwards.

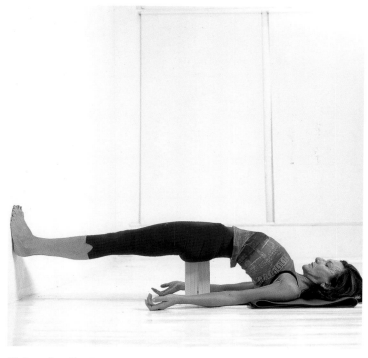

10 Setu Bandha Sarvangasana using a wooden block, feet pressing into the wall.

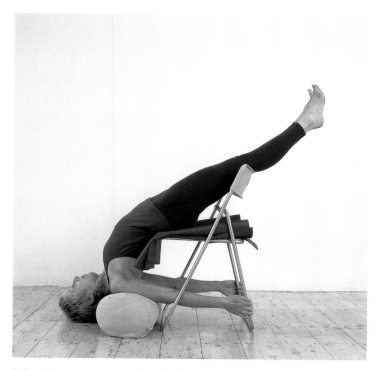

9 Chair Sarvangasana using a bolster to support the neck and shoulders.

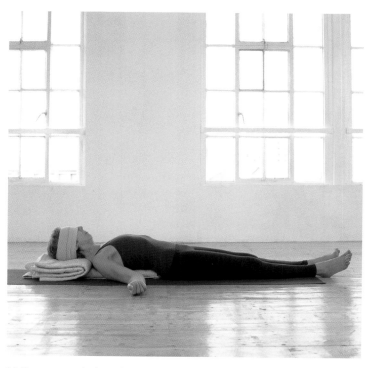

11 Savasana relaxing with a blanket supporting the head and neck, and the eyes loosely covered.

Tense Shoulders and Neck

These postures, which tone and stretch the trapezius muscles and release tension in the neck, must be done with attention to rolling and extending the muscles at the back of the neck down the back, and drawing the shoulders away from the ears.

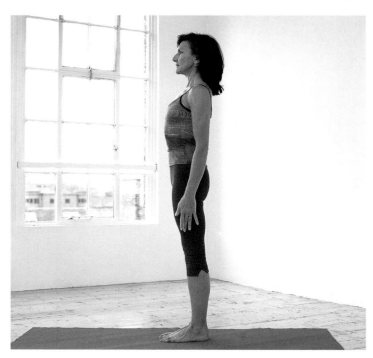

1 Tadasana standing up straight and moving the shoulders towards the body. Keep the feet together, tuck in the bottom and sacrum, and keep the legs strong and active.

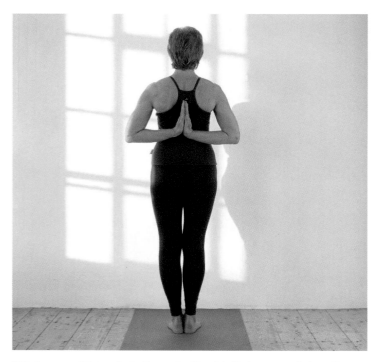

2 Tadasana with hands in Namaste Stand in Tadasana and place the palms of the hands completely together behind the back. Move the shoulders into the body, keeping the hands as high as possible.

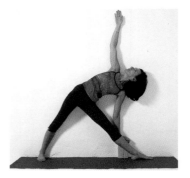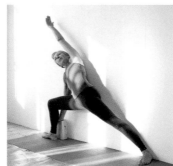

3 Utthita Trikonasana against a wall with a wooden block for support.
4 Utthita Parsvakonasana against a wall with a wooden block.

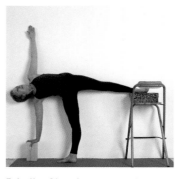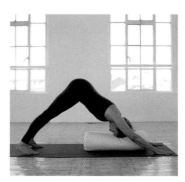

5 Ardha Chandrasana against the wall, with the foot supported by foam blocks on a stool.
6 Adho Mukha Svanasana with the head supported on a bolster.

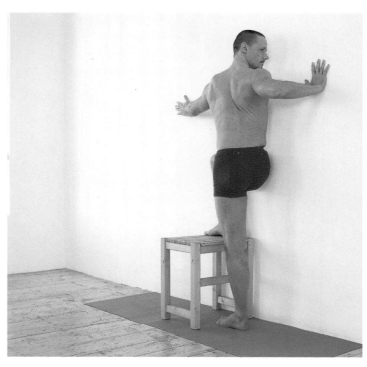

7 Standing Maricyasana using the stool, raise one foot up, and use the wall to turn the spine.

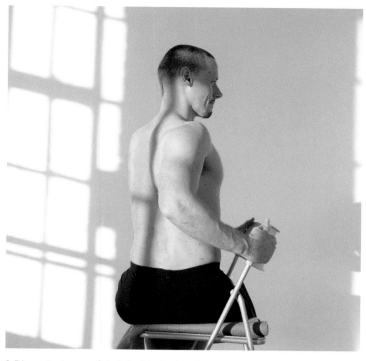

8 Bharadvajasana (chair) with the hands on the chair back to increase the turn in the spine.

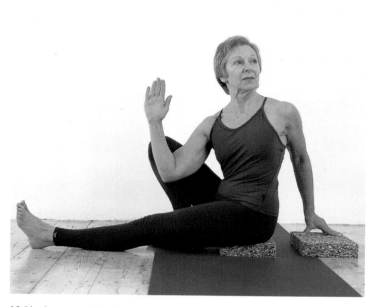

10 Maricyasana I sitting on a foam block as a support and using another block to support the back hand. Press into the block to turn the spine.

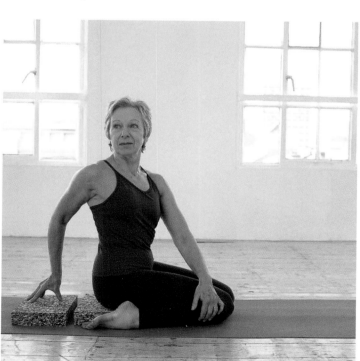

9 Virasana (twist) sitting on a support, and using another foam block for the hand if necessary.

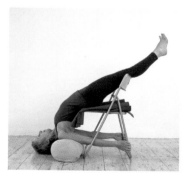
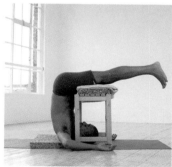

11 Chair Sarvangasana holding on to the back legs of the chair.
12 Ardha Halasana with the thighs supported on a stool.

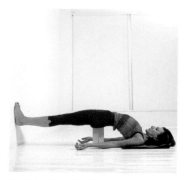
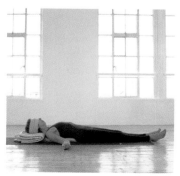

13 Setu Bandha Sarvangasana using the wall to raise the legs.
14 Savasana with the head and neck supported on a blanket and the eyes covered.

Knee Problems

These postures bring flexibility to the knee joint. Distortions of the knee joint caused by tears in the cartilage or knee injuries will be relieved. When practising the postures, try to concentrate on creating space in the knee joint.

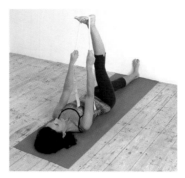

1 Supta Padangusthasana I & II with a strap around the raised foot.

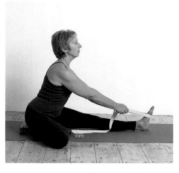

2 Janusirsasana (concave) with a strap around the foot.

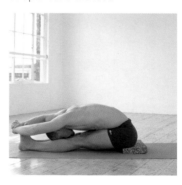

3 Pascimottanasana with one hand holding the other wrist.

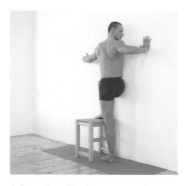

4 Standing Maricyasana using a stool and the wall to help twist.

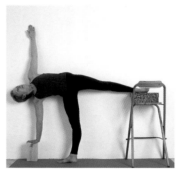

5 Virasana using as much support as necessary to relieve the knees.

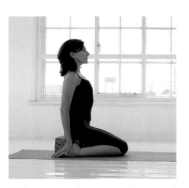

6 Upavistakonasana leaning against the wall and using straps.

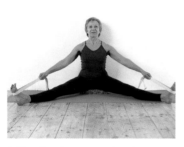

7 Baddhakonasana sitting on a support, with the feet together.

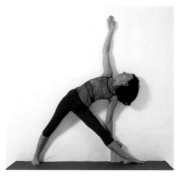

8 Utthita Trikonasana against a wall, and using a wooden block.

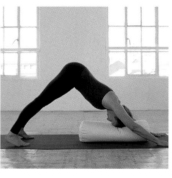

9 Ardha Chandrasana against a wall, the foot supported by a stool.

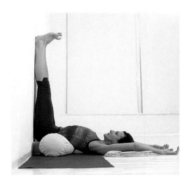

10 Adho Mukha Svanasana with the head supported on a bolster.

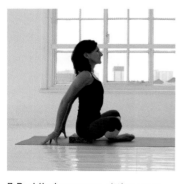

11 Ardha Halasana with the thighs supported on a stool.

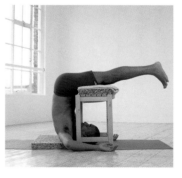

12 Chair Sarvangasana supporting the shoulders.

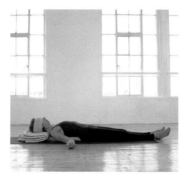

13 Viparita Karani with the sacrum on a block and bolster.

14 Savasana relaxing with the head and neck supported.

Focus
• When practising the standing postures, ensure that no sudden jerky movements are made (such as jumping).
• Draw the thigh muscle strongly up towards the top of the leg to create space in the knee joint.

Stiff Hips

The hip joint is prone to stiffness as it bears a great deal of body weight. As you get older, the spinal and hamstring muscles become stiff and the range of movement in the spine and hip joint is reduced.

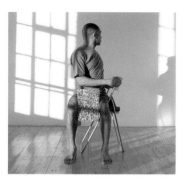 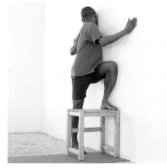

1 Bharadvajasana (chair) using a block between the knees.
2 Standing Maricyasana using a stool to raise the foot.

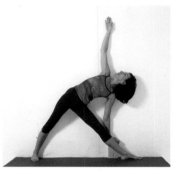 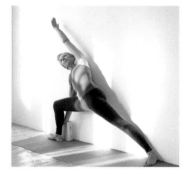

3 Utthita Trikonasana against the wall with the hand supported.
4 Utthita Parsvakonasana against the wall using a wooden block.

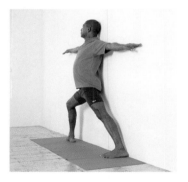 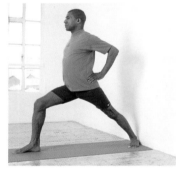

5 Virabhadrasana II using the wall for support.
6 Virabhadrasana I with hands on hips to protect the back.

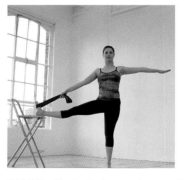 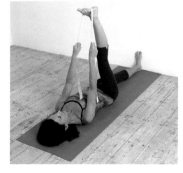

7 Utthita Hasta Padangusthasana I & II using the stool for support.
8 Supta Padangusthasana I & II using a strap to hold the foot.

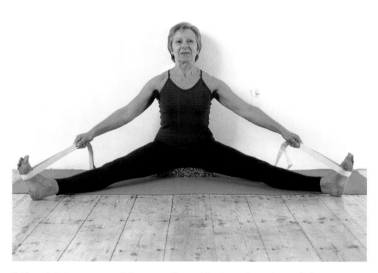

9 Upavistakonasana sitting on a foam block against the wall for support, with straps around the feet.

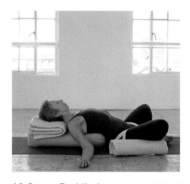 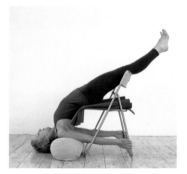

10 Supta Baddhakonasana with a bolster and blanket supporting the spine and a strap around the feet.
11 Chair Sarvangasana with the shoulders and neck supported.

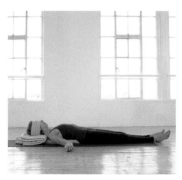

12 Savasana relaxing with a blanket supporting the head and neck.

Focus
• Flexibility is increased as a result of stretching the hamstring muscles.
• The seated postures create elasticity in the hip joints and can thus prevent the onset of arthritis.

Menstruation

Inversions and standing poses should be avoided when menstruating as you should not exert yourself physically during this time. Forward bends are extremely beneficial as they help to control the flow of blood and keep the brain quiet and passive.

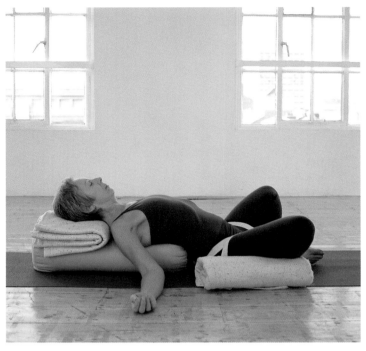

1 Supta Baddhakonasana using a bolster and folded blankets to support the head and trunk. Keep the strap around the hips to hold the feet in towards the groin and use rolled-up blankets to support the knees.

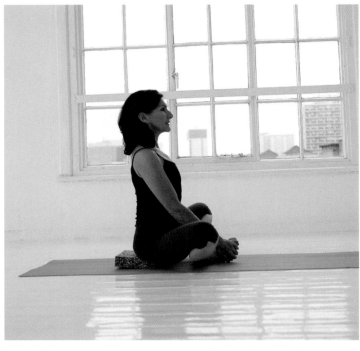

3 Baddhakonasana sitting on a support with the soles of the feet pressing together and the spine stretched up.

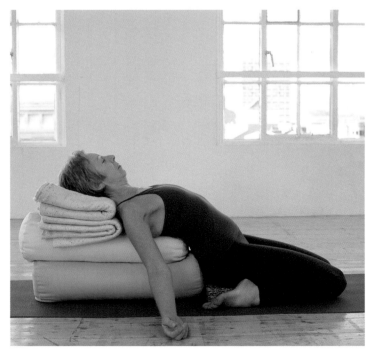

2 Supta Virasana using two bolsters and several blankets to support the head, neck and spine. The same effect can be acheived by using thick, rolled-up blankets, or cushions.

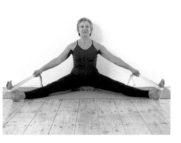

4 Upavistakonasana sitting on a support against the wall. Stretch the legs towards the heels.
5 Adho Mukha Virasana with a bolster and blanket supporting the head.

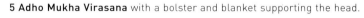
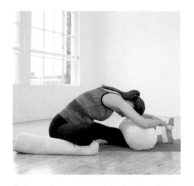
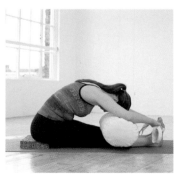

6 Janusirsasana with the head, arms and knee supported on a bolster.
7 Pascimottanasana sitting on a support, the forehead on a bolster.

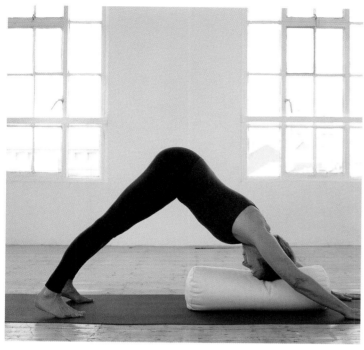

8 Adho Mukha Svanasana using a bolster or a pile of cushions to rest the head. The sitting bones should be stretched towards the ceiling, with the heels extending towards the floor.

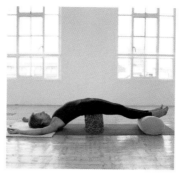

10 Setu Bandha Sarvangasana using four foam blocks to support the sacrum and raised feet.

Focus

•Menstruation is not an ailment but may cause discomfort in the form of backache, stomach cramps and bloating of the abdomen. Forward bends regulate menstrual flow, massage the reproductive organs, keep the brain passive and increase blood supply to the pelvic area.

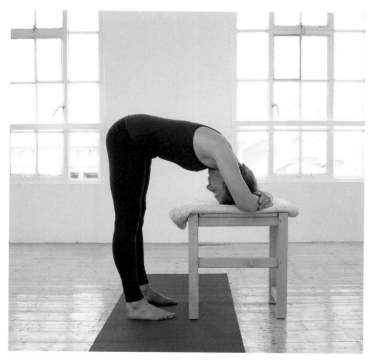

9 Uttanasana I with the head and arms supported on a blanket and stool. If the back is uncomfortable, or the hamstrings painful, increase the height of the support.

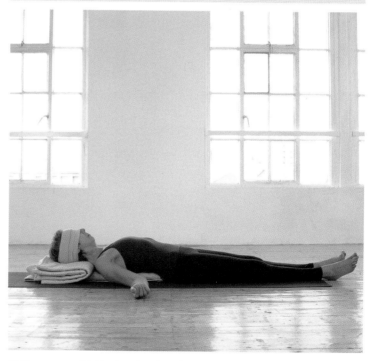

11 Savasana with the head and neck supported on a folded blanket and the eyes covered to keep the brain quiet. You can use a specialist bandage, but a scarf or small bean-bag would be adequate.

Prolapsed Uterus

A prolapsed uterus occurs when muscles and ligaments of the pelvis weaken and the uterus changes position. The postures listed below strengthen the supporting ligaments and the forward bends create space in the pelvic area.

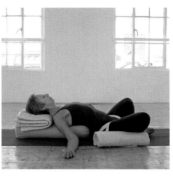
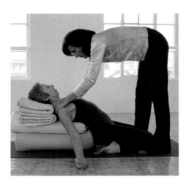

1 Supta Baddhakonasana with a bolster to support the body and rolled blankets under the knees.
2 Supta Virasana with bolsters and blankets to support the spine.

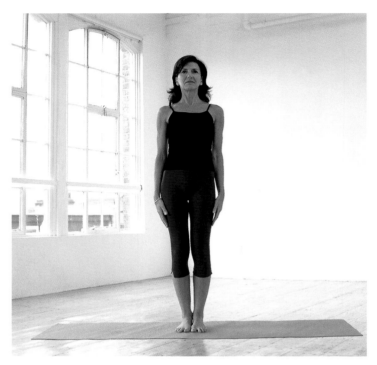

6 Tadasana stand up as straight as you can, drawing the crown of the head towards the ceiling. Keep the feet together, and the legs strong, knees lifted. Raise and open the chest, keeping the shoulders down.

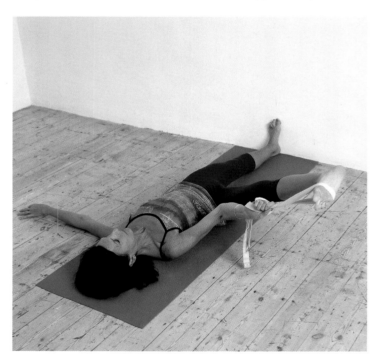

3 Supta Padangustasana II using a strap in one hand to reach the foot, keeping the opposite arm outstretched to keep the body flat on the floor.

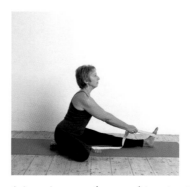
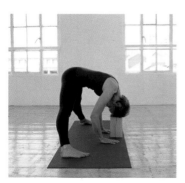

4 Janusirsasana (concave) keeping the back arched.
5 Prasarita Padottanasana with the head supported on a block (use more support if necessary).

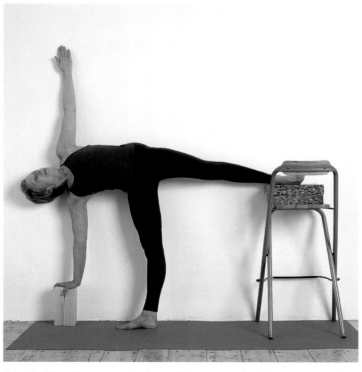

7 Ardha Chandrasana using the wall for support in this posture, keeping the foot supported on a stool with foam blocks raising it to the correct level for your height. The hand is supported on a wooden block.

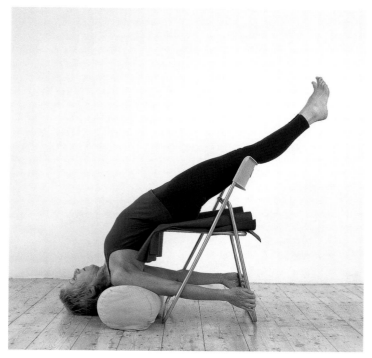

8 Chair Sarvangasana with the neck and shoulders on a bolster and the head on the floor. Reach the hands through to the back legs of the chair and use the pull to open the chest further.

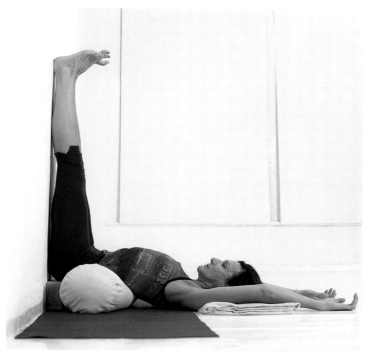

10 Viparita Karani pressing the legs against the wall and supporting the lumbar spine and sacrum with a block and a bolster. Arms stretched over the head, palms up.

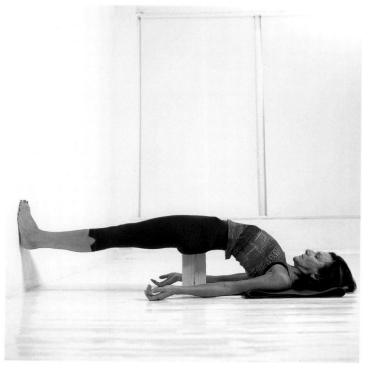

9 Setu Bandha Sarvangasana using a wooden block to support the sacrum, with both feet pressing into the wall. Make sure that the block is under the tailbone, not in the lower back.

Focus

• Symptoms of a prolapsed uterus include a dragging sensation in the pelvic area and backache. In this sequence, the abdominal muscles are strengthened and the body is inverted, which improves this discomfort.
• The forward bends, done with a concave back, create space in the pelvic area and lift the uterus.

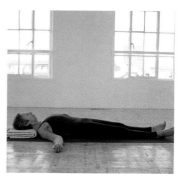

11 Savasana relaxing with a folded blanket to support the head and neck.

Menopause

The menopause occurs with changing hormonal balance. The following postures create a soothing sensation in the nerves, keep the brain passive, improve the flow of blood to the pelvic area and help to lessen many of the symptoms.

yoga therapy

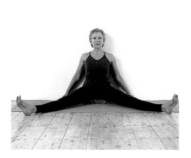
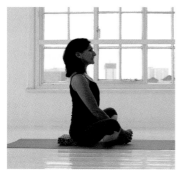

1 Upavistakonasana sitting on a support against the wall. Keep extending inner legs to heels.
2 Baddhakonasana sitting on a support with the soles of the feet together.

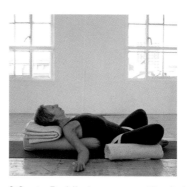
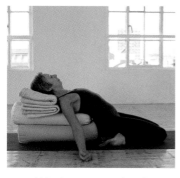

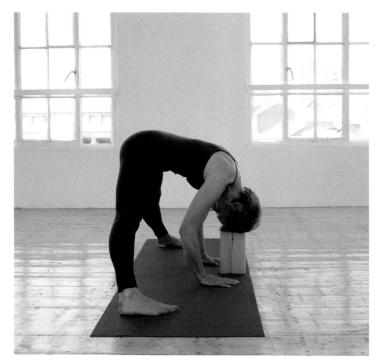

6 Prasarita Padottanasana with the head supported on a wooden block. If the hands do not reach the floor, put foam blocks under the hands so that the palms can press down.

3 Supta Baddhakonasana with a bolster and blankets supporting the head, spine and knees.
4 Supta Virasana supporting the body on bolsters and blankets.

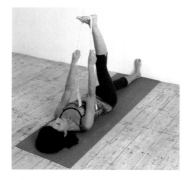
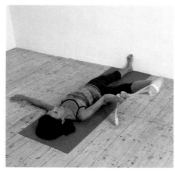

5 Supta Padangusthasana I & II holding a strap in one hand to reach the foot, stretching the leg up first, then out to the side for the second of the postures, while keeping the other foot against the wall.

Focus
• The menopause usually takes place between the ages of 45 and 55 and is accompanied by changes in the hormonal balance of the body. Symptoms include mood swings, depression, insomnia and hot flushes. Forward bends and inversions can be particularly beneficial.

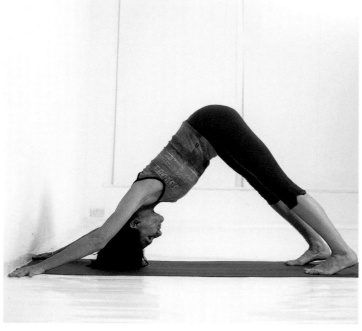

7 Adho Mukha Svanasana against the wall. Turn the hands out so that the thumbs and index fingers are pressing into the wall. Support the head with a bolster if necessary.

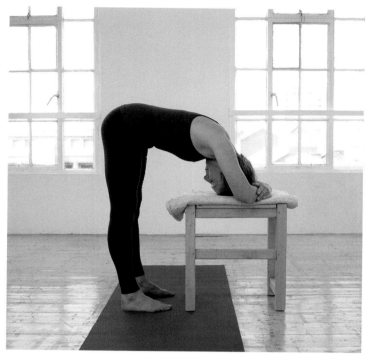

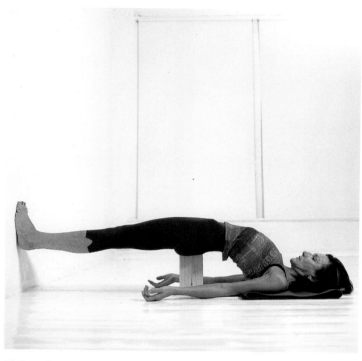

8 Uttanasana I with the head and forearms supported on a blanket and stool. Keep the feet parallel and hip-width apart, legs strong with the knees lifted.

13 Setu Bandha Sarvangasana with a wooden block under the sacrum and the feet raised on the wall. Support the head and neck on a folded mat or blanket.

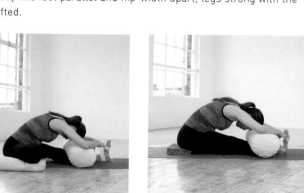

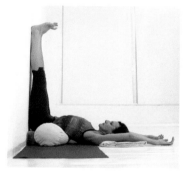

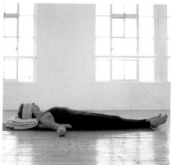

9 Janusirsasana sitting on a support and resting the head on a bolster.
10 Pascimottanasana with the head and arms supported on a bolster, and a strap around the feet.

14 Viparita Karani with the legs raised and pressing into the wall. A wooden block and bolster support the lumbar spine. The arms are stretched along the floor, palms facing upwards.
15 Savasana relaxing with the head and neck supported on a folded blanket and the eyes covered.

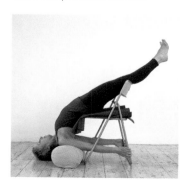

11 Chair Sarvangasana with the shoulders and neck on a bolster.
12 Ardha Halasana with the thighs supported on a stool.

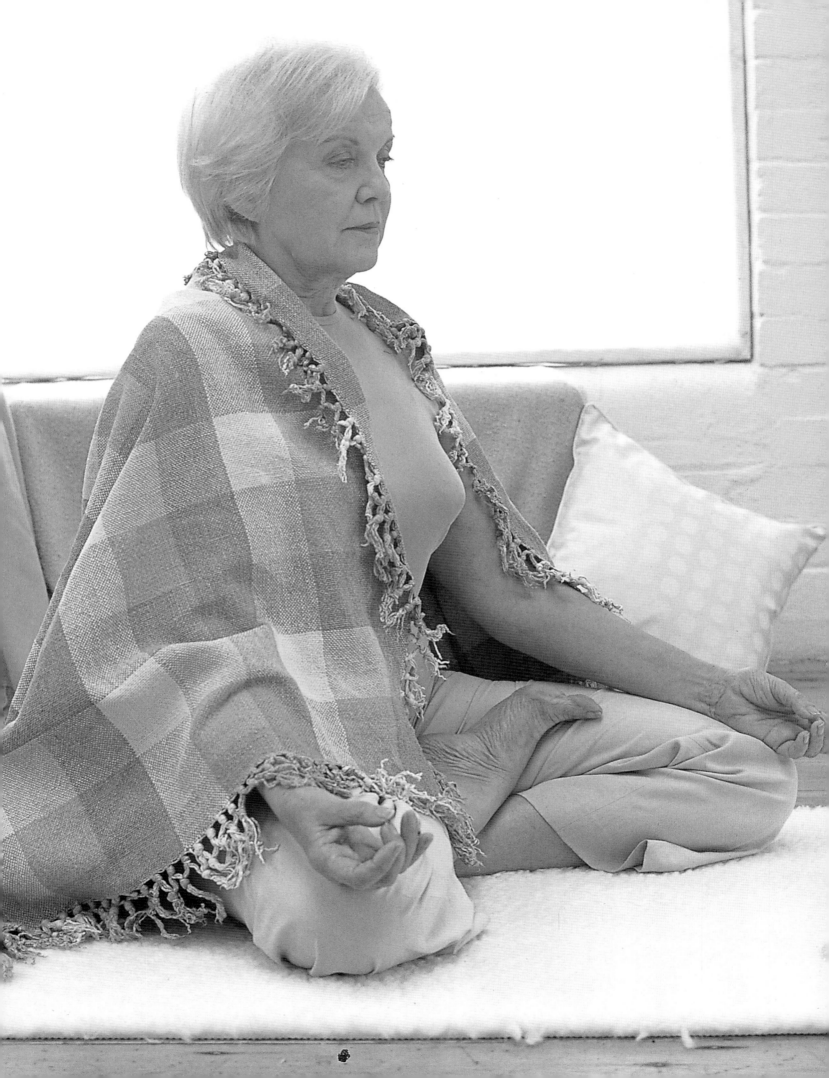

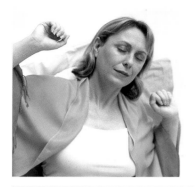
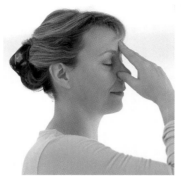
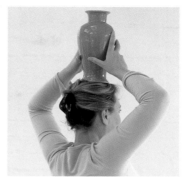
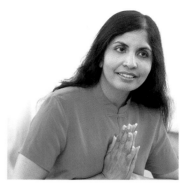

Meditation

Taking time to meditate either on your own, or with a group, is a beneficial and uplifting experience. Meditation helps us focus on the present, quietens the mind and creates serenity.

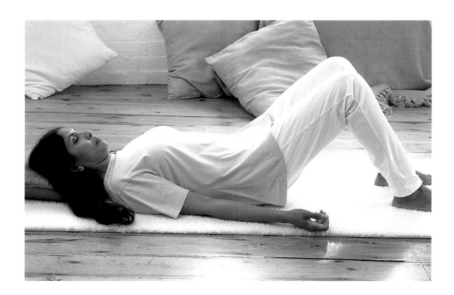

Doriel Hall

What is Meditation?

Human beings have many levels: our physical bodies, energy flow, instinctive responses, thinking processes and wisdom each play a vital part in our overall functioning, and all need to be in balance to ensure health and well-being. All too often, however, a hectic modern lifestyle can unbalance these levels, making us feel jaded in body, mind and spirit. The regular practice of meditation helps us to rebalance ourselves so that all the levels are able to work together in harmony.

Meditation has three aspects: the regular practice of techniques that enable us to reach the meditative state, the experience of the state of meditation, and recreating this state in daily life. There are traditional meditation techniques appropriate to all temperaments and levels of attainment. They all involve symbolically "going up into the solitude of the mountains" so that we can then "return to the bustle of the marketplace" and live a changed life as a result of our experience.

We practise meditation because we believe (with Robert Browning) that:

There is an inmost centre in us all,
Where Truth abides in fullness…and to know
Rather consists in opening out a way
Whence the imprisoned splendour may escape.

Meditation allows us to experience that splendour for ourselves and live our lives in the glow of our own inner radiance.

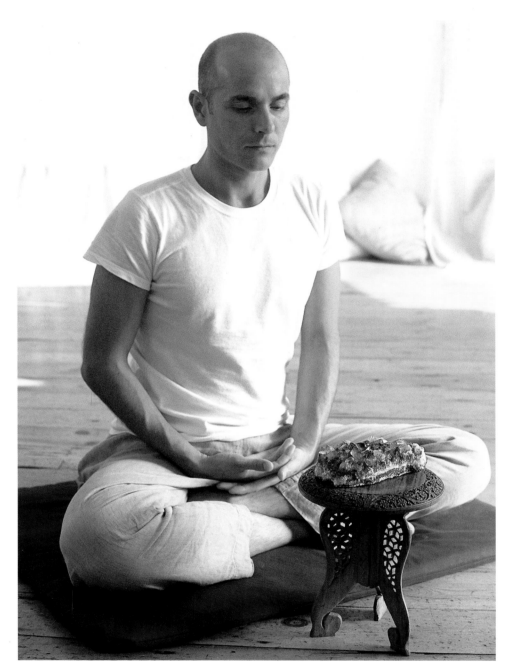

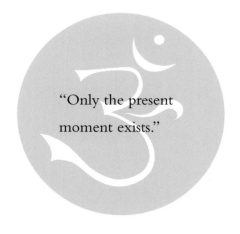

"Only the present moment exists."

Removing inner obstructions

The path to and from our "inmost centre" may be obstructed by lack of awareness, self-obsession, the stress of an unbalanced lifestyle, or by negative attitudes and thought patterns.

Most of us try to crowd too much activity into our lives, and lack the stillness and silence that are necessary to rebalance the nervous system. Regular meditation

above Meditation is practised with the spine erect and the body motionless. The mind is still but alert, vibrant and focused inward.

practice establishes a healthy rhythm of activity and rest for both mind and body. Our minds are constantly active, mulling over current problems, planning anxiously for a future we cannot control, regretting past actions or creating personal doctrines

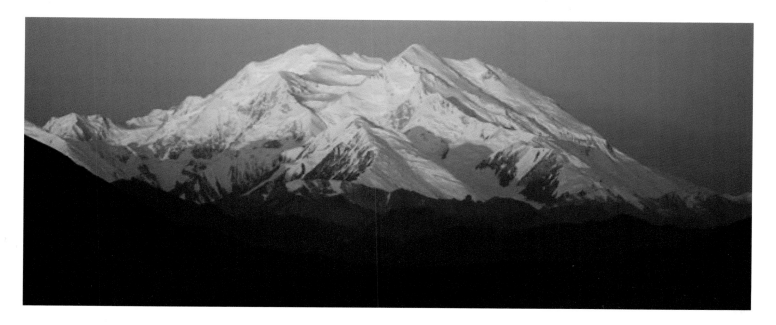

above Symbolically compared with the solitude of the mountains, meditation involves a withdrawal from the bustle of human activity.

right These traditional clay figures in a circle of friendship represent the unity nurtured by the meditative way of life.

and dogmas, opinions and prejudices. These mental "games" draw us, like magnets, away from the present moment. Meditation teaches us to live in the moment, and grow through the experiences of here and now. When we are inclined to wallow in negative emotions such as anger or resentment, and to see insults and dangers where none exist, meditation helps us to replace defensive energy-sapping reactions with open and trusting responses that enable us to build loving relationships.

Reducing stress

If you practise the meditation techniques outlined in this book regularly and with enthusiasm, you will soon start to feel the benefits, as both the causes and the effects of stress diminish.

Stress is a normal part of life, and a certain amount is essential to motivate and develop humans, but the pace and complexity of life in modern Western society can overburden our systems and block our natural ability to manage stress. Human beings are (as far as we know) the only animals with brains that are constantly

thinking – but the result may be that we allow ourselves to remain stuck in negative thought patterns, squandering our precious energy and unbalancing the nervous system.

Like that of any other animal, the human nervous system operates instinctively and is programmed to deal physically with threats to survival. Stress is a natural reaction that enables us to respond to danger, either by fighting or running away. Once the threatening episode is over the nervous system should rebalance itself as we return peacefully to our normal activities. Unlike other animals, however, humans are apt to remain in a state of arousal, because we go on feeling anxious about past and future events, as well as preferring to be continually active and stimulated in the present.

Because stress hormones make us feel excited, it is easy to become addicted to activities and challenges that trigger their release. This is why we want to watch exciting programmes on television and take part in testing activities. But if we remain in a constant state of arousal, we deny our bodily systems the chance to rest and renew themselves. Stress accumulates until the system reaches breaking point – and the result is illness and malfunctioning of the body or mind. By practising the techniques of meditation, we can reverse this build-up of stress by learning to stop and consciously clear the mind and emotions of negative attitudes the moment we become aware of them.

Stress and your health
Meditation practice can help to reduce the unpleasant effects of prolonged stress, protecting you from symptoms such as:
- muscle tension and pain in the joints
- tension and migraine headaches
- the inability to concentrate or think clearly
- digestive problems, which may include diabetes
- interrupted sleep patterns
- breathing difficulties
- cardiovascular problems
- allergic reactions
- physical fatigue
- nervous exhaustion
- weakness of the immune system
- other auto-immune problems

below Regular meditation gives you the energy and clarity you need to deal with the multiple demands of daily life.

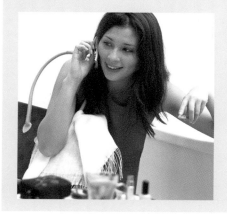

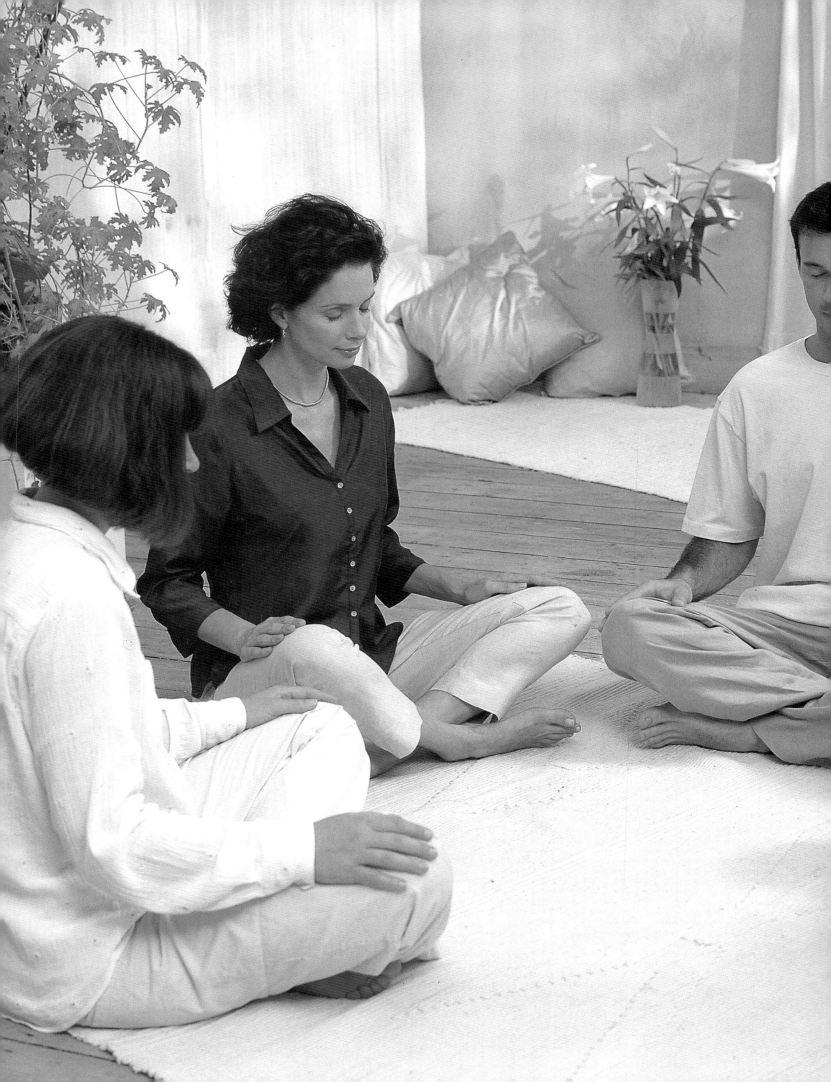

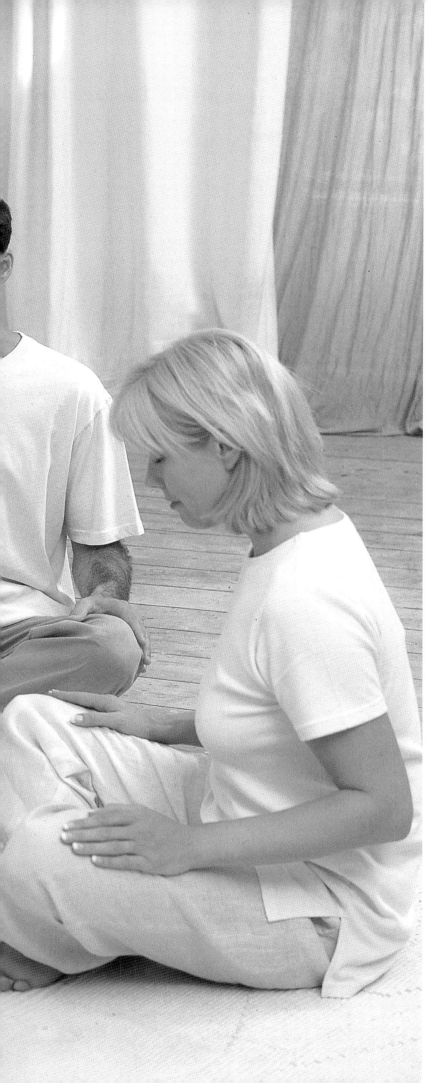

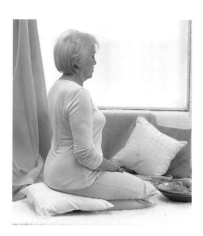

the practice of
Meditation

There are many routes to the meditative state: it can be reached in stillness or movement, with sound or in silence. The sage Patanjali saw hatha, or physical, yoga as a preparation for this transformation of consciousness. His teachings on yoga as the path to meditation still form the basis of most of the yoga practised today.

Universal Meditation Techniques

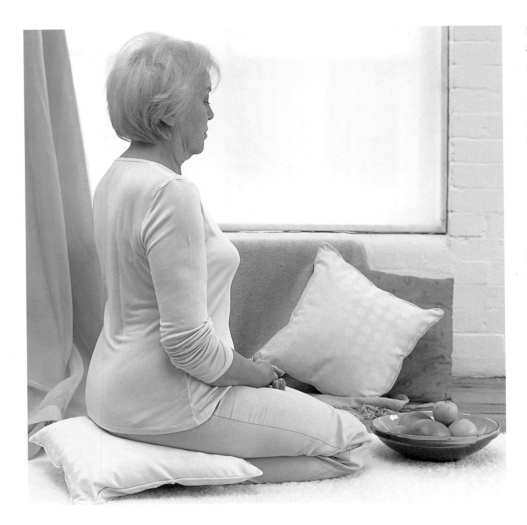

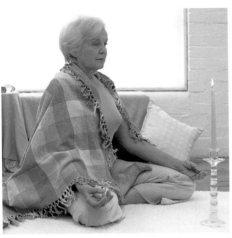

left The postures traditionally used for meditation allow the body to stay motionless while keeping the spine erect.

below Wrap a shawl or blanket around your shoulders so that you stay comfortably warm while sitting still to meditate.

Most classical meditation techniques are common to all the great spiritual traditions, although their forms may vary. Whatever the methods used, the meditation will follow a similar pattern.

For meditation practice to bear fruit in daily life there are four essential elements: detaching the attention from competing distractions outside and within; returning the mind to a single focus in order to enter a state of expanded awareness (the state of meditation); recalling and reflecting on the insights gained while in the meditative state; learning to apply these insights to daily life. The final stage of mastery is to live constantly in the meditative state, "enlightened while still embodied". It is said that the effects of meditation are cumulative and that "no effort is ever wasted".

Stilling the body

Settling into a position that can be held without effort means that the body can cease to occupy our attention. Hindus, Buddhists, Zen Buddhists and yogis usually sit on their heels or cross-legged on the floor. Christians may kneel and many Westerners prefer to sit upright on a firm chair. Classical yoga postures are designed to hold the body upright and still for long periods. The eyes may be closed to avoid outside distractions or open to gaze upon a specific object.

Breathing and chanting

Slowing and deepening the breath induces relaxation of the nervous system. Chanting aloud is a traditional way to lengthen each breath and the repetition of a mantra or prayer is soothing and uplifting. Buddhists, Christians, Hindus and yogis all practise chanting and repetition, either aloud or silently. A string of beads — such as the *mala* used by yogis or the Christian rosary — is often used for counting the repetitions of a mantra or prayer.

Focusing on a single object

When the attention is focused, the incessant chattering of the mind quietens naturally, and we become oblivious to outer or inner distractions. Sound is a universal focus, and may take the form of music, the note of a Tibetan singing bowl, a mantra or *nada* (the mystical sounds of our inner vibration).

Gazing — often upon a flower or lighted candle — is another universal practice. Christians may choose to focus on a picture of Christ or a saint, Hindus and Buddhists on an image of a divine being or incarnation of God. If you prefer an impersonal image, you might choose the Sanskrit symbol of OM, the *shri yantra* or a *mandala* (both of which are pictorial

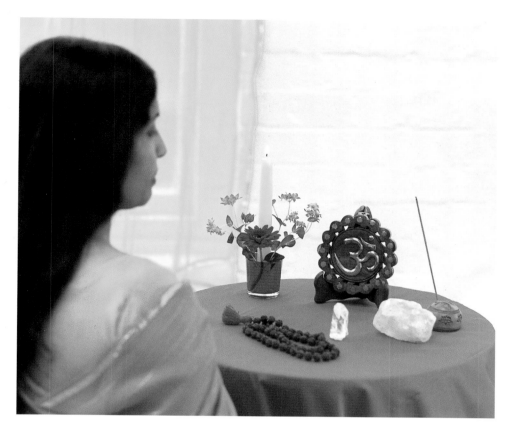

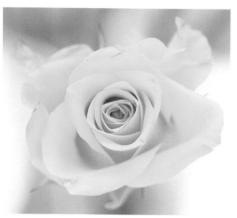

left You may wish to sit for meditation before a low table holding natural or symbolic objects on which to concentrate your gaze.

below One of the most basic focusing techniques involves gazing at a single object: focusing on a flower helps you to feel at one with creation.

representations of universal energies). The focus may be something touched or felt, such as mala beads or the breath within the body. Even the senses of smell and taste may serve as focal points for meditation.

Observation and acceptance

"Witnessing impartially" consists of relaxed observation and acceptance of what is, without any reaction of liking, disliking, criticism or judgment. After watching the contents of the mind in this way we can record them truthfully in a diary. Once we stop reacting instinctively we can start to respond from the heart and open ourselves to life as it is. This is the aim of both Western and Eastern psychotherapies.

Mental visualization

Visualization is the intentional creation of a mental image or series of images, which may be of objects, feelings or symbols, as a focus for meditation practice. Informal visualizations are often used by Western psychotherapists and might, for instance, involve experiencing a walk by the sea or in the countryside using all five senses. Skill in visualization enhances the ability to create and maintain healthy and happy attitudes, thoughts and emotions, replacing former negative feelings.

Healing through love

"Placing the mind in the heart" is an essential step, for love is an attribute of the heart – or feeling nature – and not of the mind. Love should serve our highest aspirations. When loving feelings and thoughts radiate out from the heart like light from a lighthouse, both the meditator and those meditated upon receive healing.

Living in loving kindness

When we live consciously from the highest we can glimpse in meditation, we are living from the heart. We feel strong, relaxed, focused, accepting, creative and joyful.

People in all ages and traditions have achieved this goal. The Hindu tradition has always perceived the divinity in everyone – hence the Indian greeting of "*Namaste*", meaning "The divine in me greets the divine in you". Both Buddhists and yogis practise the meditation of loving kindness, in which love is beamed from the heart to all sentient beings, including those who cause pain and distress. Jesus said, "You shall love the Lord your God with all your heart and soul and mind and strength, and your

right The Buddha is represented in contemplation of a lotus, the symbol of enlightenment, with his right hand raised in a gesture of reassurance.

neighbour as yourself." St Francis of Assisi included all of nature in his love, and the English monk who wrote *The Cloud of Unknowing* declared that "God can be known by thought never – only by love can he be known." This wisdom is available to us all: we can find it for ourselves through the practice of meditation.

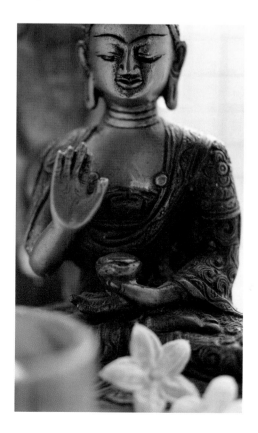

Peeling Away the Layers

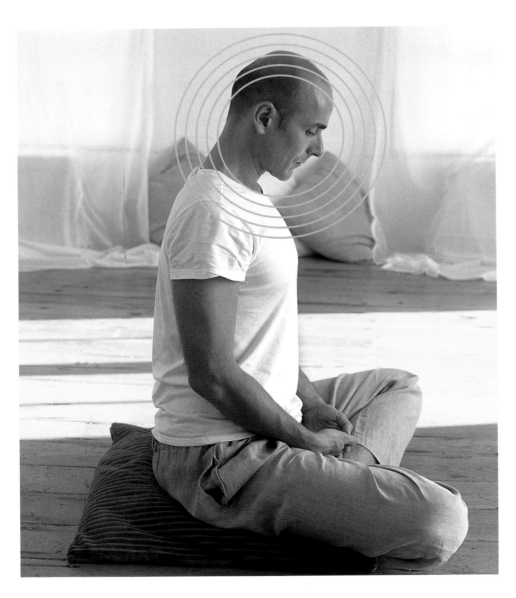

left The concept of the five koshas gives us a mental map to help us on the spiritual journey inwards during meditation.

The line of command through the Koshas

Through meditation we can influence the levels above, as well as the levels below, the one that is the focus of our meditation.

- At soul level (called *ananda maya kosha*, or sheath full of bliss) we form our life's purpose and express this through our attitudes
- which influence our conscious choices (in *vijnana maya kosha*, or sheath full of intellectual understanding)
- which influence our unconscious mental programming (in *mano maya kosha*, or sheath full of mental activity)
- which directs our flow of vital energies (in *prana maya kosha*, or sheath full of life force)
- which move our physical bodies (*anna maya kosha*, or sheath full of food) to perform our actions and behaviour, such as thinking and communicating.

According to the ancient Hindu philosophy of Vedanta, a human being consists of five bodies, each contained within the next, which hide the immortal spirit as if with a series of veils of varying density. These bodies are known as the *koshas*, or "sheaths".

Our progress towards self-realization through meditation can be seen as a journey inwards, through each of these five sheaths, from the outermost layer – the physical body – to the deepest "soul body" of unchanging consciousness, where we are in loving touch with all souls.

The five koshas

The further from the physical body they are, the finer the veils become. The most dense of the koshas is perceived by the senses as the structure of the physical body, which can be weighed and measured by scientific instruments.

The next is the energy body, perceptible to clairvoyants, which can be detected by Kirlian photography (a technique that uses a high-voltage, low-current

left The koshas can be visualized as the layers of an onion, forming a series of sheaths around the centre.

electric charge to represent the body's energy in visual form). This is the level at which we are aware of the presence of someone entering our "space" before we see them. It contains a web of energy channels meeting at the *chakra* points, or energy centres, that correspond to the concentrations of nerves, or plexuses, of the brain and spinal cord. All physiological processes interact through these channels.

Next comes the "lower" or instinctive mental body. This contains the "mental computer" that is programmed to react

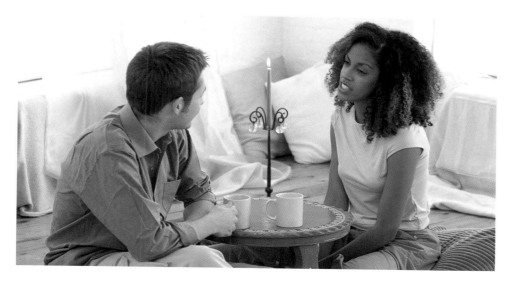

right Learning to understand your own nature and shedding negative feelings of fear through the practice of meditation puts you at ease with yourself and makes for trusting, open relationships with others.

according to the input keyed in by our temperament and previous conditioning. The nervous system operates this computer, mostly at instinctive and tribal levels below conscious awareness.

The next level is the veil of the intellect, involved in thinking, discrimination and choice. It can choose to override mental programming, and to respond consciously rather than reacting instinctively.

The finest veil of all, often called the soul body, is linked with the spiritual dimension and survives death. If we can reach this level in meditation, we can change our whole attitude to life and the way we live. This is conscious evolution, opening up the dormant areas of the brain.

Instinct, interaction and reasoning

It often seems that different forces co-exist within us, pulling us in opposing directions. This is because we have three distinct brains governing how we behave, feel and think. Our ancient reptilian brain is tiny but very powerful. Situated at the top of the spinal cord, it controls the primitive instincts and urges that ensure physical survival in animal bodies. It drives the basic needs that ensure

our physical and species survival – food, safety, shelter, sleep and procreation. The mammalian brain, above the reptilian brain at the back of the skull, evolved later and processes herd, tribal and social instincts. The rest of the skull contains the most recent development, the neo-cortex. This uniquely human brain enables us to think, reason and evolve spiritually.

The neo-cortex is so new that we use less than ten per cent of it, and it cannot easily override our older brains. However altruistic our intentions, we feel frightened and angry, and may indulge in self-centred behaviour, whenever we consider our basic needs are not being met. We actually need very little to survive, but modern society depends on inflaming our instinctive fear and addictive greed, so that we keep buying the products that keep the wheel turning – unsustainably in the long term.

Trusting more, needing less

The practices of meditation help us to balance our evolved and primitive natures. The tradition of Vedanta claims that all creation arises from the desire of the one absolute reality to experience itself as life (nature) and light (consciousness or spirit) in relationship (love) with each other. This relationship is continuously enacted within us, and is seen as the purpose of human existence. The attributes of life, light and love (sat-chit-ananda) are immortal, and therefore so are we, as part of the one indivisible whole. Trusting in the divine process of life-light-love creates joy rather than fear and makes the accumulation of things seem less important than expressing our true nature. It is like being protected from negativity by a shield that beams out goodwill to all, while hiding a glory we cannot yet understand.

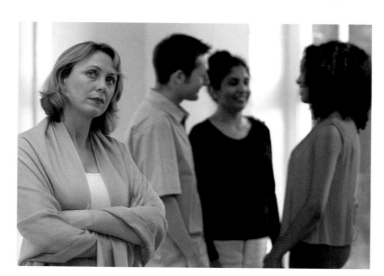

above Fear of isolation and exclusion from the crowd can be a result of feeling unhappy with yourself at a fundamental level.

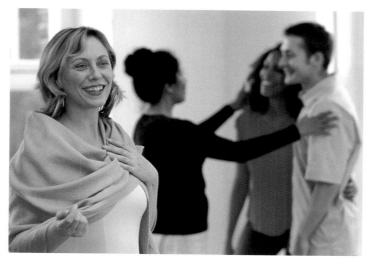

above Reaching a state of inner content means that you can be happy and relaxed whether you are alone or part of a group.

Freeing Vital Energies

"It is just as unbalanced to be held fast by material concerns as to be too heavenly to be any earthly use."

In the Eastern traditions (and also in many modern therapeutic systems) it is assumed that our vital energies – or "life force" – flow through the energy channels (*nadis*) of the second kosha (prana maya kosha), or subtle body. Techniques that operate at this level are aimed at healing, balancing and increasing our energies. Yoga postures can get energies flowing when they are sluggish or blocked, while breathing techniques clear and balance the energy channels.

The chakras and granthis

One of the major energy channels follows the spinal cord and links the seven main chakras. The chakras can be thought of as spinning vortices of energy. Breathing with awareness (pranayama) is practised to influence the energies in the chakras and to weaken the three *granthis* (knots of attachment) that bind us to our negative attitudes and prevent us from experiencing the fullness of life-light-love. Although the granthis are seen as obstacles on the path of spiritual awareness, they also act as safety valves, protecting us from surges of vital energy and misplaced enthusiasm for changes we are not ready for. We need to practise well-tried and tested methods (such as meditation) to open them slowly and naturally, rather than forcing them with drugs or stimulants.

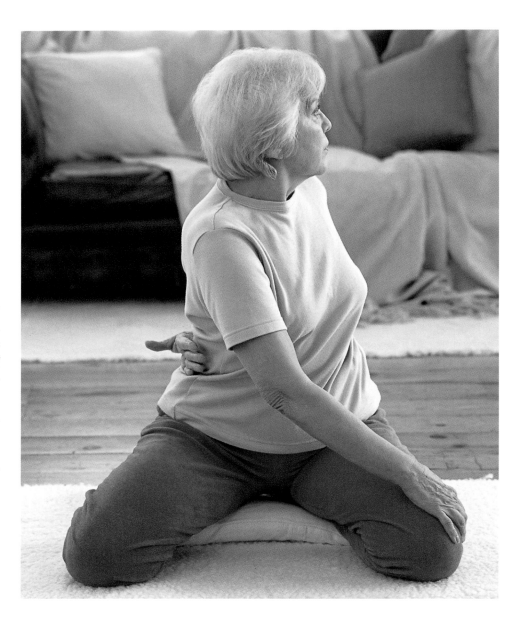

above Yoga postures use movement and stretches to tone the physical body and stimulate the chakras and the connecting energy channels.

right The chakras are often described as lotus flowers; meditation makes them bloom and perfume our lives with their positive attributes.

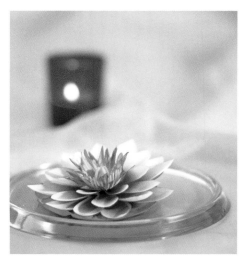

The energies of all the koshas are expressed in each chakra. We can behave spiritually in practical ways from the base chakra, or serve the divine efficiently from the crown chakra. However we behave, feel or think we cannot help bringing life and

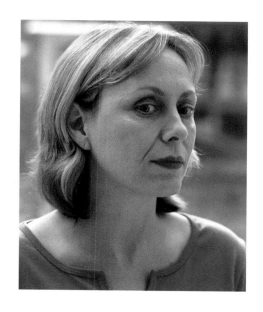

light together in the relationship of love – even if we can perceive only conflict and fear. Awareness is the key to all meditation practice, so we must first "switch on the light" in the brow (mind) chakra before doing anything else, through breathing techniques that quickly "light us up".

Life chakras and the life granthi

The life chakras correspond to the positions of the nerve plexuses attached to the spine behind the abdomen. Their energies are concerned with our survival in the physical human body (the base chakra, connected to the legs and feet), our role in human society

(the sacral chakra) and our sense of self-esteem as a human personality (the navel chakra). The life granthi that binds us is our attachment to material well-being, physical comforts and luxuries, and the amassing of things. Patanjali teaches self-discipline for regulating the energy through the life chakras and life granthi.

Love chakras and the love granthi

The love chakras are situated in the chest (the heart chakra, connected to arms and hands) and neck (the throat chakra, connected to voice, mouth and hearing). In this area self-concern gives way to sharing with others. The heart chakra energies are concerned with relationship – especially unconditional love – and the throat chakra with expressing the truth and hearing what others are telling us. The love granthi that binds us is our attachment to emotional excitement and the desire to be the hero of every drama, so that we are not receptive to the needs of others. Patanjali teaches

self-surrender for increasing the energy through the love chakras and love granthi.

Light chakras and the light granthi

The light chakras are situated in the skull. They are the brow chakra (connected to the mind) and the crown chakra (connected to the spirit). "Taking the mind into the heart" is an essential element of meditation, bringing the realization that relating, not thinking, is the purpose of life. The light of divinity is received through the crown chakra and is present in us as "the eternal flame burning in the cave of the heart". The light granthi that binds us is our attachment to our own opinions, prejudices and fantasies. It is hard to relinquish treasured opinions and pride in our own intellect, yet it is not our minds but the light and love in our hearts that make us divine. We cannot claim ownership of universal life-light-love. Patanjali teaches self-awareness to dissolve pride and those mental habits that obscure divine light.

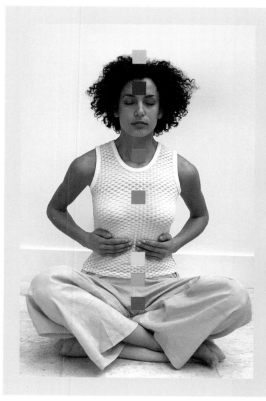

The chakras

The base chakra (*muladhara*) is concerned with survival.

The sacral chakra (*svadisthana*) is related to our role in human society.

The navel chakra (*manipura*) is related to energy and self-esteem.

left The seven main chakras are represented in a line running up the spinal column. Each is traditionally associated with a colour.

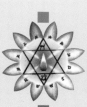
The heart chakra (*anahata*) is concerned with relationships.

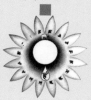
The throat chakra (*vishuddhi*) is related to communication.

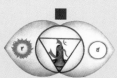
The brow chakra (*ajna*), also known as the third eye, is related to intuition.

The crown chakra (*sahasrara*) is related to spiritual understanding.

Breathing Techniques

Focusing on the breath is a universal technique for enlightenment and healing, and many traditions use breathing practices either as a way to prepare for meditation or as meditation techniques in themselves. Conscious control of the breath, or pranayama, is the fourth of Patanjali's eight limbs of yoga. The technique of holding the breath – either in or out – is beyond the scope of this book, as accomplishing it safely requires one-to-one teaching, but becoming aware of the breathing process and directing the flow of the breath is within the capacity of everyone.

Slowing down the breathing and lengthening the breath out (which is what happens when we sing or chant) switches the nervous system into its peaceful happy mode, allowing stress to be dissolved and rest, digestion, absorption and healing to take place at every level of the five koshas.

Patanjali's path to enlightenment

This use of the breath fits in perfectly with Patanjali's philosophy. He describes three vital steps (which have been called "preliminary purificatory practices") that encapsulate his path to enlightenment. The steps are as follows (quoted words are from the translation of Patanjali's *Sutras* by Alistair Shearer, Ch 2, v 1/2):

"Purification" [through self-discipline]
"Refinement" [through self-awareness]
"Surrender" [through self-surrender and continual letting-go]
"These are the practical steps on the path of yoga. They nourish the state of samadhi" [absorption/ecstasy/expansion]
"And weaken the causes of suffering."

The whole process of self-development starts with taking conscious control over our own nervous system, so that we experience more "expansion" and joy and less stress and unhappiness. Our circumstances influence the outcome of events far less than our own basic attitudes, and these can be changed from negative to positive by the simple act of changing our breathing pattern.

The breath forms part of the energy system and the physiological processes in the energy kosha, while nervous energy runs the mental computer in the kosha of unconscious programming. All the koshas meet and blend in the chakra system in the energy kosha and all can therefore be consciously influenced through the practices of breathing and meditation.

Although some translations of the *Yoga Sutras* describe Patanjali's three "purificatory steps" as "preliminary", there is really no end to our need of them. We always have to maintain our discipline and keep our attention focused – and we never stop needing to let go of something or other.

"Those who see a glass as half empty feel deprived, whereas those who see it as half full feel blessed."

Viloma: focusing on the breathing muscles

This useful focusing technique can be practised anywhere, sitting with the spine erect and the hands and eyes still.

1 Place your hands on your knees, palms either up or down, with thumb and index fingers touching to close the energy circuits. As you breathe in deeply, feel your ribs expand and your diaphragm contract downwards against your stomach. Notice how these movements cause air to flow into your lungs.

2 As you breathe out, count "One and two and...", then stop your breath in mid-flow for the same count. Repeat until you have slowly and comfortably expelled enough air, then repeat this cycle four times more and rest. Then reverse the cycle, breathing in counting "One and two and..." and out slowly for five breaths. Use the fractional breath in to start your day or whenever you need energy, and the fractional breath out to relax before meditation.

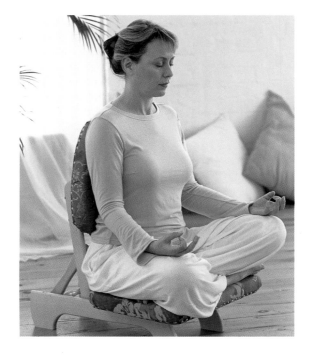

Watchpoints for breathing practice

Regular practice will calm the mind and raise your energy levels. As the lungs strengthen, their capacity will be increased. Practise little and often – a few rounds of the breathing exercises now and then throughout the day will prepare you for longer sessions during meditation practice.

• Avoid any breathing practices after meals – when your stomach is full it presses against your diaphragm, constricting your lungs.

• Keep your spine stretched and as straight as possible (allowing for its natural curves) whether you are standing, sitting, kneeling or lying down to practise breathing. This allows maximum lung expansion and helps the free flow of both air and energy.

• Keep your breastbone lifted to open your chest and give your diaphragm room to move freely. Keep it lifted even when breathing out, letting your diaphragm and rib muscles do all the work.

• Always breathe in through your nose, as it is the filter that protects your lungs from cold, dust and infections from outside. Breathe out through your nose unless you are making sounds.

• Develop your focus on, and conscious awareness of, your breathing patterns, so that you constantly monitor their effects upon you. Develop the habit of watching yourself breathing.

• Slow your breathing down – especially your breath out – whenever you feel agitated or anxious, in order to gain conscious control over your autonomic nervous system.

• Stop your breathing practice and rest for a few natural breaths the instant you feel breathless. Start again when your nervous system has settled down and relaxed. It is not used to being watched and controlled, as breathing is usually an unconscious process.

Alternate nostril breathing

This universally popular exercise quickly balances the nervous system, so that you feel calm and centred after just a few rounds – ready either for meditation practice or to get on with your day refreshed.

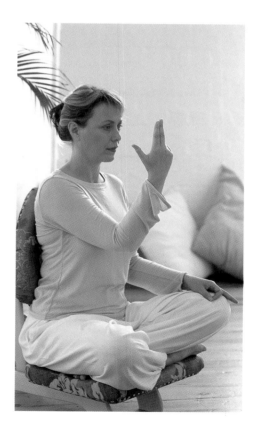

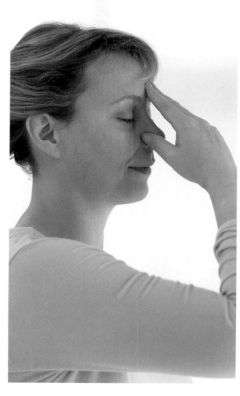

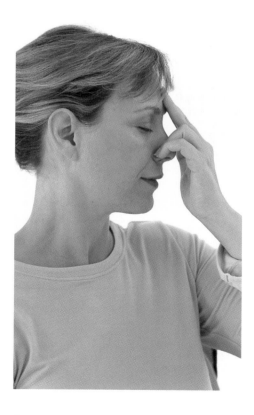

1 Sit erect with your left hand on your knee or in your lap. Raise your right hand to place it against your face. Your thumb will close your right nostril, your index and middle fingers will rest aginst your forehead at the brow chakra and your ring finger will close your left nostril.

2 Your eyes may be closed, or open and gazing softly ahead. Keep your eyeballs still, as quiet eyes induce a quiet mind. Close your right nostril with your thumb. Breathe in through the left nostril.

3 Release the right nostril and close the left with your ring finger. Breathe out slowly, and then in again, through your right nostril. Then open the left nostril, close the right and breathe out. This is one round. Do five rounds, breathe naturally to rest, then repeat a few times.

Choosing a Posture

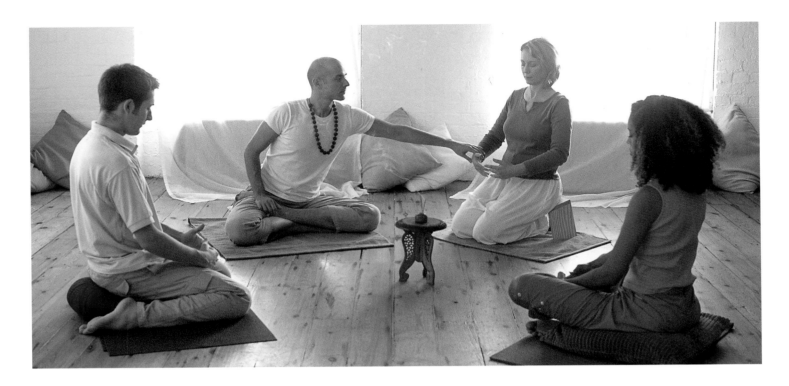

Regular practice is the best teacher, as your body quickly gets used to the new routine and settles into it more and more easily. When you find a position that is comfortable for you, practise sitting in it until you can remain motionless, relaxed yet alert, for half an hour or more. It is helpful to vary your position when you sit at home, or to change purposefully from one position to another without disturbing your inner focus whenever your muscles begin to ache. This is much better than focusing on the complaints coming from your body when you push it to sit too long without moving.

above You may find it helpful to attend a meditation class, where you can be shown different ways to sit and try out the various props available before buying any of them for yourself.

Simple cross legs (Sukhasana)

This involves sitting erect with hips loose and knees wide. Each foot is tucked under the opposite thigh so that the weight of the legs rests on the feet rather than the knees. Place cushions under each thigh and/or under the buttocks if you feel pressure in the lower back. The tailbone (coccyx) should hang freely, letting the "sitting bones" take the weight of the trunk. Place your hands on your knees or rest them in your lap with palms facing up.

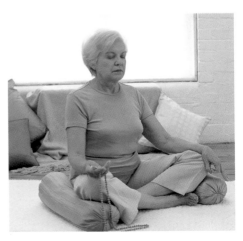

left If the hips are not sufficiently flexible for the knees to rest on the floor when sitting cross-legged, support them with a couple of cushions. Resting the hands palms up enables you to hold a mala, or rosary.

right This low chair, which folds for easy carrying, is specially designed for meditation. It supports the back when sitting in the cross-legged pose. The hands are in gyana mudra, with the tips of thumb and forefinger joined to complete the energy circuit.

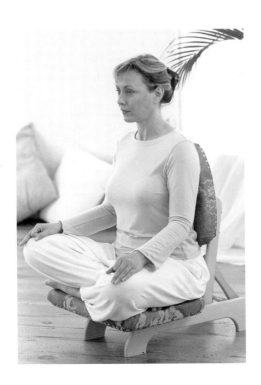

Buddhist position

The Hero pose (Virasana) is sometimes used as a position for meditation. Buddhists often choose to sit on a very firm cushion that lifts the hips, with the knees resting on the floor on each side of the cushion and the shins and feet pointing back. Lifting the hips in this way helps to keep the spine correctly aligned, and this position can be very comfortable as long as your knees are fairly flexible.

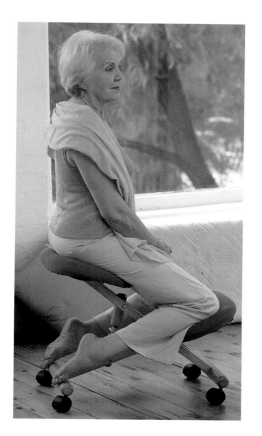

left Using a "kneeling" chair helps to keep the spine straight and gives a good, well-supported position that is similar to the Buddhist kneeling pose.

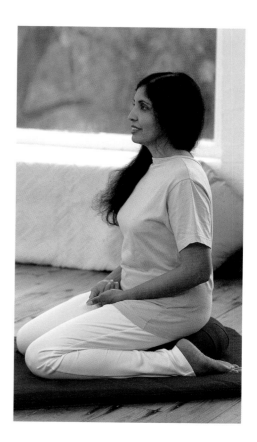

right While sitting on a firm cushion in Virasana, the knees and feet can also be supported on a larger cushion. The meditator sits between the feet, rather than on the heels. The hands are in the gesture called bhairavi mudra, to focus the energy for meditation.

Early morning meditation

Many people like to meditate first thing every morning, while the mind is quiet and before the events of the day have a chance to distract it. If you meditate in bed, use a V-shaped pillow or ordinary pillows to support your back, so that you can sit erect in a cross-legged position. Wear a shawl round your shoulders and pull up the bedclothes so that you feel warm while you are doing your meditation practice. Choose a practice that energizes rather than relaxes you, such as chanting or repeating a mantra using a mala. You may prefer to keep your eyes open in a soft gaze.

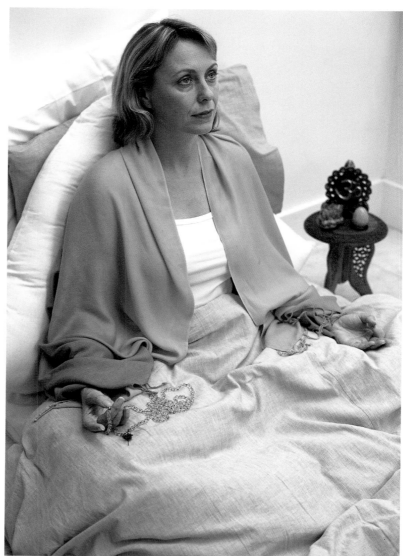

right Your bed can be a haven of peace and warmth if you prefer to meditate on waking in the morning.

below A V-shaped pillow helps you to maintain an erect posture while meditating in bed. A mala, used for counting the repetitions of a mantra, is traditionally kept concealed in its special bag when not in use.

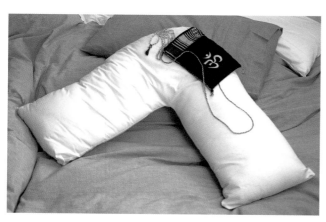

The Time, the Place

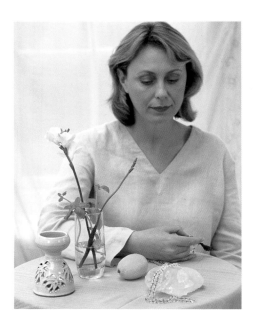

It takes determination to establish a new habit and to make room in your life for a new regular activity. It helps if you train your mind to meditate routinely at a specific time and place. You may still be tempted sometimes to skip your meditation slot and do something else instead, but you will begin to feel uncomfortable when you miss your practice. There will be days when you have to forgo your normal routine, but that will be a conscious decision rather than simply forgetting or procrastinating.

left Your "meditation corner" may contain a number of objects on which to focus: any object can act as a trigger to put you in the right frame of mind for your practice.

right A crescent-shaped "moon cushion" is often used as support when sitting for meditation.

Meditating at a regular time

It is helpful to place your meditation practice in the context of long-established habits – such as before showering in the morning, or after cleaning your teeth, or before lunch or supper. Since you do all these things daily you will meditate daily as well. A good time is when you wake up or before a meal – after meals people are apt to feel sleepy – or in the evening after a brisk walk or listening to soothing music. You might read an uplifting book in bed and then meditate before going to sleep. Choose a time when you are normally alone and undisturbed – the fuller your day, the more rewarding and de-stressing your meditation session can be. Couples often meditate together at a mutually convenient time, or get up early before the household is awake. Whatever time you choose, stick to it to establish your meditation habit.

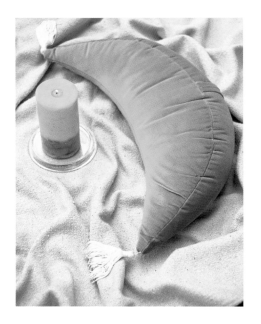

Creating a meditation corner

If you always do your practice in the same place this will also help to establish your meditation habit. Choose a quiet and uncluttered space so that the moment you sit there your mind becomes calm and focused. Make sure you will be warm enough, as body temperature drops when you relax and turn inwards.

Your "meditation corner" might consist of a special chair in a peaceful part of your home, or perhaps you might sit on a

Meditation in bed

If you practise meditation in the early morning your bed (with a warm shawl around you and the covers pulled up) can become your "meditation corner". Have a wash, a drink and a good stretch to really wake you up first – and make sure you sit with your spine erect.

If you regularly meditate in bed in the morning, and this is the place where you are in the habit of turning your mind inwards, it can also be very soothing to perform simple meditation techniques before you go to sleep at night.

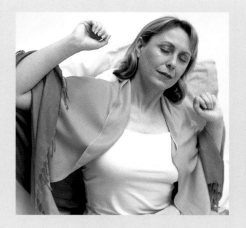

above When you wake up, have a relaxed, "releasing" stretch before starting your early morning meditation.

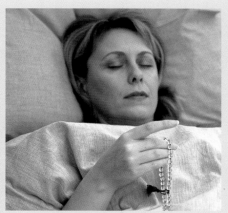

above Last thing at night, relax with your mala and repeat a mantra or simple prayer before you go peacefully to sleep.

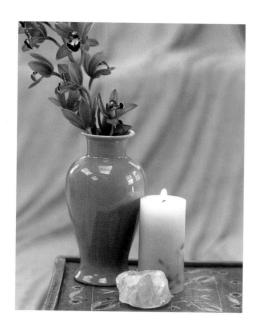

above If you choose to meditate sitting on the floor, a low table is useful for holding objects on which you wish to focus your gaze.

favourite cushion, or spread out a lovely rug. The corner might contain a table holding a candle and flowers, or anything you find soothing and inspiring.

Objects of devotion

The things you keep in your meditation corner can be used for the classic technique called *tratak* – or "gazing". This involves sitting erect and motionless while focusing your gaze upon an object.

The point of focus is often a lighted candle. If you practise this form of meditation, check that there are no draughts to move the candle flame, as this can give you a headache. (Epileptics and migraine sufferers should avoid gazing at a flame.) After gazing softly, without staring, for a while, close your eyes and keep the image in your mind's eye. When it fades, gaze at the candle again and repeat the visualization. Your mental image will gradually become firmer and your concentration deeper.

You may like to light a candle before starting meditation practice and blow it out with a "thank you" as a final gesture. A flame is a universal symbol for the presence of the divine, and you may like to develop a greater awareness of this presence dwelling within you and surrounding you.

There are different forms of tratak. A flower can be held and turned around in the hand, as you observe every detail of its

Postural stretch

If you have been sitting all day in a car or at your desk, you may want to regain a strong upright posture before you start an evening meditation session. You could try standing with a weighty object on your head to strengthen the spinal column and improve your sense of balance. Previous generations learned "deportment" by walking around the room balancing piles of books on their heads, and porters the world over have strong straight backs, developed by carrying loads on their heads.

right Stretching your spine up against the weight of gravity makes your meditation pose "firm and comfortable", as Patanjali recommends.

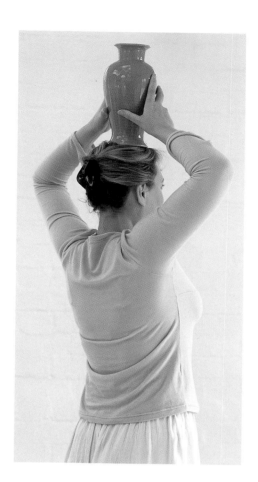

beauty and structure. Holding a crystal in your hands and feeling its contours and coolness is another form of tratak – in this case the eyes are closed throughout and the "gazing" is accomplished through the sense of touch. You could equally well choose to gaze at any object that inspires you.

Relaxing horizontal stretch

Stretching out on your back is the perfect preparation for meditation. Ten minutes lying stretched out on the floor on your back, with your mind gently but firmly focused on the movement of your breath while your body relaxes, is an instant restorative.

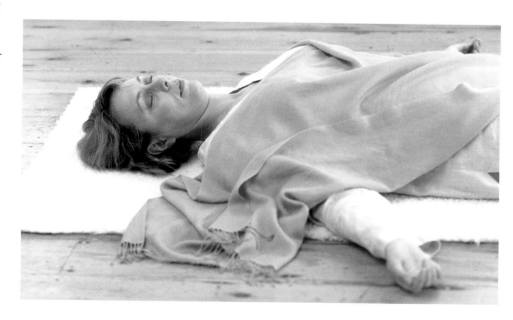

above Keep alert and warm while you relax on your back. Stretching in this position prepares you for keeping your spine erect – the spine should always be as straight as possible when meditating. While you lie on your back and relax your body, many meditation techniques can be used to keep your mind alert and focused, such as counting your breaths from one to ten and back again, visualizing energy moving through the spine, repeating a mantra, or visualizing a tranquil scene in the country or by the sea. After your relaxation take a few deep breaths, move your fingers and toes, stretch and yawn and sit up very slowly. You are now ready for meditation practice.

The Art of Visualization

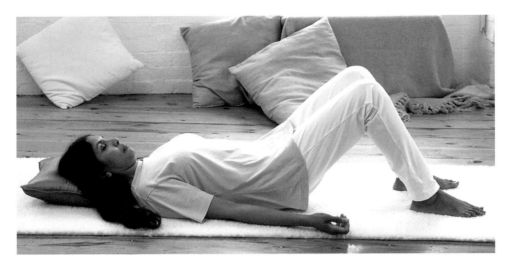

Visualization is a technique that brings the senses into full play, and enables us to build up a happy inner world. Relaxed visualization is a tool used in many different types of therapies. Its aim is to help us change our perception of the world by changing the way we feel inside ourselves. It can be done lying down or reclining just as well as sitting in an upright meditation pose. This means that we can help ourselves to feel better when we are tired and depleted, or ill in bed, or needing to create a calm and relaxed state to prepare for a peaceful night's sleep.

Choosing an affirmation

You can use your relaxation time for your own greatest long-term benefit by using affirmations to create lasting change. The first step is to decide on an affirmation or resolve, known as a *sankalpa*, to repeat when you are in a state of deep relaxation.

You need to ask yourself what positive changes in your behaviour (life), perception (light) or attitude (love) would make you more like the person you would wish to be. The answer requires reflection and an honest appraisal of your personal qualities. Having decided on your sankalpa, you can set about creating a suitable visualization by using your imagination and all five senses to become fully present in a place of your choice where you feel naturally safe and relaxed. Once this scene is set you can go

above For relaxation adopt a comfortable position lying on your back with your knees raised and feet flat on the floor. A cushion under your head keeps your neck from contracting at the back.

below Once you are deeply relaxed, focus your imagination and all your senses on being present in the place you want to be.

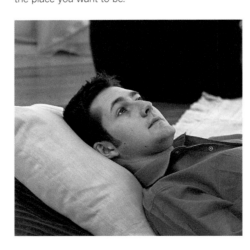

deeper and reinforce the changes in attitude, outlook and purpose that you have already decided to adopt. The unconscious mind is happy to respond to the suggestions put to it by the conscious mind, provided your nervous system is in a thoroughly relaxed and trusting state and that you express your intention in the following ways:

- Phrase your affirmation as clearly and as briefly as possible, with no "ifs" and "buts", descriptions or qualifiers.

Creative imagining

It has been said that nothing can be imagined that we have not already experienced – either at first or second hand. We have an almost infinite variety of memories to choose from. Our life happens in our heads, so we should create as harmonious an inner world as we possibly can. There is no need to put up with a haphazard and chaotic inner world once you know how to change it. The choice is yours and meditation techniques are the tools.

- Mention just one change. When that change has occurred you can replace your sankalpa because it will have become redundant.
- Describe the change you wish for in the present tense, such as "I am…[happy, healthy, confident, successful at…, or forgiving of…]" or, "I am becoming more and more…day by day." The unconscious mind lives only in the present and ignores the past or future. Tomorrow never comes and is of no interest to it.
- Express your sankalpa in positive terms only, for the unconscious mind becomes confused by negative words such as "not" and "never".
- Avoid any words like "try" or "work at" or "difficult" because they immediately put the nervous system on guard and undo all the good relaxation you have achieved up to now
- Repeat your sankalpa three times slowly and decisively, so that your unconscious mind knows you mean business. In this way you are programming it to carry out your intentions all the time – even when the conscious mind is busy with other things. This is why the sankalpa has such a powerful effect.

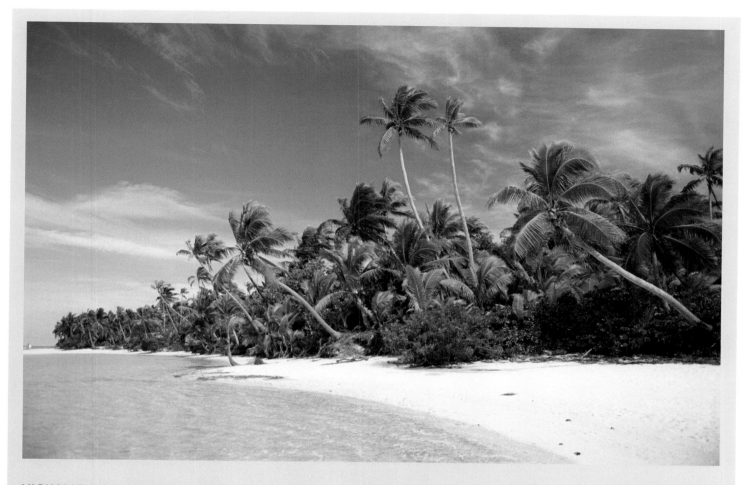

VISUALIZING A BEACH SCENE

You have become deeply relaxed, perhaps after some stretching and deep breathing exercises. Sit or lie down in a comfortable position and start to imagine yourself reclining on a beautiful beach. You are lying on soft sand near the water's edge on a pleasant sunny day. Use all your senses to appreciate all the details of the scene, so that you experience it fully.

You can feel the texture and dampness of the sand beneath you, dig your toes into it and let it run through your fingers. Look at the scenery around you, the deep blue of the sea and sky, the pale sand, the distant horizon, a few fluffy white clouds, seagulls flying overhead. You can hear the seagulls calling, the wavelets lapping across the sand and the sound of a gentle breeze moving the leaves of the trees behind you. You can smell the salt air and taste it on your

above The beauty, warmth and peace of a tropical beach make it pleasing to all the senses, so it is an ideal subject for a visualization to help you create your happy inner world.

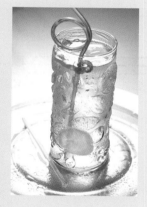

right The more detailed your visualization the more completely you will be able to experience the scene. Taste and feel the coolness of an iced drink on a hot day.

left Feel the sand between your toes and visualize the soft sheen of seashells.

lips. What else can you feel, see and hear? Perhaps the air caressing your body, the intricate patterns of individual grains of sand and tiny shells, the sound of children laughing in the distance. Can you smell the sea, taste a half-eaten peach, feel the welcome coolness of the wind lifting your hair?

When you have built up all the details of this lovely scene, stay in it for a while feeling peaceful and contented, grateful and relaxed. The whole purpose of this visualization is to bring you to this inner place where you know that "all is well", now and always. Before you decide to leave the beach repeat your sankalpa (the affirmation or resolve you have already decided upon) slowly and clearly three times. Then gradually let the whole scene dissolve, knowing that it is always there for you to return to, no matter what is going on in the external world.

Meditation in Daily Life

Many people think of the meditative state as being rather "otherworldly", something that they can only achieve if they divorce themselves from daily life. Although regular meditation practice requires that you set time aside to turn the attention inwards, it can also be woven into daily life. You can turn mundane chores into a form of meditation by practising "mindfulness" – focusing all your thoughts on them; you can experience a sense of spiritual enlightenment from appreciating the beauty of everything around you; you can use meditative practices when trying to engage with and understand your emotions; and you can introduce meditative elements into the ways in which you relate to others.

right By focusing all your awareness on everyday activities such as eating, you can turn them into a form of meditation.

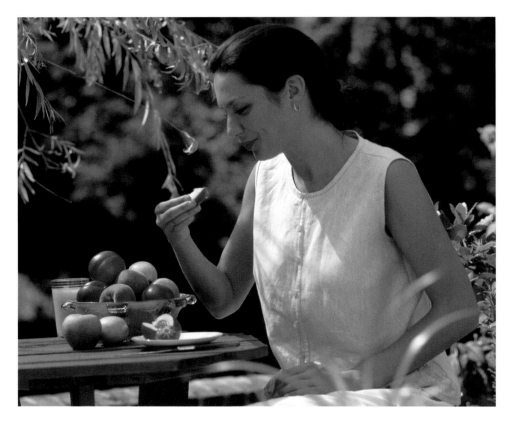

Key elements

There are many ways in which you can bring meditation into every aspect of your day-to-day life:

- Focus your mind and body entirely on what you are doing at this moment, letting distractions wash around you.

- Live in the present moment as much as you can.
- Try to perceive the beauty and worth in everything (and everyone) around you, and in everything you do, no matter how mundane the task.

- Learn to use your senses to the full.
- Develop self-awareness, and work with the interplay between your emotional and physical self – noticing how certain breathing practices and positions affect your mental state, for example.

Working with your feelings

The following traditional technique, based on experiencing "opposites", allows you to become impartially aware of your feelings (many of which are usually below consciousness):

- Relax deeply – sitting, reclining or lying on your back.
- Imagine various "pairs of opposites" and notice the physical sensations that arise.
- Start with pairs that have little or no positive/negative emotional associations – such as hot/cold, hard/soft, light/dark – and observe how you feel in your body while remaining deeply relaxed.

- Move on to a more emotionally challenging pair, starting with the positive side, and observe what feelings are evoked: birth/death, spacious/confined, happy/sad, delighted/angry and welcome/ excluded are some examples.
- Still deeply relaxed, observe what feelings arise in your body as you contemplate the negative half of the pair – so that you can recognize and identify them from now on and understand what "pushes your buttons" and how you feel out of sorts when your emotions are negative. You can then take appropriate action to make you feel better and defuse tension in and around you.

- Repeat the positive half of the pair before moving on to the next pair of opposites.
- End with your sankalpa and some gentle deep breathing before coming out of relaxation with a grounding ritual.

Relating to others

This Buddhist "loving kindness" meditation helps you to relate better to those around you. Breathe in universal love and kindness to help and support yourself, then breathe it out, directing it to a specific person or group. Repeat this meditation often, until it becomes second nature both to receive and to give loving kindness. Make it part of your daily life: any part of it can be used in any situation to promote peace and harmony.

• Relax deeply in a seated position with your spine erect.
• Breathe in, drawing "loving kindness" from the universe into yourself.
• Breathe out, directing that loving kindness with gratitude towards a particular person, or to all those who have taught you (given you light in many ways). Breathe more loving kindness into yourself.
• Breathe out, directing loving kindness with gratitude towards a particular person or to all those who have nurtured and nourished you (given you life in many forms). Breathe in…
• Breathe out, directing loving kindness with blessings towards a person or people you love dearly. Breathe in…
• Breathe out, directing loving kindness with blessings towards acquaintances, neighbours, people you work with. Breathe in…
• Breathe out, directing loving kindness with forgiveness to people who annoy or obstruct you, who are unkind or dismissive. Breathe in…
• Breathe out, directing loving kindness with forgiveness to anyone who has ever hurt or injured you in any way. Breathe in…
• Breathe out, radiating the prayer, "May all people everywhere be happy." Breathe in and give thanks for all the loving kindness you receive. Pause before coming out of your meditation and grounding yourself with a ritual.

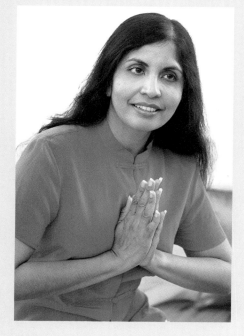

above The traditional Indian greeting "Namaste", spoken with a bow while bringing the hands together at the heart chakra, acknowledges the presence of the divine in the heart of each person, conveying the sense that everyone is part of the unity of creation.

How are you feeling?

As a way of linking the physical and non-physical, it is important to get into the habit of noticing consciously what your senses are telling your mind. This makes it much easier to monitor your emotions as they arise, because you can feel them through your senses. In fact, there is no other way to feel how you are "feeling". For every emotion there is a corresponding physical sensation: we "see red" when angry, our legs "turn to jelly" when we are frightened, sadness makes the heart "ache" or we are "in the dark" when confused.

Once you learn to recognize how you are actually feeling you can avoid reacting negatively to everyday situations. Whenever you notice a negative feeling arising, pause for an instant (the proverbial "counting to ten"), relax and visualize the positive, opposite feeling. You can then respond in a positive manner instead, bringing what you have learned through the regular practice of meditation into your daily life.

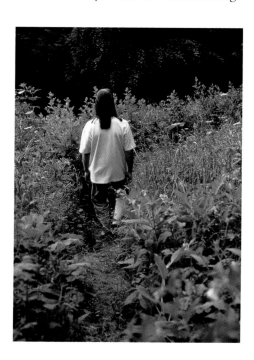

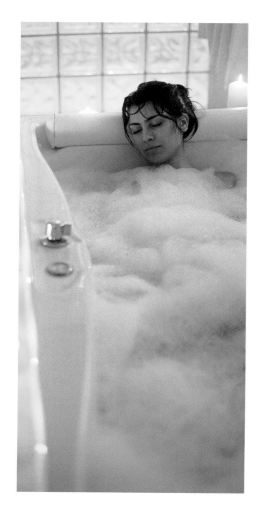

right Use the time you spend in the bath or shower each day to relax and enjoy the present moment.

left When you take a walk among plants and trees, focus your whole mind and all your senses on the experience, noticing the beauty of everything you pass along your path. Plants teach us how to "just be".

Meditating on: the OM Mantra

Patanjali begins his list of meditations with: "Complete surrender to the almighty Lord…who is expressed through the sound of the sacred syllable OM. It should be repeated and its essence realized." (From Alistair Shearer's translation of the *Sutras*.) OM, or Aum, is recognized in many cultures as the primordial sound, whose vibration brought the universe into being. Repetition of the OM mantra on a daily basis, chanted aloud, whispered or repeated silently, has a cumulative and profoundly beneficial effect.

When chanted aloud (intoned rather than sung), the OM sound – pronounced as in "home" – should be deep and full, with the vibrations resonating in the life chakras, then moving up into the chest and the love chakras, and finally closing with a long,

humming "mmm" in the head and the light chakras – all on one deep steady note. Overtones may sometimes be heard. These are the faint sounds of the same note at higher octaves, as when groups of Buddhist monks chant in a deep resonant rumble, with the overtones wafting above like celestial choirs.

a–u–m

The syllable can also be divided into three sounds – A (the created beginning), U (the sustained now) and M (the dissolution of creation). This trinity corresponds to sat-chit-ananda. A is the beginning of life, time and forms; U is maintained through the relationships of cosmic love; M comes when we experience personally that all is spirit – and the rest is mental illusion.

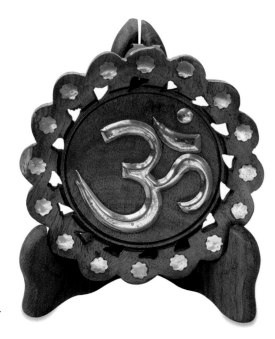

above The Sanskrit symbol of the sacred syllable OM is often used as an object on which to focus. Place it on a low table so that you can concentrate your gaze on it during your meditation practice.

Chanting with a mala

The mala has 108 beads. It should always be held in the right hand and passed between thumb (representing universal consciousness) and middle finger (representing sattva guna). One bead is passed with each repetition of the mantra. Start from the larger bead (*sumeru*) and, when you come round to it again, do not cross it but turn the mala and go back for another round.

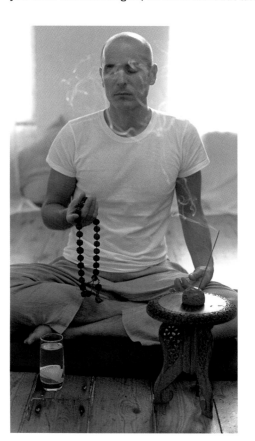

1 Sit in a meditation pose and settle your body and breathing.

2 Hold the mala in a comfortable position (traditional positions are near your heart or on your right knee).

3 As you breathe in chant OM silently. As you breathe out chant OM aloud (or silently), then move to the next bead on the mala and repeat 107 times. If your mind wanders bring it back gently to the mantra.

4 Sit for a few moments and feel the vibrations of the sound within you, before grounding yourself. The sensation of these vibrations creates a trigger for you – recalling them at other times will take you back instantly to the harmonious state you were in while chanting.

"This Self, beyond all words, is the syllable OM.
This syllable, though indivisible, consists of three letters – A–U–M [representing three states of being]…The fourth [state], the Self, is OM…the supreme good, the One without a second. Whosoever knows OM, the self, becomes the Self."

Mandukya Upanishad

Chanting the mantra in a group meditation

This meditation is particularly effective when done in a group. Each person sounds his or her own note, all taking a breath in together (as indicated by the leader) and then chanting A, U, or M on the slow breath out. The meditation ends with everyone chanting OM on their own note and in their own rhythm, so that the sounds mingle together until a natural pause occurs. Silence follows until the meditation ends with a grounding ritual. The more people who join in the OM chanting the more powerful the effects become and the longer the subsequent silence is likely to continue.

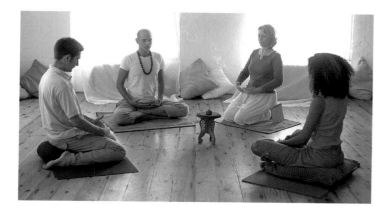

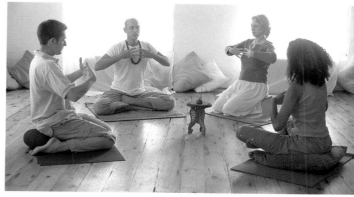

1 Sit in a circle in a comfortable meditation pose with spine erect and sternum lifted. Place the hands in front of the body with palms facing the lower abdomen and fingertips just touching. Breathe in together and chant A (aah...) on a deep note on the breath out, to resonate in the life chakras in the abdomen. Repeat this sound at least twice more, to energize and remove blockages.

2 Move the hands up, with palms in front of the heart and fingertips just touching. Breathe in together and chant U (oooh...) on the breath out to resonate in the love chakras. Notice the different quality of the sound and the vibrations. Repeat twice more, feeling your own sound resonating within you.

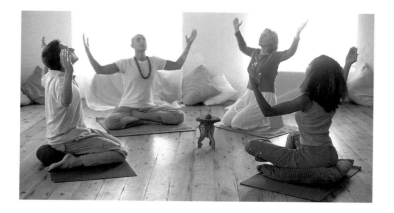

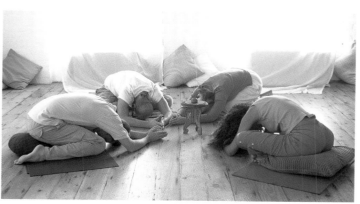

3 Move the hands overhead, stretching up and out in a joyful expression of complete freedom, palms facing forwards. Look up (without compressing the neck) and breathe in together. Breathe out to chant M (mmm...) into the skull cavity and the light chakras, experiencing the sound within. Repeat twice more, then bring your hands down and remain silent. Finally chant OM, each in your own rhythm and pitch, until the group naturally falls silent. Sit in this silence for a while.

4 Finish by bringing hands and forehead to the floor in a gesture of grounding and complete surrender.

Dharma and Karma

OM is said to be the sound of creation, harmony and order. The eternal being expressed through the sound of OM is not the personal deity of any religion but the super-conscious organizing principle that sustains the divine order (*dharma*) by means of cause and effect (*karma*), and whose wisdom is available to all human beings as "the teacher of even the most ancient tradition of teachers".

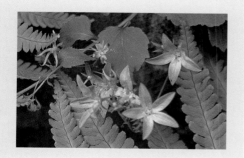

right OM is the sound vibration that underlies every part of the universe, down to the smallest detail.

Meditating on: the chakras

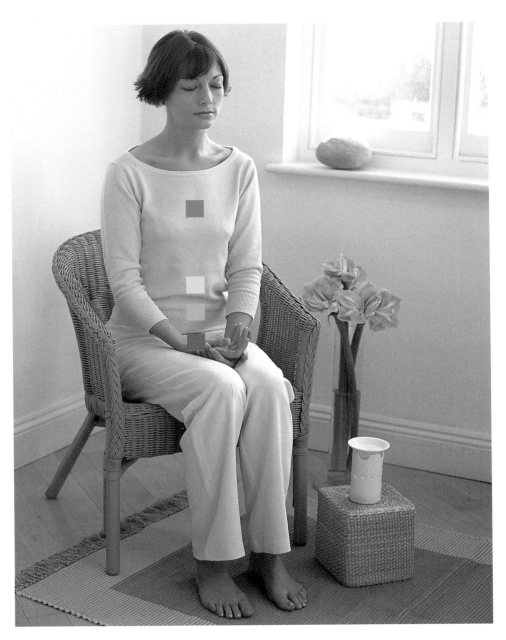

left **left** Most of us have a dominant type of chakra energy, and traditional correspondences can help to define the basic character of the chakras. Each of the four lower chakras corresponds to one of the four elements.

The chakras, which exist at the energy level, can be thought of as transformers that process the energy from all the koshas through our bodyminds into the physical world. The body, mind and emotions are all extensions of chakra function. Changes at one level will bring automatic changes at every other level.

The chakras are vortices of energy within our own being that we can become aware of for ourselves and then work with to balance and activate all levels of our being. We can gain a wealth of psychological insight by using meditation to explore the qualities traditionally attributed to each of the major chakras.

Awareness of the chakras

To gain true insight into yourself, you need to understand the current state of your own chakra system – and this means becoming aware of it. To help you do this, work through the series of three meditative breathing routines that follows. You should bring focused awareness and discrimination to your exploration, so that, whatever your meditation may reveal, you can remain an impartial observer and learn from the experience, rather than getting carried away by it – especially if emotional responses catch you unawares.

As you explore your chakras during the meditation, try to feel each one's individual brightness or dullness. All the chakras spin, giving off light, colour, sensation and sound, and it is by picking up these subjective phenomena that you can assess if or when a particular chakra is under- or overactive within the system as a whole.

"Balance comes when we can accept and get along with everyone without compromising what we believe in. The balancing of the chakras and the flowering of each one brings us to Patanjali's "state of unclouded truth" and heaven on earth."

Chakra Correspondences

Each of us has a mix of influences, but one particular influence is usually dominant. Like each sign of the astrological zodiac, each chakra is associated with an element, which can help us to recognize its basic character. The four lower chakras display the following characters:

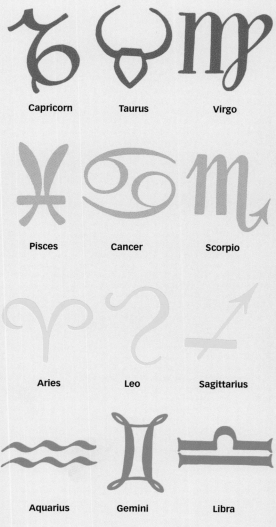

Capricorn   **Taurus**   **Virgo**

Pisces   **Cancer**   **Scorpio**

Aries   **Leo**   **Sagittarius**

Aquarius   **Gemini**   **Libra**

1 The base chakra (muladhara) corresponds with the element of Earth – as do the star signs of Capricorn, Taurus and Virgo. Their characteristics ensure survival, and among them are practicality, reliability, tenacity, logic, and a generally materialistic and no-nonsense approach to life. An Earth weakness can be a rigid and unimaginative outlook, unless it is tempered by other influences. If Earth is blocked we fail to ensure that we have the wherewithal to survive and if it is overactive we are obsessed with protecting ourselves by acquiring possessions.

2 The sacral chakra (svadisthana) corresponds to the element of Water – as do the signs of Pisces, Cancer, and Scorpio, whose characteristics ensure social bonding. Among them are empathy, enjoyment, sensuality, homemaking and caring for others. A Water weakness can be a tendency to tearfulness, emotional sensitivity and slipping into overindulgence to avoid facing facts. If Water is blocked we may become outcasts from society, upon whose acceptance our lives depend, and if it is overactive we may become addicted to substances, pleasures or people.

3 The navel chakra (manipura) corresponds to the element of Fire – as do the signs of Aries, Leo and Sagittarius, whose characteristics enable us to achieve personal success. They include warmth and friendliness, enthusiasm and zeal to inspire others to believe in themselves and their opinions. A Fire weakness is the tendency to burn out through overconfidence and ignoring obstacles. If Fire is blocked we lack the energy to plan or achieve anything and drift helplessly through life, and if it is overactive we develop inflated egos.

4 The heart chakra (anahata) corresponds to the element of Air – as do the signs of Aquarius, Gemini and Libra. Their main characteristic is to reach beyond the ego to other people, beauty and harmony, ideas and ideals. Air is a property shared by all, and Air signs understand that we are all interactive parts of a greater whole. An Air weakness is a tendency to be disorganized and unrealistic, though well-meaning. If Air is blocked we are imprisoned by our ego and if it is overactive we do not recognize boundaries.

Chakras 1–3 are the life chakras that combine to maintain physical life for the individual. Chakras 1–4 can be perceived as forming the base that supports the three "higher" elements: Ether (or communication), Mind (the organ of consciousness) and Spirit (the link with the whole).

1 Chakra awareness: "switching on the light"

First, settle yourself into a suitable position for meditation practice to promote a sattvic state. Awareness is a function of the brow (ajna) chakra, so this meditation begins by "switching on the light".

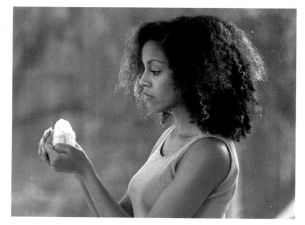

right A good "switching on" practice is tratak – focused gazing for a few moments upon an object such as a candle flame, flower or crystal. This balances the nervous system and focuses energy in the centre of the head to light up the mind. Alternatively, you could perform a short breathing practice, such as alternate nostril breathing.

▷

2 chakra awareness: breathing up and down the spine

This sequence will make you sensitive to the energy pathway upon which the chakras are located, like roundabouts or junctions on the busy highway that lies within the spinal cord.

1 First breathe in and "drive" up the motorway from the tailbone to the top of the head.

right 2 Breathe out and drive back down again. Alternatively, you can imagine drawing light up on the breath in and letting it release back down on the breath out – like mercury rising and falling in a thermometer. You may like to feel the flow of breath with your hands as you practise this exercise.

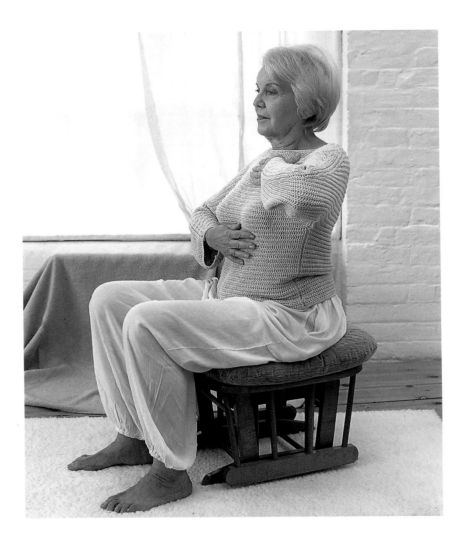

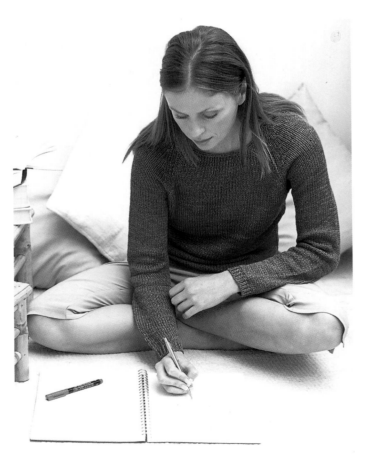

3 chakra awareness: stopping at each chakra

You should really feel the quality of each major chakra as you practise the following meditation.

1 At the base of the spine breathe in and out of the base chakra. Energy is concentrated at this point on the breath in and radiates outward as it is released on the breath out. Repeat twice more before moving up to the next chakra point, the sacral. Again, breathe in to focus energy in the chakra and breathe out to allow it to radiate outward.

2 Continue up the spine with three breaths to activate each chakra point. After breathing into the crown chakra three times, pause and rest, letting its energies inspire and heal you, then start the downward journey, beginning with the crown chakra. After reaching and breathing in and out of the base chakra three times, pause and rest again – feeling the nurturing support and safe solidity of the physical plane upon which you live. The aim is to restore balance between the chakras by understanding and putting right what is causing imbalances.

3 Repeat the whole process once or twice more in a slow, relaxed and observant manner. Then come out of your meditation gently and ground yourself throroughly.

left 4 Once out of the meditation, you may like to record your experience to help you reinforce your increasing sensitivity to the different "feel" of each chakra.

chanting the chakra bija mantras

Once you have located your chakras and can breathe in and out of them easily, you may like to explore chanting to brighten them up or nourish them. Each chakra has its own sound (see box below). These are bija, or "seed" mantras, which have no literal meaning but are designed to plant the seed of a concept in the mind. They should each be chanted three times on a low, slow note that vibrates in tune with the chakra's own vibratory rate. The Sanskrit sound "AM" is soft – somewhere between "ham", "hum" and "harm".

right 1 Start at the base chakra and chant in each chakra all the way up. Pause after chanting in the crown chakra, then start again at the crown chakra and move down, pausing again after chanting into the base chakra.

2 Repeat the whole cycle twice more before coming out of the meditation. The bija mantras are represented by Sanskrit letters placed within a symbol that you may also like to visualize.

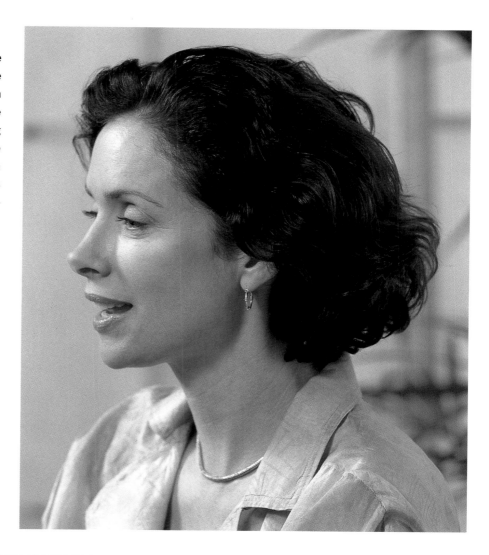

The Sounds of the Chakras

As you chant these sounds, think of the qualities of each chakra, expressed perfectly by their particular symbol.

- **LAM** for the **base chakra (muladhara)**, placed within a **yellow square** (the compact quality of earth).

- **VAM** for the **sacral chakra (svadisthana)**, placed within a **white crescent moon** (the moon governs the waters).

- **RAM** for the **navel chakra (manipura)**, placed within a **red triangle pointing downward** (fire spreads upward and outward from a single point).

- **YAM** for the **heart chakra (anahata)**, placed at the centre of **two interlaced triangles** (the colour varies, as does the colour of air, which joins heaven and earth together).

- **HAM** for the **throat chakra (vishuddhi)**, placed within a **white circle** (ether or space pervades the entire universe).

- **AUM** for the **brow chakra (ajna)**, placed within a **grey or mauve circle between two petals.** This is the "command centre" where all opposites (the two petals) merge and are transcended through awareness and understanding.

- **OM** for the **crown chakra (sahasrara)**, placed at the **centre of a sphere of light** radiating in all directions – spirit pervades all creation.

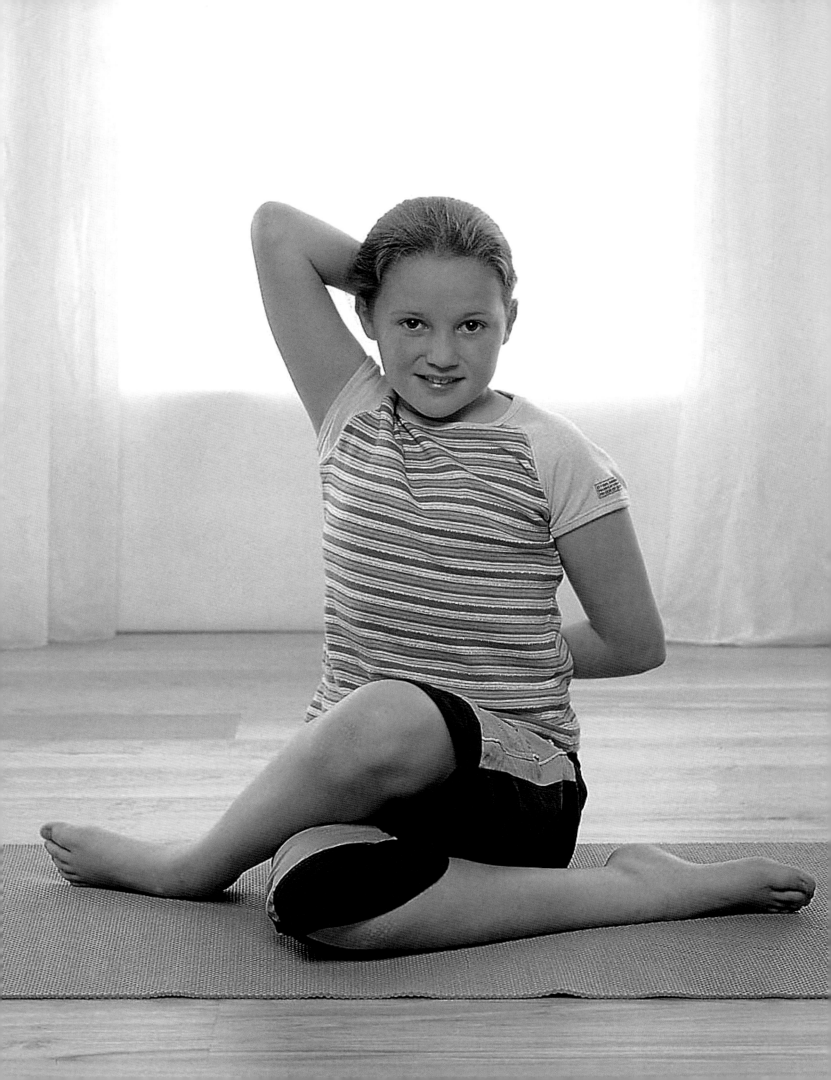

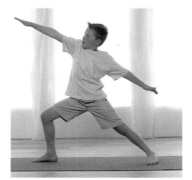
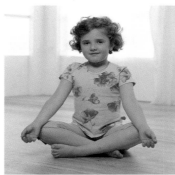
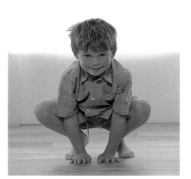
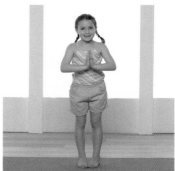

Yoga for Children

Making yoga a fun activity for children is easy. Here are exercises designed to develop an understanding of yoga practice, and there are plenty of fun ideas too.

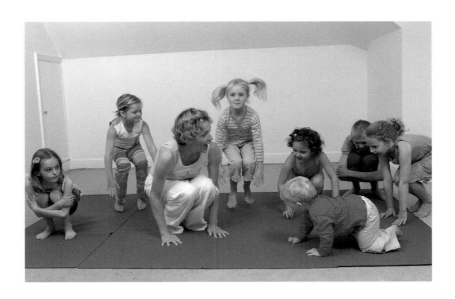

Bel Gibbs

How is Yoga Suitable for Children?

Adults have been practising yoga for many centuries, and while many people complain that children today are growing up too fast, they're never too young to start enjoying yoga. Introducing the concept and practice of yoga and a yogic lifestyle to your children means that you are giving them the very best start in life.

Yoga for children

Childhood is a vibrant time when natural energy and creativity are high, also when eyes and minds are open and learning is fun. This makes it the perfect time for children to explore and enjoy their bodies, while putting them in touch with how their minds work and introducing them to the idea of an inner self, or soul.

We all have the potential to develop our inner self, and yoga can show us how. Yoga is expressive, and this is

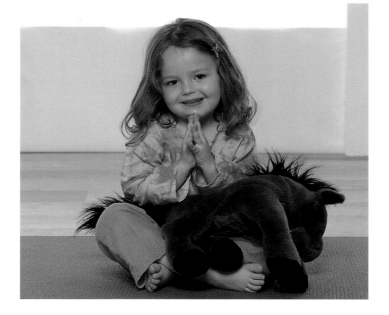

left Yoga encourages us to find quiet time and to enjoy being rather than doing.

what makes it so appealing to children. There are countless benefits of yoga for children, but the principal focus is to nurture a strong, healthy body, a calm, contented mind and, with commitment, a sense of inner peace.

What's in it for parents?

This chapter is primarily aimed at children between the ages of 3 and 11 years, but in a sense it is for children of all ages. As you demonstrate the yoga postures to your children, you will be rekindling your own sense of fun, putting you in touch with your inner child. You will also be increasing your motivation as a parent by taking an active role in the well-being of your child, physically, emotionally and spiritually. By practising yoga as a family, you will be spending valuable time together, learning new skills and having fun, and all without having to go near a television or the car!

What's in this chapter?

This chapter is written with a sense of fun and adventure. It is bursting with animals and objects from the natural

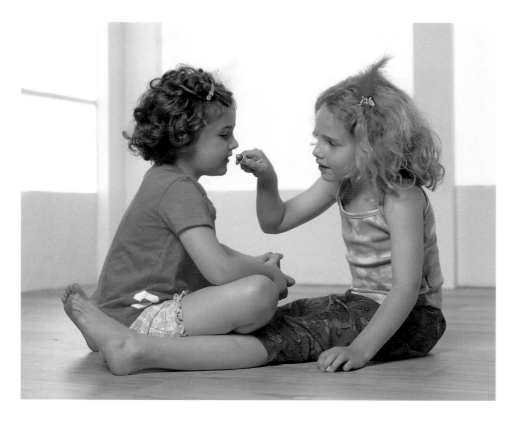

left Enjoying spending time with family and friends is an important part of growing up and will help us to build lasting relationships later on in life.

world, all of which will appeal instinctively to a child's imagination. So this is where we start. Encourage your children to "become" an animal from the colourful, easy-to-follow Animal Parade chapter. As they become adept at the animal postures, try some of the other fun poses and encourage your children to make up their own, or link them together in the themed story sequences in the Putting It All Together chapter. Try some of the yoga games, and even act out a yoga play.

In addition, learn how yoga breathing exercises can alter your children's moods and how peaceful postures, chanting and meditating can soothe away tension and nurture quiet time and contemplation.

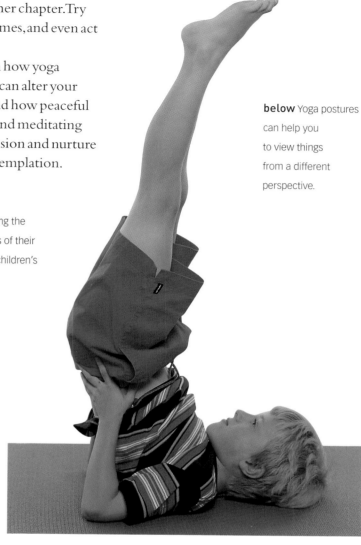

below Yoga postures can help you to view things from a different perspective.

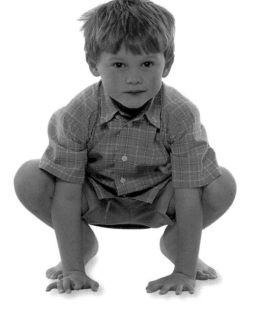

left The thought of imitating the behaviour and movements of their favourite animals is most children's idea of a lot of fun!

below Crow walking helps to physically strengthen our legs, and teaches us not to take everything too seriously.

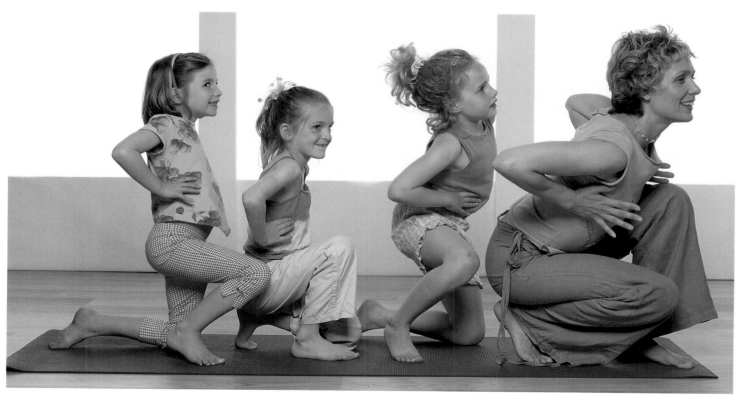

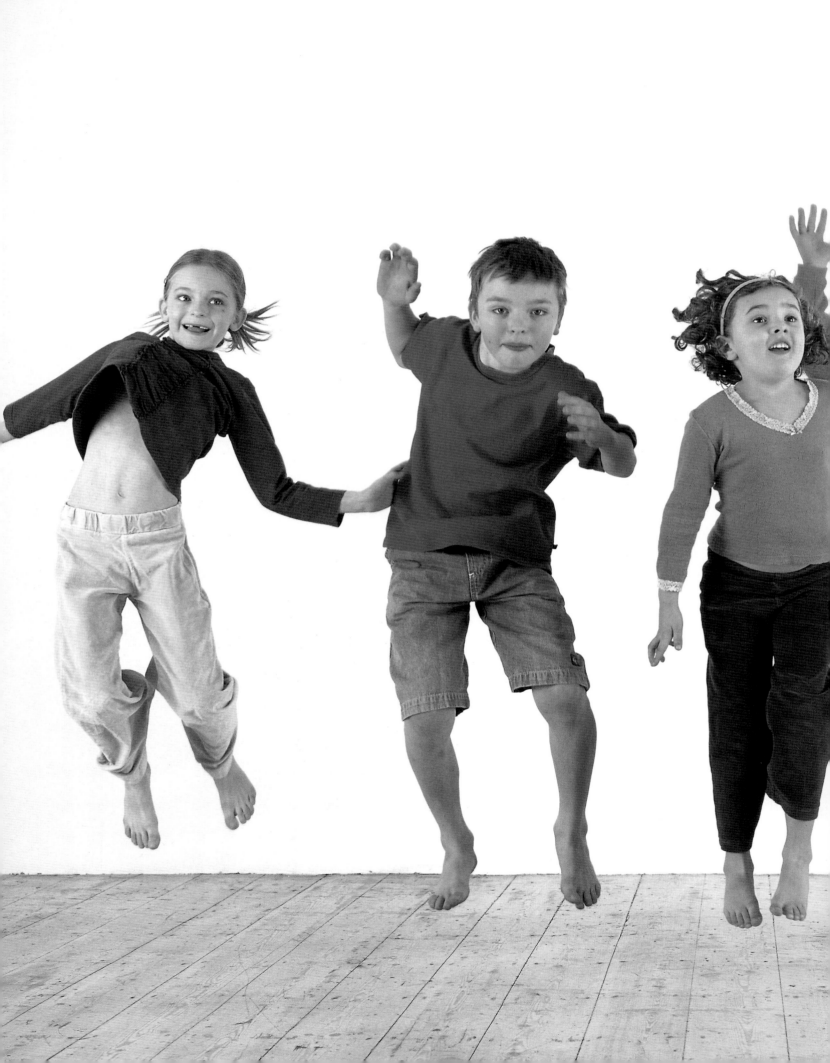

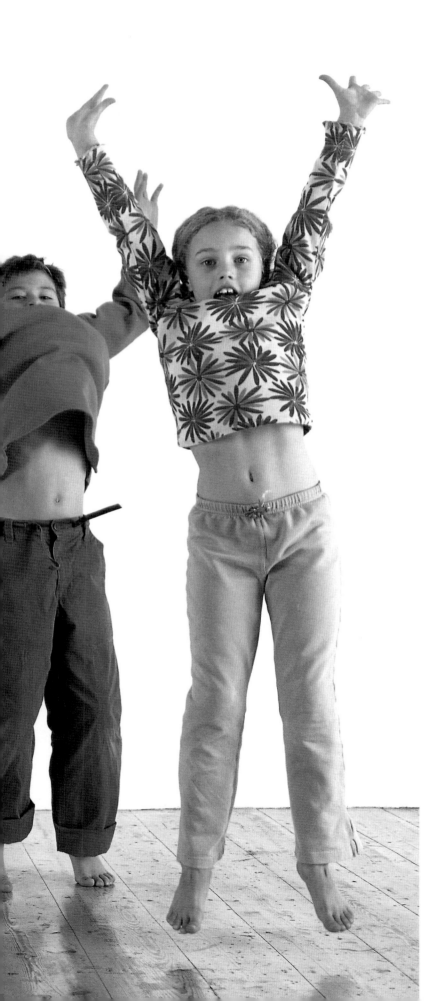

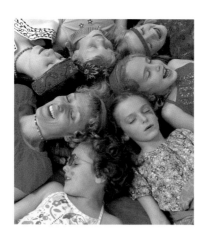

what's it all
About?

The following pages will inspire you to put yoga firmly on your family agenda. A brief "history lesson" explains how yoga began and why it is still relevant to our busy lives today. We all have a special place inside us that holds the key to our inner potential, like a treasure chest of precious jewels, and here we show children how to unlock their own inner powers.

Where Does Yoga Come From?

Yoga evolved several thousand years ago, in India, as a system of self-enlightenment. Today, in spite of all the benefits of 21st-century living, more and more people are turning to yoga for inspiration, confirming its timeless appeal.

The meaning of yoga

Originally, yoga evolved as a way of feeling closer to a higher, divine presence, and the focus of yoga practice was spiritual rather than physical. Today, yoga can be enjoyed as a physical discipline, known as hatha yoga, as well as a spiritual one. Many people still find that practising yoga can help to deepen their faith.

The Indian sages, or gurus, who first developed the idea of yoga believed that to attain spiritual enlightenment required a systematic approach. They devised a code of practice to follow in order to achieve all-round health, and believed that by training the physical body – the first step in yoga – they could tame the mind, improve the concentration, and find their inner self, or soul.

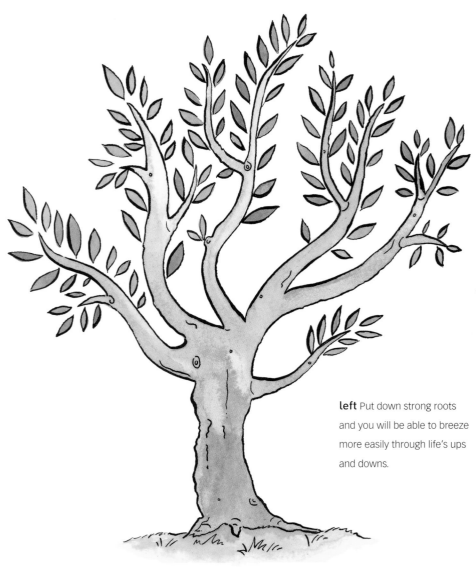

left Put down strong roots and you will be able to breeze more easily through life's ups and downs.

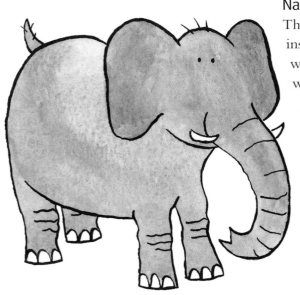

Nature knows best

The gurus sought their initial inspiration from the natural world around them. They watched and studied the patterns of nature and the behaviour of animals with a scientific passion. They marvelled at the power and focus of predatory creatures and birds as they hunted, at their ability to conserve energy and to sleep soundly when the opportunity arose.

left and below Some animals inspire us with their quick agility, while others show it pays to take things slow.

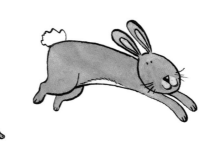

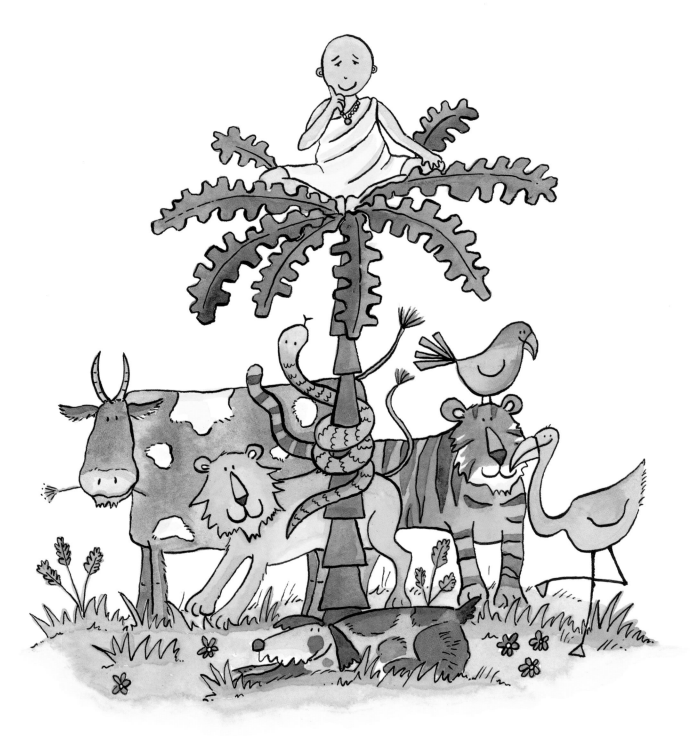

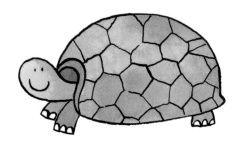

Admiring this balanced, instinctive way of living, the yogis – the gurus who developed and practised the yoga philosophy – began to imitate the way the animals moved and behaved, and soon they found themselves empowered with special qualities. And so the classical asanas, or animal postures, were born.

What the yogis learned
The gurus observed the breathing patterns of animals, and noted that animals with slow heart rates, like the elephant and the tortoise, lived much longer than agile and nervous animals with quick heart rates, such as mice and rabbits.

They saw the sun as the centre of their energy universe after watching how plants and flowers grow upwards

above Just like the yogis of ancient times, you can learn from the natural world around you. Simply open your eyes and strive to see the good in everything.

to bask in its warmth and energy. They admired the huge trees because they were at the same time strong and flexible, rooted firmly in the ground but with branches moving freely in the wind. Seeing these attributes as metaphors for a human code of living, they saw that people could be happier and healthier if they, too, could be both grounded and flexible.

Yoga and Your Body

According to yoga philosophy, a human being is made up of different layers, a bit like all the layers you can see when you cut an onion in half. These are known as koshas.

You are an onion!

The outermost layer is our physical body, called the *anna maya kosha*. This is the layer we are most familiar with because it is visible and we use it for all our everyday activities. At a deeper level is our mind or mental layer, or *mano maya kosha*. This is where our thoughts, feelings and emotions take place. The deepest layer of all is our spiritual layer, or *ananda maya kosha*, the home of our inner self or soul.

The mental and spiritual layers are more difficult to relate to because they are invisible, but the aim of yoga is to use the physical body as a way of reaching first the mental and then the spiritual layer. It is here that yogis believe true happiness resides, and if we can reach our inner self we can enjoy a whole new side of our personality. Regular yoga practice can help to connect us with the inner self and develop our spiritual nature. The sooner we start on this wonderful inward journey the better.

Getting physical

The human body is made up of a brain, a heart, two lungs, trillions of tiny cells, 206 bones, 600 muscles and lots of blood. More than half our body weight is made up of water.

The brain is the body's central computer, delivering instructions and messages to the limbs and internal organs, while the heart is a powerful pump pushing blood around the body.

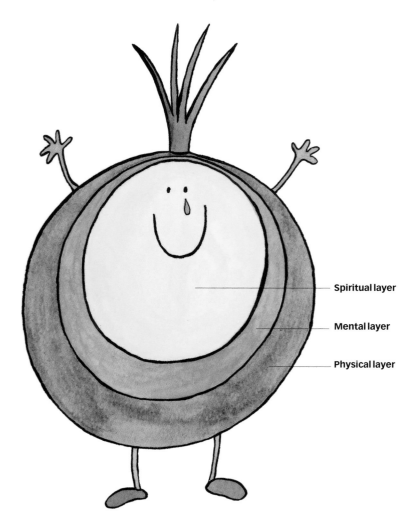

Spiritual layer

Mental layer

Physical layer

The blood is our body's "river of life", transporting its precious cargo of oxygen and nutrients to where they are needed, and relaying waste and carbon dioxide back to our lungs to be breathed away. Our lungs are like two big sponges that soak up oxygen from the air we breathe to keep us alive. As for all that water inside us, this is vital as every bodily function, from swallowing and blinking to breathing and moving – including reading this book – needs water.

Our bones are like scaffolding bound together by bandage-like muscles that literally stop us from falling apart. If our muscles are too tight, we feel stiff and our movements are limited. If left for long periods of

above Think of all the parts that go into the layering of an onion. The more parts you unravel, the more there seems to be. This is the wonder of you too!

time, tight muscles can affect our physical posture and how we carry ourselves, locking our bodies into uncomfortable positions and leading to rounded shoulders, stiff necks and knock knees. The good news is that muscles can be retrained through gentle, regular stretching, which helps them to regain their elasticity. This allows us to straighten our shoulders and open up our chests, stand tall with our heads up, touch our toes with ease, avoid injuries and generally feel in good physical shape.

Why it is wise to exercise

The benefits of physical exercise are enormous. Exercise strengthens the heart, and this promotes good circulation, which increases the flow of oxygen- and nutrient-rich blood to all parts of the body. Boosting the circulation speeds up the elimination of waste products, improves digestion, and helps to relax tense muscles, releasing mental stress and negative emotions. Exercise also strengthens bones, and tones muscles and ligaments, keeping us trim and fit. It increases energy levels and leads to the production of endorphins, the body's natural feel-good hormones, which enhance mood and well-being.

All types of exercise are good in moderation, but a variety of activities will work a wider range of muscles. Introducing yoga as a complement to regular exercise is manageable because it can be done at home and it doesn't cost anything. Because yoga can involve all members of the family, it offers valuable bonding time while teaching important new life skills.

Hatha yoga

Physical or hatha yoga relates to the practice of special postures called asanas. These asanas have evolved to work all parts of the body. They fall into families of postures, including forward bends, backward bends, standing poses, seated poses, twists, side-bending postures, balances and inverted postures. As you work through the book you will see that the groups of postures have different physical and emotional effects. Some are calming and grounding, while others are energizing and uplifting.

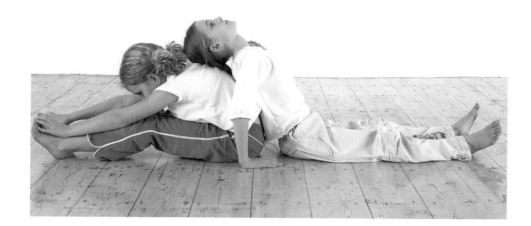

above We can use our bodies in so many ways. This assisted Sandwich pose quietens the mind as you fold your upper body forwards, and it gives your partner a nice back stretch at the same time.

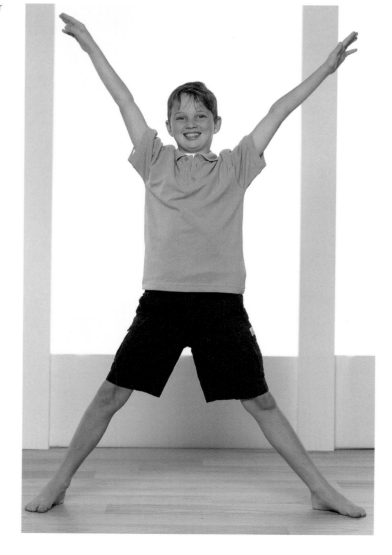

right The body is your temple and physical activity makes your body an exhilarating place to live in.

What's on Your Mind?

According to yoga philosophy, the mind is the force that both drives the physical body and feeds our inner world or soul, where the yogis believe our true nature is to be found. The mind plays an essential role in determining whether our journey through life will be smooth or bumpy, or whether we will see our glass as half full or half empty.

The guru Patanjali defined yoga as "the mastery of the stilling of the mind". He believed in training the mind to focus completely on one thing at a time and therefore become as useful as possible.

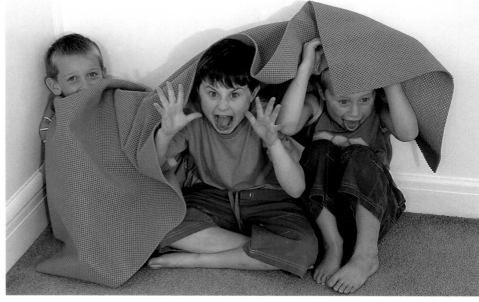

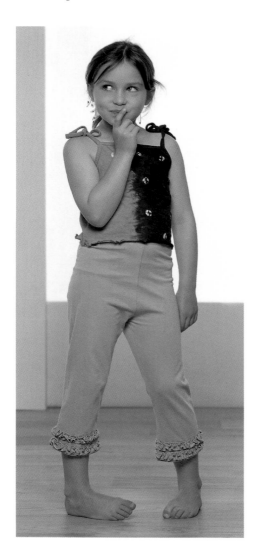

left Thinking before you speak or act helps you to behave appropriately.

Five ways of thinking

The gurus who developed yoga philosophy believed that our thought processes functioned at five different levels, from muddled and irrational to clear and focused. The latter, superior level of thinking is attainable by all of us, but we first have to conquer the lower thought processes that govern our irrational or base behaviour.

Our least refined level of thinking is likened to a drunken monkey swinging from branch to branch, where thoughts are random and jumpy with no common thread. Moving up, the second level resembles a lethargic water buffalo standing in the mud, inactive and uninspired. The third level – which is the most common mental state – is a mobile mind that flits endlessly between doubt and conviction, knowing and not knowing. The fourth level reveals a relatively clear mind that has direction but lacks attention. The fifth and highest level is where the mind is linked exclusively with the object of its attention. Here, mind and object merge to become one.

above Give it a rest! A mind that is always busy can become physically exhausting.

Minding the mind

Learning to refine our thinking processes is one of the rewards of regular yoga practice. The yoga techniques outlined in this book concentrate on yoga postures, breath awareness and learning to enjoy stillness and silence. Getting to grips with these essential techniques will help you to improve your ability to concentrate. This is the first stage in learning to control the endless fluctuations of the mind.

Why concentrate?

The art of concentration is being lost. It is being undermined by the desire to be permanently busy and a notion that we must always be achieving, producing and progressing. So involved are we in multi-tasking that we risk becoming a jack of all trades but master of none. The absence of concentration makes it difficult for us to sit still, or think before we speak, or plan before we act. Those unruly monkeys take over our mind and our physical body responds with restless behaviour and hyperactivity.

Present and correct

Concentration helps us to enjoy the "bloom" of the present moment and to think about tomorrow only when tomorrow comes; this is how it feels to be absorbed in a good book or enjoy an interesting conversation with a friend. Concentration makes for attentiveness in school and the ability to understand and retain information. It lets us fully engage with the people around us, and helps to cement relationships. It allows us to put 100 per cent of ourselves into everything we do, and means we will always do our best. In the same way that the sun's rays can be intensified through a magnifying glass, our fragmented thoughts can be harnessed together to make a powerful tool.

above Left to its own devices the mind can become as unruly as these monkeys.

Meditation

Once we have learned how to concentrate and focus our mind and energies on one thing at a time, we can begin to talk about meditation. Meditation is simply concentration in a more *concentrated* form. Think of concentration as a flow of water that stops and starts. Meditation is simply a flow of water that continues unbroken in an endless stream.

One way or another, we are all looking for the peace of mind that this deeper level of concentration brings. When our attention is fully engaged, our mind becomes silent, worries are temporarily forgotten and an inner contentment replaces all else.

left The inner contentment that a quiet mind brings is available to all of us.

Your Invisible Friend the Breath

Breathing is our most important daily activity and, alongside eating, it is one of the two ways in which we provide our body with the energy it needs to live. That said, we can live for a few days without eating but only a few moments without breathing. Learning to be aware of, and improve, our habitual breathing patterns can dynamically enhance our physical, mental and emotional well-being.

Regular breathing encourages the exchange of old air for new. Breathing in and out through the nose involves complete in and out breaths, which encourage the diaphragm to contract and relax, massaging the heart and all of the abdominal organs respectively.

Shallow breathing, on the other hand, robs the lungs of oxygen and the diaphragm of its potential range of movement. With the lungs unable to function properly, stale air can become trapped and the body is deprived of oxygen. This is when our resistance to illness drops.

Posture

Diaphragmatic breathing, or tummy breathing, opens up the chest and allows the lungs to expand. We all have to stand tall or sit upright to breathe in this way. This means that our chest opens, our shoulders drop and overall posture is modified for the better. All in all, good breathing habits produce a stronger respiratory system, improved posture and a happier frame of mind.

Prana

In yoga philosophy, the other function of breathing is to increase our vital life energy, known as *prana*. The yogis believed that this in turn would lead to control of the mind.

Prana is controlled by special breathing exercises or *pranayama* (*ayama* meaning to lengthen or add a new dimension to). These exercises are designed to enhance our life energy and help us connect to our quiet inner self.

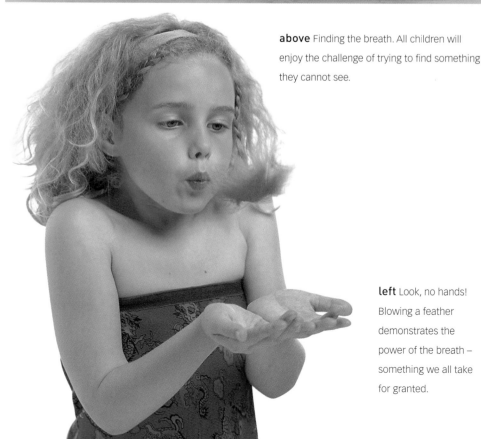

above Finding the breath. All children will enjoy the challenge of trying to find something they cannot see.

left Look, no hands! Blowing a feather demonstrates the power of the breath – something we all take for granted.

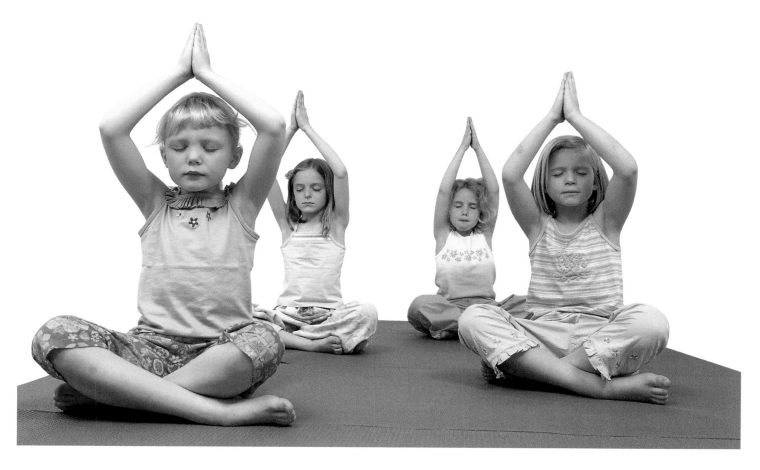

The breath as a bridge

The breath acts as a bridge between the mind and the body. You can see this in action by synchronizing simple stretches with your breathing patterns. Notice how the ebb and flow of your breath soothes your mind and helps your body to stretch.

Your invisible friend
Who has seen the wind?
Neither you nor I,
But when the trees bow down
   their heads
The wind is passing by.

This poem illustrates that by seeing what the wind touches, we know it is there, even though we cannot see the wind itself. The same goes for our breath. If you blow a feather into the air, puff out a candle or watch your

above Breathing slowly and deeply through your nose as you stretch your arms is a wonderfully empowering gesture that says "I am me!"

breath condense on a frosty day, you will see your breath at work. You can find "where" your breath is by using your hands. To do this, lie on your back, with your feet flat on the floor and your knees bent. Place both your hands, palms down, on your tummy. Position your hands so that they are covering your tummy button. Now feel the rise and fall of your breath.

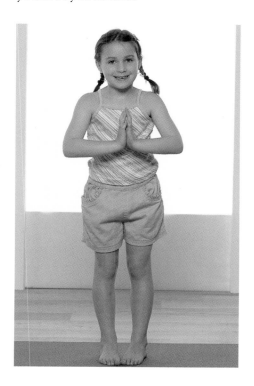

left The taller and straighter you stand, the better you breathe and the better you feel.

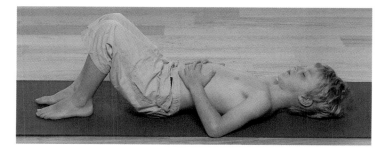

above Tummy breathing is simply breathing with your hands on your tummy. Notice how your fingers gently separate as you breathe in and come together again as you breathe out.

Getting Into the Spirit

Yoga teaches us that we are more than just a collection of muscles and bones, and that we possess an inner spirit or soul. In many developed cultures, it is the appearance of the physical body that is championed and not what we are like on the inside. Not surprisingly, many people question whether the body does have a soul. However, the committed yogi would not only confirm its presence but would add that the soul is *the* essential element of our make-up.

Our secret self

In yoga philosophy, the physical body is considered to be a vehicle for the soul on its journey towards truth and enlightenment. The soul represents our true nature and identity. It is an inner world that lies not in the body's external casing but in the deeper ananda maya kosha, also known as the bliss sheath. Like a hidden jewel, the soul is always there for us to discover. It is always with us, just as the sun is always in the sky even though it may be hidden behind a bank of rain cloud.

Reaching the soul

The regular practice of yoga can take us to this special internal place, so that we can experience the real us. Beginning to practise yoga asanas for physical reasons, to improve agility and strength or to ease a specific complaint such as backache, is the logical place to start. This gives us visible results and begins to break down our physical shell. As our awareness of our physical body grows, so too does our emotional sensitivity. We begin to experience things differently, and very soon it dawns on us that not only does yoga meet our initial expectations, but it gives us an extra something too.

> "A man travels the world in search of the answers and comes home to find them."

Showing your true colours

Yoga is a process of self-discovery, an unpeeling and unravelling, a working down through the layers until we reach our core. To begin with we may only glimpse the tranquillity of this inner sanctum, but over time, we may notice a subtle change in our approach to life. We feel more content with what we have got, rather than dissatisfied that we don't have more. We find that we have become more philosophical, more accepting of life's ups and downs, and less bothered by the little problems. This subtle, gradual evolution helps us to marvel at the spectacle of life rather than be overawed by its complexity.

Less is more

For children, getting spiritual is about learning to tap into this inner joy. Yoga encourages us to use our natural, inner resources. With guidance you will see that you have all you need to be happy within yourself.

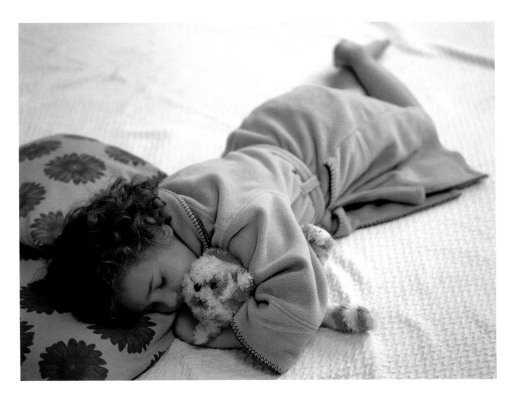

left Home is where the heart is. The security of a happy home environment makes for sweet dreams.

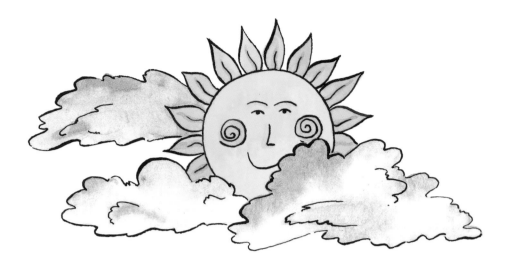

right Yoga philosophy states that we are all naturally sunny by nature. Simply blow away the clouds and see that the sun is still there, shining away as brightly as ever.

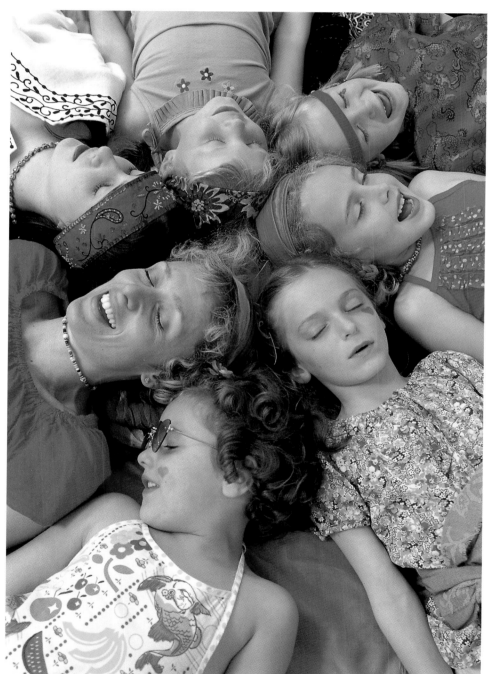

left Get your heads together! Group bonding helps you to enjoy the people you are close to, and to appreciate that life is all about giving and receiving love.

below Nothing beats the familiar feeling of a big hug from your favourite bear.

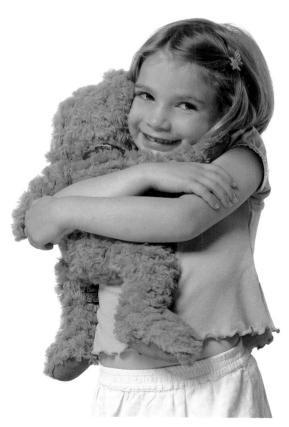

Finding the Wizard Within

All children can be encouraged to believe in themselves and to locate their inner strengths or powers. They only need to be shown how.

Positive atttitudes

One aspect of yoga has to do with our actions. It means acting so that all of our attention is directed towards the activity to which we are engaged. This starts at home as we practise the physical aspects of yoga, and can then be applied to daily life.

Patanjali, author of the classic text the Yoga Sutras, outlined a set of guidelines for living. These comprise *yamas*, which help us to check our behaviour, and *niyamas*, which help to refine our attitudes. Together they teach us to act in a conscientious and attentive manner in all that we do, making the very best of ourselves.

Yamas

Non-aggression, or *ahimsa*, is one of the principal yamas. This encourages us to avoid injury in yoga asanas by underlining the importance of being nice to our bodies.

Developing compassion for others and protecting the environment are also aspects of the non-aggression principle. Always try to help others who are less fortunate than yourself, and take your litter home with you.

The honesty yama, known as *satya*, is about not trying to be what you are not. It asks us to know our strengths and weaknesses and to be proud of who and what we are.

Openness, known as *asteya*, teaches us to be flexible and open to change, allowing time for postures, like everyday situations, to evolve rather

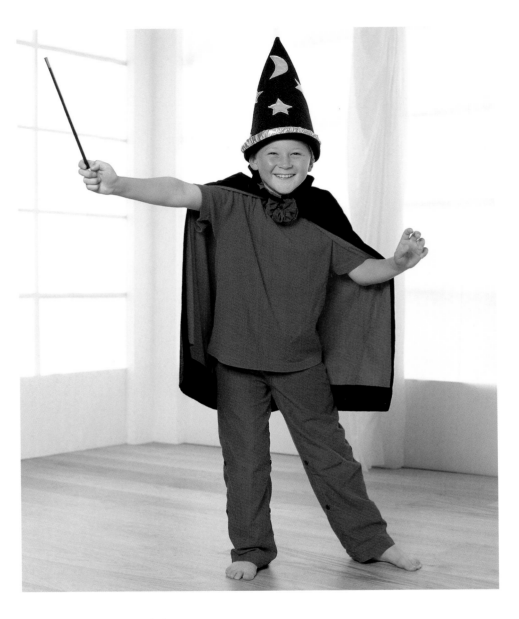

than trying to control them. *Asteya* literally means "not stealing", and it teaches us not to take advantage of others or to be jealous of what they have. It tells us to think about what we *have* got instead, and to nurture contentment within ourselves.

Niyamas

Cleanliness, or *sauca*, is about living healthily and taking pride in our appearance. One way you could do this is to keep your bedroom tidy.

above All of us have magical powers within ourselves, and with a bit of help from yoga we can learn how to unleash them.

Contentment, known as *samtosa*, is about doing what we do because we enjoy it and not because other people are doing it.

Enthusiasm, known as *tapas*, which literally means "heat", is about keeping our passion for life alive: making the best of ourselves, putting in the effort and really going for it.

Energy chakras

In yoga philosophy the chakras are invisible centres of spiritual and physical energy located in the body. They reflect our emotional state, and can affect our behaviour and attitudes. There are seven main chakras:

• Root or base (1) Feeling grounded and safe; the survival instinct

• Sacrum (2) Feelings about friends and family, social skills, and the ability to enjoy ourselves

• Solar plexus (3) Self-belief and enthusiasm for life

• Heart (4) Being open-hearted and joyful

• Throat (5) Communication

• Third eye (6) Clear thinking

• Crown (7) Wisdom and spirituality

Many yogis believe that learning to balance our chakras can help to restore harmony to our lives. Think about these energy centres and use visual imagery to bring them alive. A traditional image is the lotus flower. The idea is that when the petals of the lotus flower are closed, the chakra is closed too. Encouraging the petals to open and to be filled with a warm light is the way to bring back life and energy to the chakra. Try making up your own positive images that are relevant to you and your feelings.

Using visual imagery in this way can give all children a sense of the power of awareness. Don't be afraid to talk about your emotions. Ask yourself "where" in your body you feel sad or hurt. Describe and direct a visual image at the relevant chakra to help soothe emotional problems. Remember that a physical problem is often a sign of an underlying emotional imbalance.

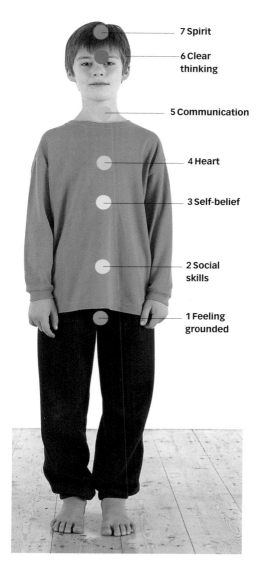

7 Spirit
6 Clear thinking
5 Communication
4 Heart
3 Self-belief
2 Social skills
1 Feeling grounded

left The seven chakras are located along the spine. Awareness of these special energy centres can enhance emotional well-being.

You could also visualize rays of warm sunlight flooding into the body in Little Buddha pose.

Standing strong and still

The inability to concentrate or sit still can suggest a lack of grounding. Feeling able to stand on our own feet relates to our root chakra. Strong poses such as Warrior or Tree develop conviction, and make us feel anchored to life. Visualize a strong, majestic tree and feel its roots anchored deep in the earth. Try Little Buddha pose to feel grounded but still.

Shout it out!

Shyness and the fear of speaking up relates to the throat chakra. Use sound to encourage self-expression and build confidence. Try Lion roar and Humming Bee Breath. Stretches that open up the chest, such as Cobra and Camel, may help too.

Open your heart

Rounded shoulders may mean that the heart chakra is closed. The heart chakra represents love for ourselves, for others and for life in general. Encourage open-heartedness and boost self-esteem by using upper body stretches that emphasize the meridians to the heart. Finger, arm and shoulder stretches are all good for this. Suitable stretches are found in the Lion, Fish and Camel poses.

right Sitting in Little Buddha pose keeps you grounded but helps your mind to think clearly.

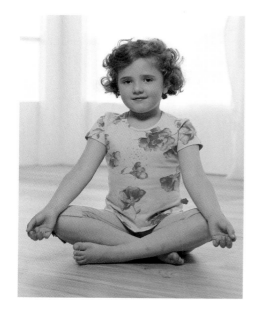

Let's Warm Up!

Warming up with gentle limbering exercises is essential preparation for your yoga practice. Spending just 5 or 10 minutes on these fun and simple exercises before you start your session will help to warm up cold muscles, focus your mind and get you in the mood. Preparing your body in this way is important as it will help you to avoid injury.

Keep the movements small to start with, working up from your feet and legs to your hands, wrists and arms, neck and head. Then move on to the body warm-ups and partner work.

Getting started

- Choose a warm, light room in a quiet part of the house. Make sure the television is switched off!
- Wait a good hour or two after a meal before you start your yoga session.
- Practise on a rug or carpet, or on your own yoga mat if you have one.
- Wear loose, comfortable clothes.
- Have some soft cushions handy and, for younger children, a few soft toys as props.
- Light some candles or mild incense to set the mood.
- Play some relaxing music for the quiet time session.
- Plan for a 15 minute session and build it up gradually to 30 minutes as you become used to it. Use your body language and energy levels as your guide, and learn to recognize when enough is enough.
- Aim to make your yoga positive not perfect. Have fun!

Planning a yoga session

- Do some of the warm-up exercises before you start.
- Practise nasal breathing.
- Come in and out of postures gently and thoughtfully – asana means "comfortable seat", and you should always feel at ease in the poses you do.
- Encourage self-expression by accompanying animal poses with sound: roar like a lion! bark like a dog!
- Balance the body by doing postures on both sides of the body.
- Erase the last posture by following it with a counter pose. For example, follow a forward bend with a backward bend, and lie down to rest after a series of strong standing poses.
- Poses that twist the spine are best done after you have stretched the back forwards, as in the Rag Doll pose (standing forward bend).

- Think about linking breath to movement and, as a general rule, breathe in when you stretch up or back and out when you fold forwards or down (the Sunshine Stretch is a good example of this).
- Sequence your session with asanas, games, breathing exercises and quiet time, and always end a session with at least 5–10 minutes in relaxation, or longer if you like.
- Keep a yoga diary using stick men to show the postures you have done. Record feelings and sensations and talk about which parts of the session you enjoyed the most.

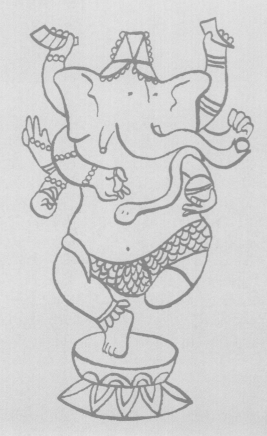

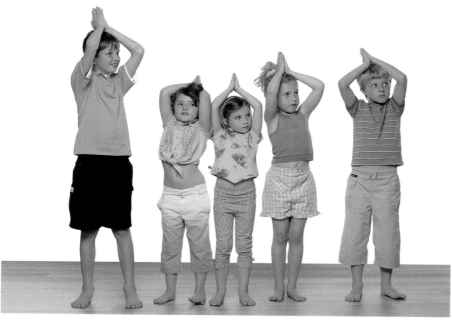

left Spinning top Make a pointy hat by holding your hands together above your head. Now draw an invisible circle with your pointy hat to wake up your waist.

right Draw circles Use your feet, your hands and your hips to draw circles in the air. Make circles of different sizes; the slower you can make them the better. If there are a few of you, you may want to hold hands to stop yourselves falling over!

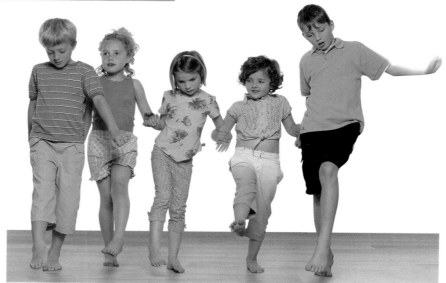

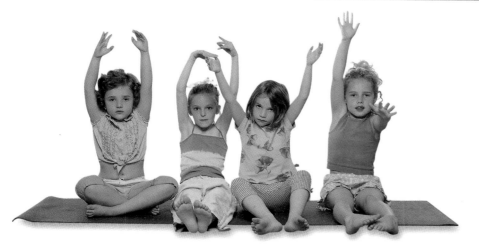

left Windmill arms Gently circle your arms like the sails of a windmill. Breathe in as you stretch up your arms, and breathe out as your arms come back down to your lap.

right Shoulder shrugs Squeeze your shoulders up to your ears as you breathe in, and round behind you and down again as you breathe out. Notice how long your neck feels now.

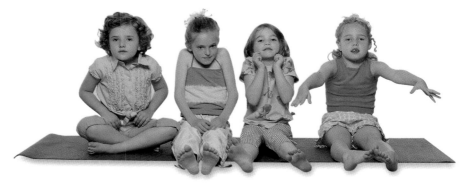

▷

Rocking the Baby

This warm-up gives a strong stretch to your hips and buttocks. Imagine your lower leg is a little baby that you are gently rocking to sleep in your arms. Cradle your lower leg as you would a sleeping child and rock from side to side, breathing deeply. Lift your foot to kiss the baby's forehead.

1 Sitting on your bottom, lift up your right leg and gently bend your knee. Draw your right foot in towards your tummy button, cradling your ankle in your hand.

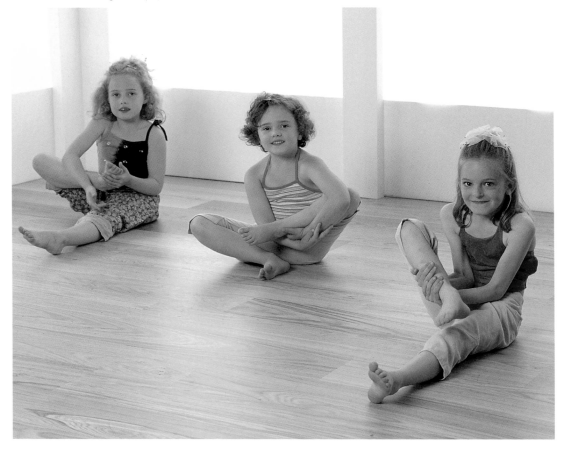

2 Hug your knee and lower leg with your arms and gently rock your baby from side to side. Finish off with a little kiss on your baby's forehead as you lift your foot towards your face.

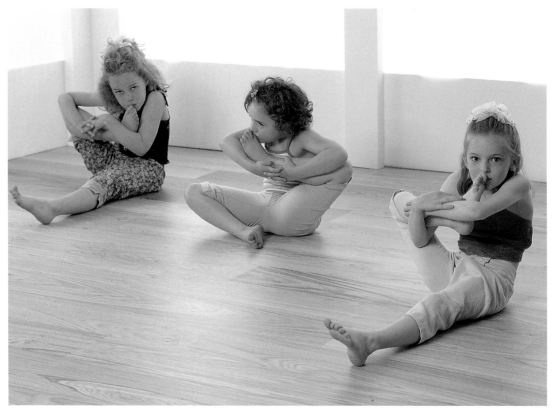

Cat, Dog, Snake and Mouse

Do as many rounds of this flowing animal warm-up sequence as you like. It wakes up your back, stretches your legs and strengthens your arms, wrists and hands. You can do the sequence on your own but it is much more fun to do it in pairs. Let each part merge into the next and don't forget to breathe!

1 Kneel on the floor in Cat pose, with your shoulders over your hands and your claws (your fingers) spread wide. Rub noses with your cat friend and breathe in deeply.

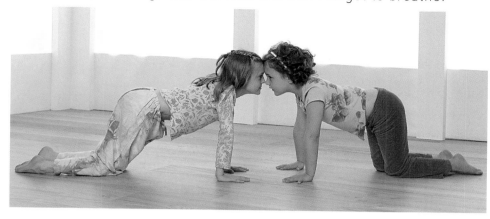

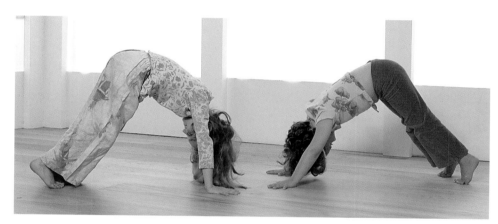

2 As you breathe out, curl your toes under and lift your knees and bottom upwards, letting your head hang forwards and down. Let your heels sink into the floor as you imagine you are a dog doing his morning stretch. Take a few more breaths.

3 As you take your next breath in, roll over your toes and let your hips and tummy drop to the floor. Point your toes behind you, stick out your tongue and hiss like a snake. Keep breathing steadily.

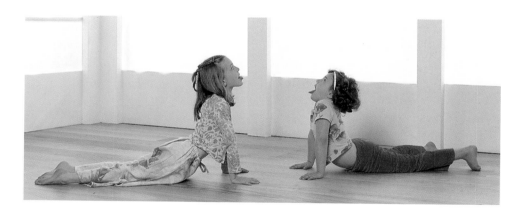

4 Lift your bottom up as you breathe out and sit back on your heels with your forehead on the floor. Rest like a quiet little mouse. Then lift your bottom up to come back to Cat pose, and start all over again.

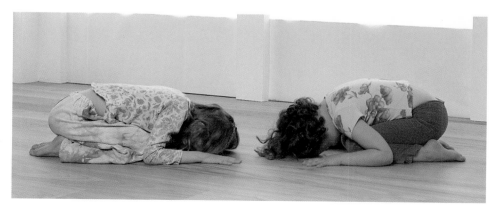

▷

Partner Work

Doing limbering exercises and yoga postures in twos gives you double the fun. You can make your stretches deeper when you have someone to help you. Working together makes you more considerate and helps you to develop responsibility for your partner. Talk to each other as you do these exercises to help each other get the most out of each movement.

At a spiritual level, partner work builds connectedness and reinforces the concept of yoga – to unite. It is a wonderful way to bond relationships and to promote the idea of sharing.

left Table top Stand facing each other and place your palms on each other's shoulders. Hold on gently but firmly and then step away from each other until the crowns of your heads come together. Keep hold of your partner's shoulders and stretch your bottom back, so that your back flattens. Breathe deeply then walk your feet in towards each other and relax.

right Rainbow In this pose the sides of your bodies create the arc of a beautiful rainbow. Kneel down about 1m/3ft away from each other, with your bottoms lifted off your heels. Extend your outside legs, and rest your inside hands on the floor between you for support. Breathe in and, as you breathe out, bring your outside arms up and put your hands together to give a lovely stretch to the upper side of your body. Picture a rainbow filling you with its vibrant light. Release and change sides.

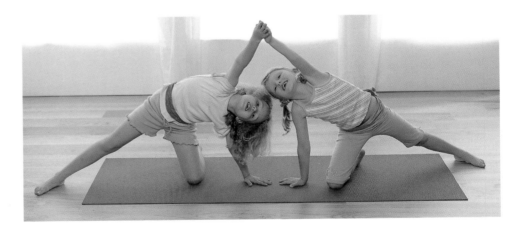

left Seesaw Sit opposite each other with your legs outstretched. One of you needs to place the balls of your feet against the inside of your partner's shins. Reach forwards and take her hands. Gently pull her forwards towards you so that she gets a lovely stretch in her back and the backs of her legs. Release and swap.

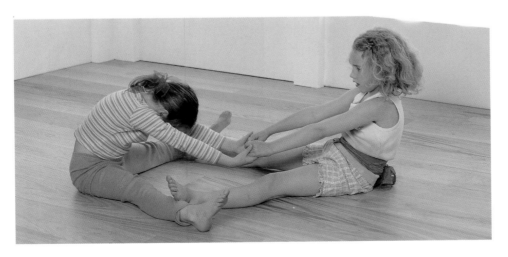

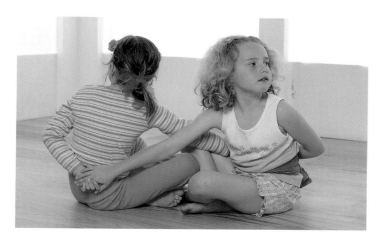

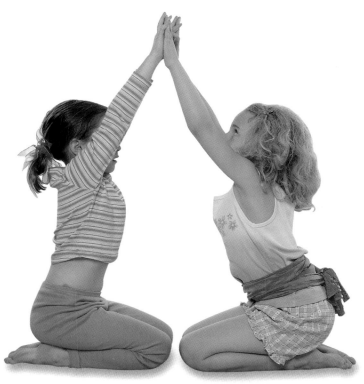

above Figure of eight Sit opposite your partner with crossed legs and your knees touching. Reach your right arm forward and down towards your partner's right arm. Fold your left arm behind you and reach round to grasp your partner's right hand. Breathe steadily and deeply and on each out-breath, gently pull your partner's left hand towards you. Hold for a few long breaths, then change arms.

above Washing windows Kneel opposite each other, raise your arms and press your palms together. Imagine you have a sheet of glass between you. One of you will guide the other's hands as you wash the window, and one of you will let yourself be guided. Draw big circles, reaching as high up and as far to the sides and down towards your knees as you can. Keep the hands together as you make the circles.

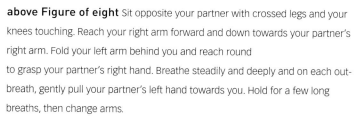

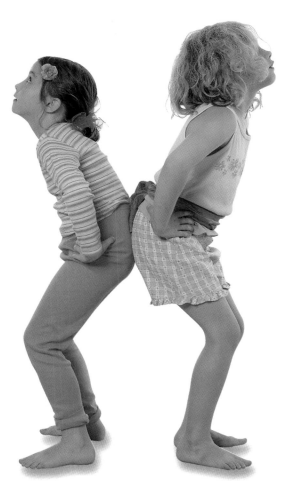

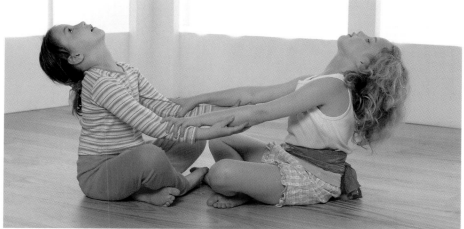

above The fountain Sit cross-legged on the floor. Hold each other's lower arms. Breathe in and, as you breathe out, lean back and allow your partner to support your body. Do this one at a time to begin with, then do it both together.

left Chair Stand with your backs to each other, feet apart. Squat down until your bottoms touch, and put your hands on your hips. Breathe deeply. When your legs begin to ache, imagine energy flowing between you so that you can hold the pose for a few more breaths. Release and relax.

Did you know that...
Ligaments and muscles need to be stretched gradually and naturally without hurry or forcing. This is especially true during childhood, when the muscles are still growing. This is what makes warm-up exercises so important.

Sunshine Stretch

This sequence was designed as a greeting to the sun god, who in Hindu mythology is worshipped as a symbol of health and immortality.

The Sunshine Stretch limbers up and energizes the whole body, particularly the back, making it flexible and strong. It also clears your mind, puts a smile on your face and makes you ready for the day ahead.

Stand in front of a window for this sequence, particularly if the sun is shining, or stand opposite a friend. Breathing deeply will help each part of the sequence flow into the next. As a general rule, you breathe in as you stretch up or backwards and breathe out when you bend forwards.

"Truly, a flexible back makes for a long life." CHINESE PROVERB

1 Stand in Mountain pose (Tadasana), looking straight in front of you – facing your partner or a window – with your legs straight and your feet together. Hold your hands in Prayer position (Namaste). Breathe deeply and imagine a cord from the crown of your head, gently drawing you upwards while your feet remain firmly grounded.

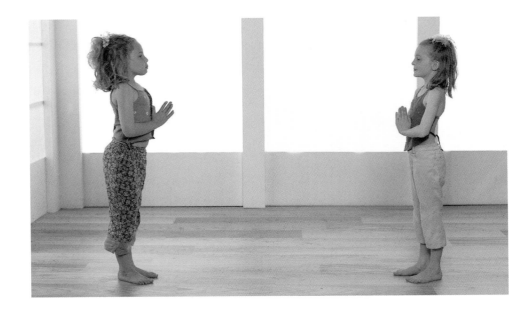

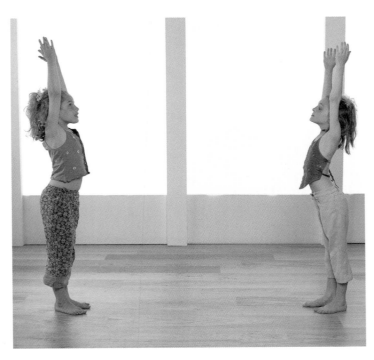

2 Stretch your arms up high above your head as you breathe in. Bring your palms together and hold for a few seconds.

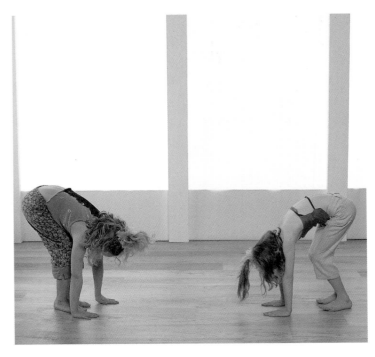

3 Now exhale and fold forwards, bending your knees, and bring your hands to the ground in front of you, keeping your palms flat.

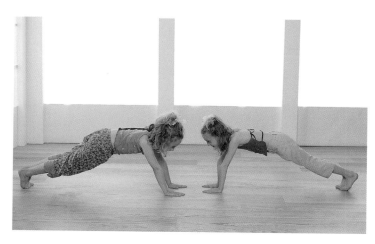

4 Step one leg back as far as you can, and then the other. Push back through your heels, keeping your legs straight. Imagine that your whole body feels like a stiff, strong plank of wood.

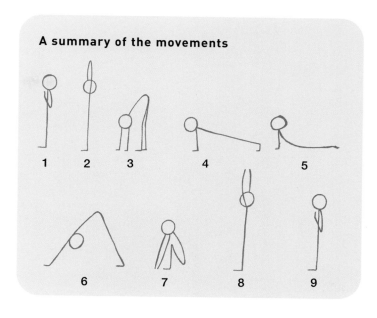

A summary of the movements

1 2 3 4 5

6 7 8 9

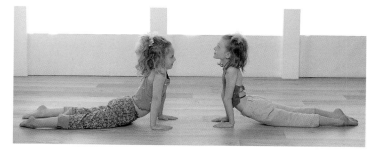

5 Lower your legs to the floor, drop your hips forwards and arch your back as you breathe out. Keep your head up. This is Cobra pose.

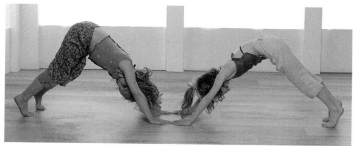

6 Breathe in and, as you breathe out, tuck your toes under and lift your bottom up into Dog pose. Hold here for a few breaths. Try to sink your heels into the floor and straighten your legs.

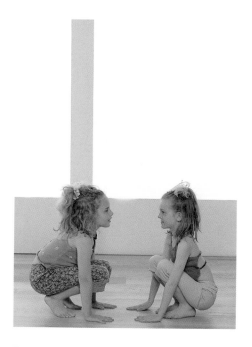

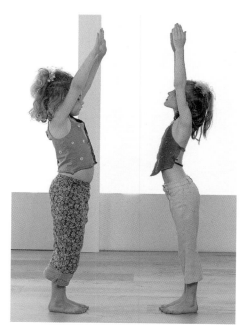

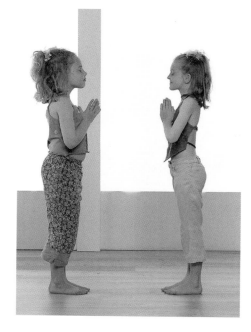

7 As you breathe out, bend your knees and look forwards so that you are facing each other. Then jump both feet forwards towards your hands and squat down.

8 Now straighten your legs and lift your arms up high above your head with palms together. Breathe in deeply. Stretch upwards to make yourself grow as tall as you can. Hold for a few breaths.

9 Breathe out and bring your hands into Namaste, or prayer position, in front of you. This completes the Sunshine Stretch. Repeat as many times as you like until your whole body feels warm and alive.

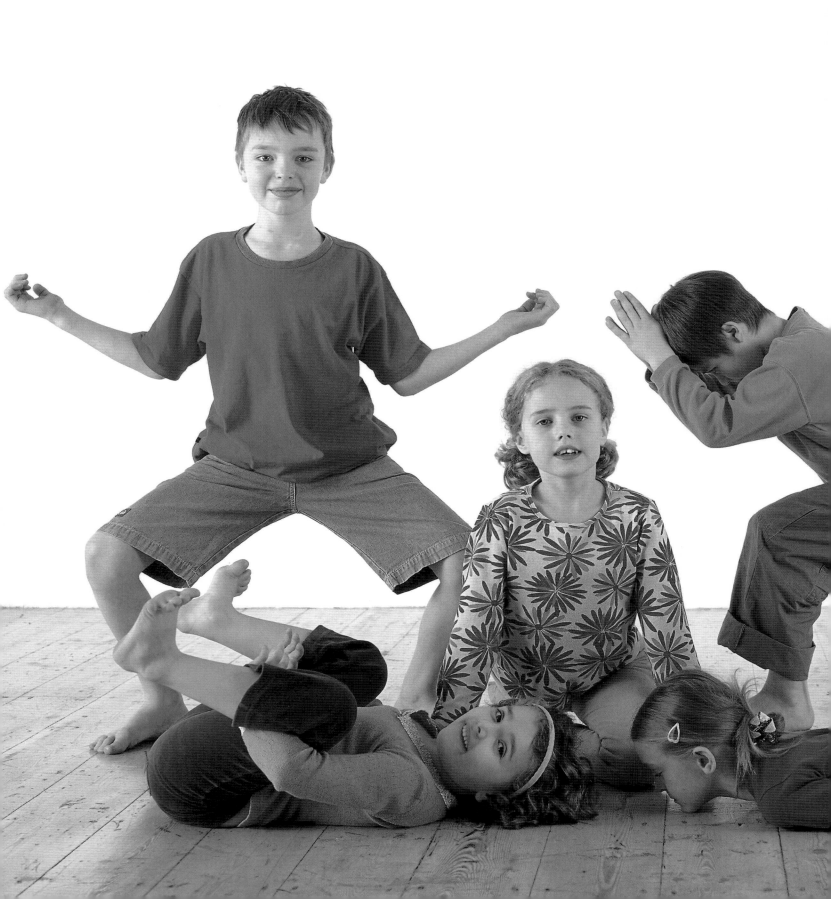

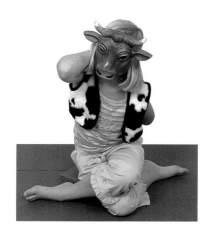

animal
Parade

This section allows you to have some fun as you come face to face with a parade of animals of all shapes and sizes. These expressive poses show you how to imitate the instinctive behaviour and movements of your favourite creatures, birds and insects, so that you can assume the characteristics of each. Feel the power and pride of the roaring lion or soaring eagle, the quiet serenity of a fluttering butterfly, the suppleness of a slithering snake and the joyful agility of a leaping frog.

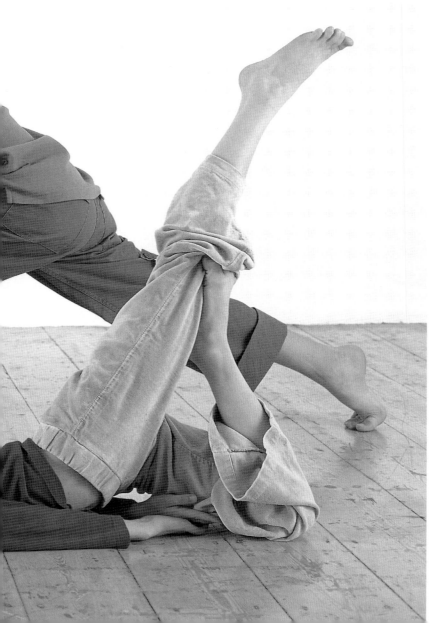

Lion Pose
SIMHASANA
Roaring Lion
SIMHAGARJANASANA

The lion is known as the king of beasts. He sleeps in the heat of the day and hunts by night, when it is cooler and his energy levels are at their highest. This is a very simple pose that all children love, and it is easy enough for even the very young or those who are new to yoga. It is lots of fun, and things can get quite noisy when everybody starts to roar!

Benefits

Lion pose energizes the body and mind. It builds self-confidence and improves communication skills. In addition, it dispels nerves and physical tension in the face, and helps to allay sore throats and problems with the eyes, ears, nose and mouth. It also clears your mind, makes you smile and gets you ready to start the day.

When to do the pose

This is a good pose for when energy levels need a boost. It can also be very helpful before an important event that may be making you feel anxious and a little apprehensive. Because it is so easy to do, it is suitable for children of all ages. It is a fun way to start a yoga session, especially if you can make a nice loud roar.

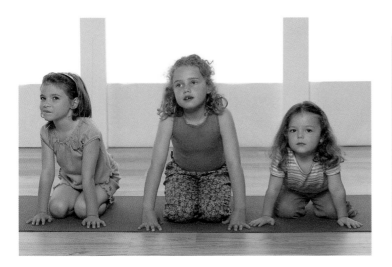

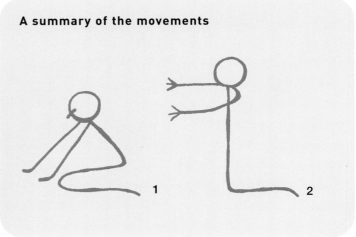

A summary of the movements

1

2

1 First, bend your knees and sit on your heels with your hands on the floor in front of you. Then rest your hands – which are now your paws – gently on your lap. Sit quietly, breathing gently.

2 Breathe in steadily and sit forwards on your knees, with your hands and arms out in front of you. Roarrrrr! Look upwards and stick out your tongue. Now sit back on your heels and roar in this way twice more to make yourself feel powerful but calm.

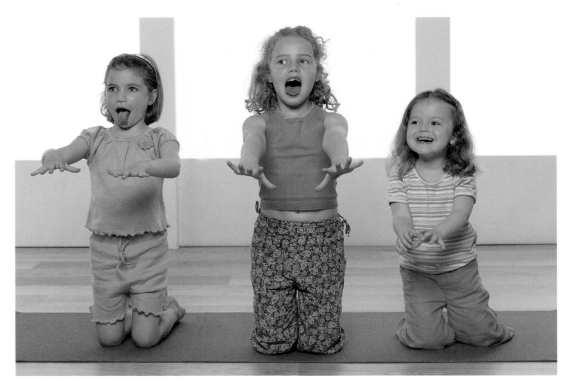

Dog
ADHO MUKHA SVANASANA

Domestic dogs have been man's best friend for thousands of years. The Downward Facing Dog is a classic pose that imitates the stretch that dogs do when they wake up. It combines an instinctive grace with a lovely elongation of the whole back.

Benefits

This pose will give you energy. It also stretches the back from the tailbone to the top of the neck, and strengthens wrists, hands, arms and shoulders. It brings fresh blood to the head and helps to release stiffness in the neck.

When to do the pose

Do this gentle stretching pose when you get out of bed in the morning, or as part of your warm-up sequence before a yoga session. It is particularly good as preparation for the Sunshine Stretch.

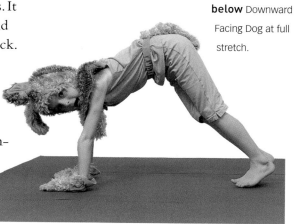

below Downward Facing Dog at full stretch.

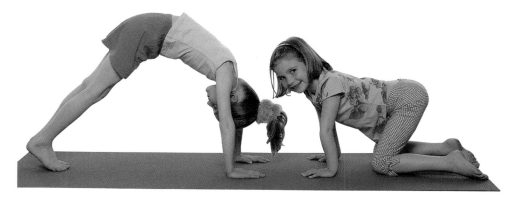

1 Rest in cat pose on all fours. Your knees should be under your hips and your hands under your shoulders. Spread your fingers wide and spread your body weight evenly into each hand. Curl your toes under.

2 Breathe in, and as you breathe out, lift your knees off the floor and push your bottom upwards. Keep the legs a little bent to begin with and push your chest gently back towards your thighs. Walk your heels up and down a few times. Then try to release both heels to the floor, straightening your legs as much as you can. Imagine someone lifting you up by your tailbone so that your body resembles the two sides of a capital "A". Look back towards your tailbone, allowing your head to feel really heavy. Breathe deeply. To come out of the pose, drop to your knees and sit back on your heels, with your forehead on the floor. Relax.

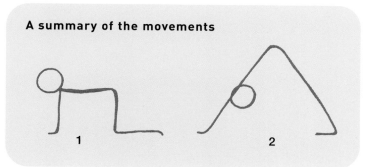

A summary of the movements

1

2

Variation

Now try the Upward Facing Dog, which turns the pose into a back bend. From Downward Facing Dog, bend your knees and rest them on the floor. Push your hips forwards, but keep them off the floor. Push into your hands, lift your chest and look up as you gently arch your back.

Cobra
BHUJANGASANA

In this strong, energizing back bend, let your legs feel really heavy and keep them still so that the top half of your body can rear up strongly, like a cobra poised to strike. Feel free to hiss as loudly as you like.

Benefits
Cobra pose keeps the spine supple and healthy, and tones the nerves, improving communication between the brain and the body. It also helps to stimulate the appetite.

When to do the pose
Practise Cobra when you are feeling floppy and in need of an energy boost. It is also good for when you want to feel strong and powerful.

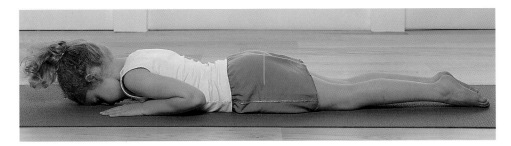

1 Lie on the floor with your forehead touching the ground. Tuck your elbows in at your sides and place the palms of your hands under your shoulders. Concentrate on keeping your legs and hips heavy. Push your feet into the floor.

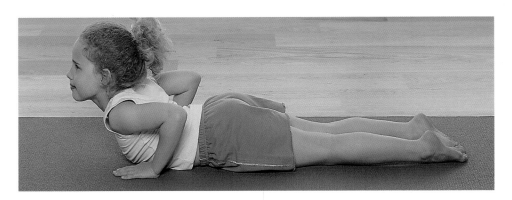

2 Breathe in deeply and, as you do so, slowly lift your head off the ground. Begin to look upwards as you push your hands into the floor. Keep your legs out straight behind you, with your toes pointed and your feet pushed into the floor.

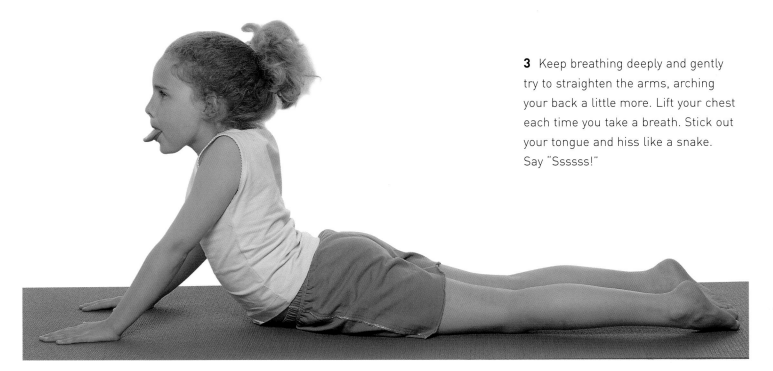

3 Keep breathing deeply and gently try to straighten the arms, arching your back a little more. Lift your chest each time you take a breath. Stick out your tongue and hiss like a snake. Say "Ssssss!"

4 If you fancy scratching your head with your tail, simply widen your knees and arch your back a little more as you raise your feet towards your head. Gently lie down again and curl yourself up in Child's pose, sitting on your heels and resting your forehead on the floor in front of you, with your arms lying relaxed by your sides. This is a counter pose to "unsnake" your back.

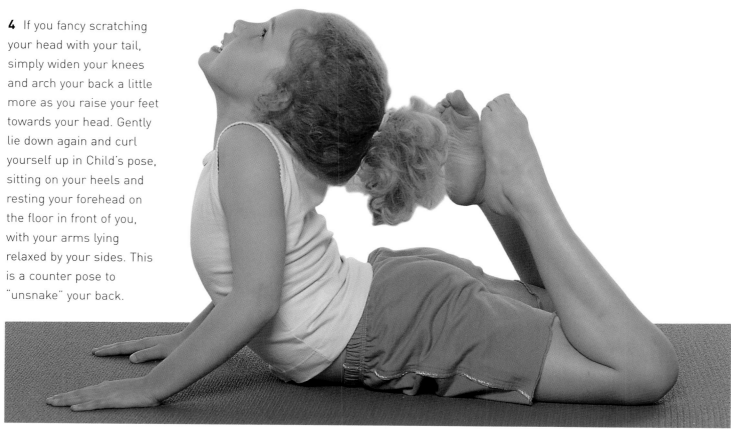

A summary of the movements

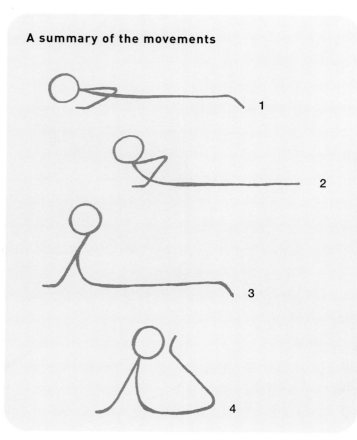

1

2

3

4

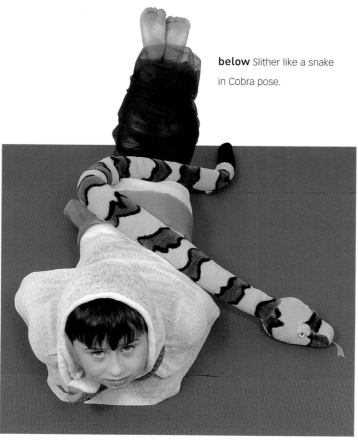

below Slither like a snake in Cobra pose.

Eagle
GARUDASANA

One minute the golden eagle can be standing motionless, high on a mountain top, scanning the landscape. The next minute he can summon all his energy, stretch out his enormous wings and plunge through the air at speed in the search for prey. Eagle pose is a standing balance that mimics the poise and strength of the golden eagle.

Benefits
Eagle pose is very good for nurturing determination and inner conviction. It also helps you to concentrate and makes your legs feel really strong.

When to do the pose
This is a good movement for when you are feeling uptight or unsure, and need to find some inner strength.

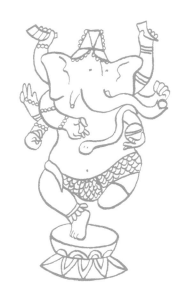

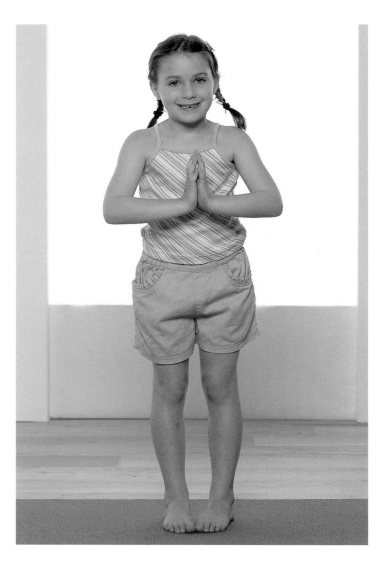

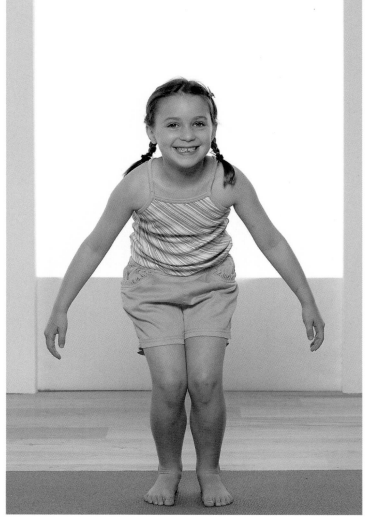

1 Stand in Mountain pose (Tadasana), looking straight in front of you with your legs straight and your feet together. Put your hands in Prayer position (Namaste). Visualize a beautiful golden eagle perched high on the peak of a mountain, looking down majestically on to the valley below. Steady your breath.

2 As you breathe out, bend your knees and spread your arms out to your sides like a pair of wings. Feel yourself firmly rooted in the floor. You are the eagle high on the mountain peak.

A summary of the movements

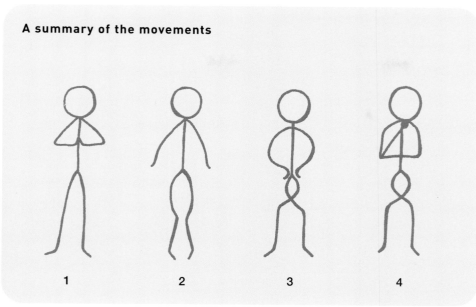

1   2   3   4

4 Make a soft fist with your right hand and place it under your chin. Support your elbow with your left palm. Breathe steadily for a few moments. Release the pose, shake out your arms and legs, and repeat on the other side.

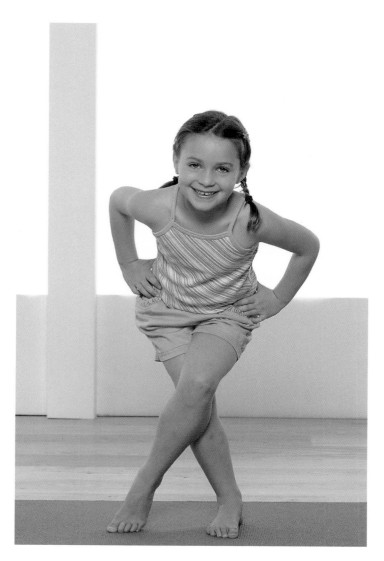

3   Keeping both of your knees bent, cross your left leg over your right so that the ball of your left foot makes contact with the floor just to the side of your right foot.

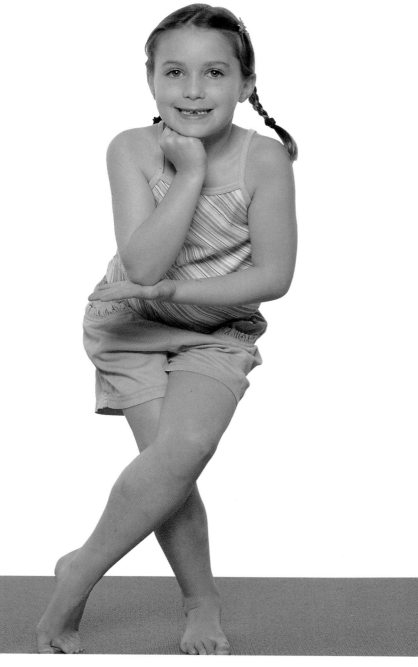

Fish

MATSYASANA

In Hindu mythology the God Vishnu turned himself into a fish, or *matsya*, to save the world from the flood. Fish pose is a gentle yet powerful back bend in which the raised chest mimics the rounded back of a fish. In the pose you lie on the floor with your knees bent and your back arched.

Benefits

Fish encourages deep breathing and can give relief to mild symptoms of asthma and bronchitis. The graceful arching of the back opens up the chest, keeping the heart chakra open and releasing positive feelings of love and well-being.

When to do the pose

Use Fish to improve posture and chase away negative feelings. You can do it after Shoulder Stand, Candle or Dragonfly pose too. The very young may find this pose a bit too much for them. They can try Crocodile instead, which has many of the same benefits.

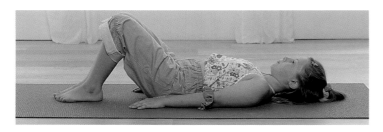

1 Lie on the floor with your knees bent, legs together and feet flat on the floor. Your arms should lie straight by your sides.

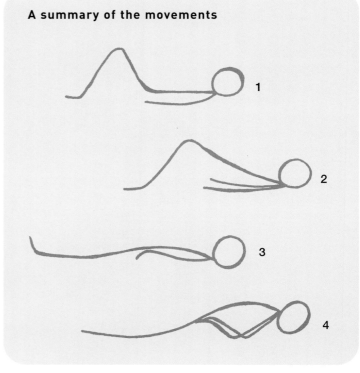

A summary of the movements

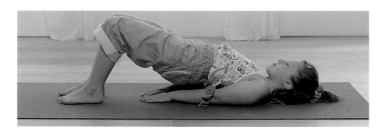

2 Breathe in and, keeping your knees bent, lift your bottom off the floor and slide your hands underneath. Bring your hands close together so that the fingers touch.

4 On a breath in, push up your chest, letting your back arch and the top of your head roll on to the floor. Push your elbows down. Take five deep breaths, then release to the floor, slide out your hands and hug your knees.

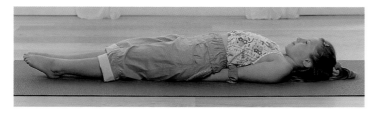

3 Lie down on your hands. Extend your legs and allow them to feel heavy. Let your breath become steady.

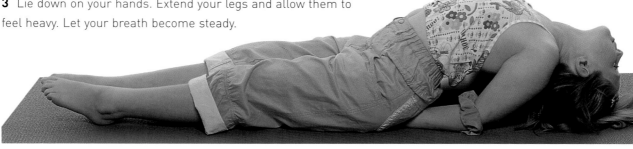

Frog
MALASANA

Frogs are cold-blooded amphibians that start life without any limbs at all. They develop arms and legs as they grow older, and by the time they are adult frogs their legs are strong and very springy. This is a fun action pose that grows from a quiet squat into an explosive leap upwards into the air.

Benefits
Frog is good for strengthening the upper and lower legs and making them more flexible. It also helps to tone the ankles and feet. It is a fantastic way to raise energy levels quickly if you are feeling tired but still have lots of things to get done.

When to do the pose
Leap like a frog when you feel tired and lethargic and want a quick boost of energy, or if you feel over-excited and need to let off some steam. Because this is quite a sudden, jerky movement, it should only be done after the warm-up exercises.

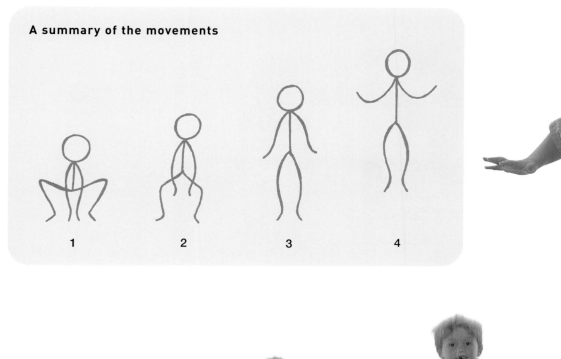

A summary of the movements

1   2   3   4

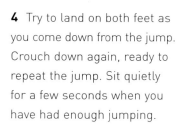

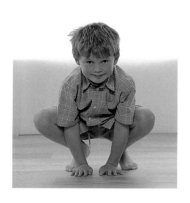

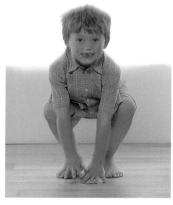

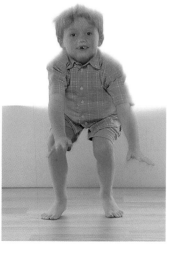

1 Crouch down on the floor with your knees wide and the palms of your hands flat on the floor in front of you. Breathe steadily and visualize your legs becoming strong like a frog's.

2 When you feel ready, push down into your hands and feet and spring upwards.

3 Stretch out your body and jump as high as you can. Make frog noises as loud as you can – "Grribbiid!"

4 Try to land on both feet as you come down from the jump. Crouch down again, ready to repeat the jump. Sit quietly for a few seconds when you have had enough jumping.

Crocodile
MAKARASANA

This playful posture will encourage self–expression and is fun to practise in a group. Look out for it later on in the book in the children's game called Snap and Snack.

Benefits
Crocodile pose strengthens the back and gives you energy. If you find yourself in a bad mood, Crocodile can help release anger and aggression.

When to do the pose
When you feel low or cross, Crocodile helps you to get rid of negative feelings and will brighten your mood.

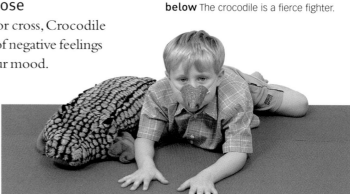
below The crocodile is a fierce fighter.

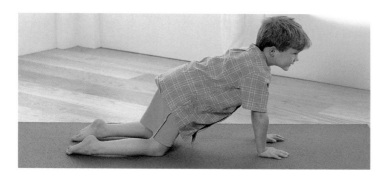

1 Kneel on the floor in Cat pose, with your shoulders over your hands and your fingers spread wide. Stretch out your legs behind you.

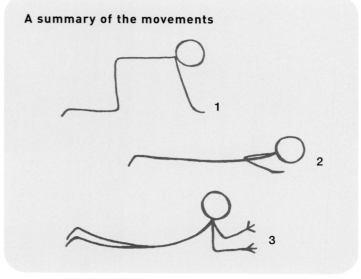

A summary of the movements

2 Lie down on the floor and bring your hands underneath your shoulders with your elbows tucked into your sides. Spread your fingers like claws. Make a heavy tail by bringing your legs together. Rest your forehead on the floor and visualize yourself as a crocodile.

3 As you breathe in, lift your legs and rear up your head. Keep swishing your tail from side to side to help you slither forwards and sideways. When you have had enough, curl up in Child's pose to release your back.

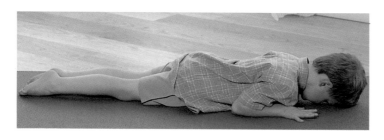

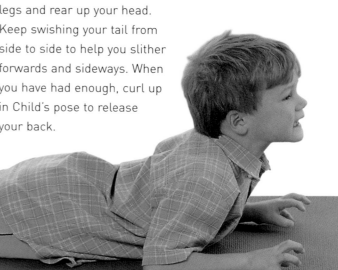

Crow
KAKASANA

The black crow is the largest of the songbirds. He has strong feet and legs to enable him to move swiftly and purposefully on land, and broad wings that help him to soar powerfully in the air. In this pose your hands turn into the crow's feet and your back becomes his body. This pose requires strength, confidence and concentration. Imagine the beady eye of a crow to help you concentrate on the position.

Benefits
Crow pose focuses the mind. It also strengthens the wrists, arms and upper body, and helps to develop physical balance and co-ordination.

When to do the pose
Do Crow when you feel apprehensive about something and your mind is jumpy. It will help you feel in control and will strengthen inner conviction.

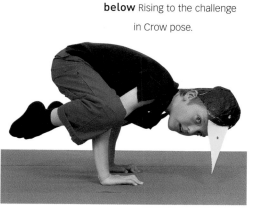

below Rising to the challenge in Crow pose.

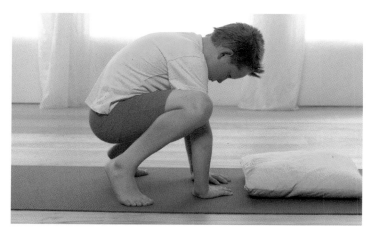

1 Place a cushion on the floor, and then squat down with your feet hip-width apart and the cushion in front of you. Place your palms on the floor with your fingers spread out and turned slightly inwards.

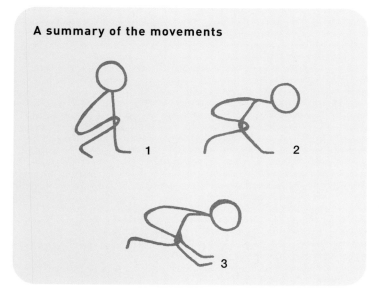

A summary of the movements

1

2

3

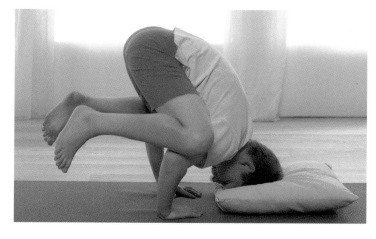

2 Press your upper arms against the inside of your knees. Start to rock forwards until you feel your body weight spreading on to your hands. Rock back to transfer the weight to your feet. Use the cushion for support and don't worry if you lose your balance, just keep trying.

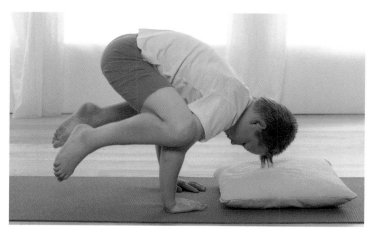

3 With practice you will be able to balance on your hands for longer and longer. Then bring your feet together to make your crow's tail. Hold for as long as you can and then lower your feet and release.

Blue whale
SETU BANDHASANA

The yogis called this Bridge pose because it makes your tummy look like a bridge. But being a big blue whale is more fun!

The blue whale is the largest living animal and even though it weighs as much as 15 elephants, it still manages to be graceful. Blue Whale pose is an energizing back bend. The lower part of the body makes the back of a big blue whale – imagine your navel is its blowhole. Start off from Dead Man pose, lying on the floor with the feet hip-width apart, the arms away from the body and the eyes closed.

Benefits

Blue Whale pose is very good for strengthening the back and leg muscles, and it gives a nice stretch to the back of the neck. It helps to keep the spine supple and opens up the heart, chest and lungs.

When to do the pose

Practise Blue Whale pose when you need a little lift after something has upset you. Not only can this help to calm you down, it will also help to relieve backache.

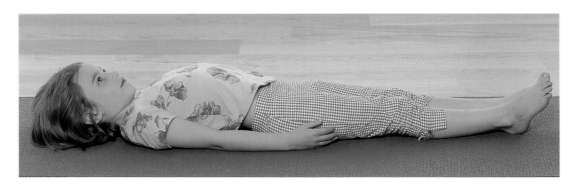

1 Lie down on your back in Dead Man pose (Savasana). Rest your arms by your sides and steady your breathing.

2 Bend your knees so that your feet are flat on the floor, hip-width apart and a little away from your bottom. Keep your arms at your sides.

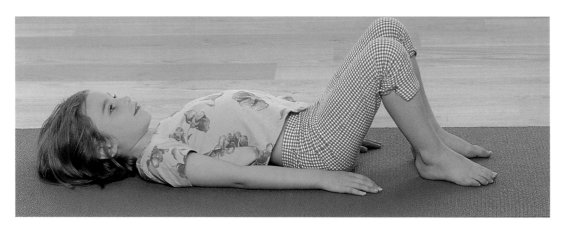

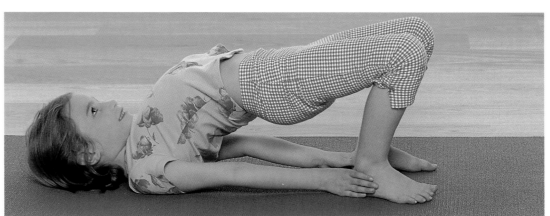

3 Breathe in and slowly peel your back off the ground. Breathe out and imagine you are spurting water out of your tummy button – just like the whale's blowhole.

A summary of the movements

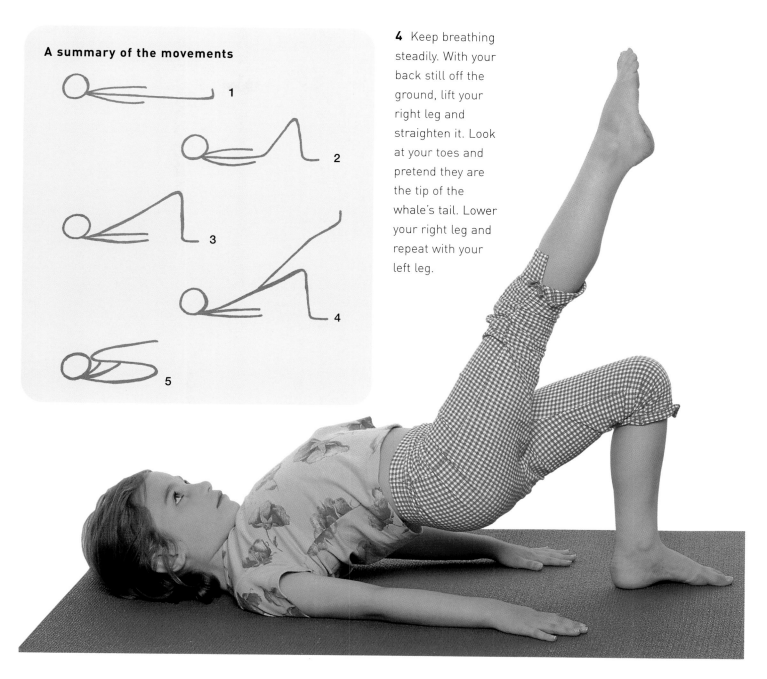

4 Keep breathing steadily. With your back still off the ground, lift your right leg and straighten it. Look at your toes and pretend they are the tip of the whale's tail. Lower your right leg and repeat with your left leg.

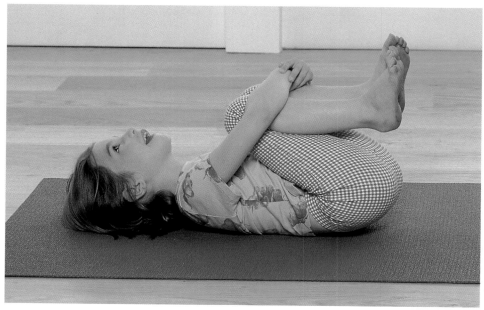

5 As you breathe out, roll slowly back down to the floor again and hug your knees to your chest like an upturned beetle. This is a counter pose to release your back.

Butterfly
BADDHA KONASANA

The butterfly is a wonderful example of transformation. It starts its life as a humble caterpillar and evolves into a beautiful, winged creature. This simple seated pose will help your hips to become more flexible, allowing your spine to elongate. Try sitting on a cushion if you find it hard to sit up directly on the floor.

Benefits

This will give your inner thighs a lovely gentle stretch, and will help to improve your posture when seated. It will also help you to feel grounded.

When to do the pose

Practise Butterfly in preparation for Little Buddha pose and to relax your legs after Rocking the Baby, as part of your warm-up sequence.

below Learning Butterfly pose will help you to sit up straight.

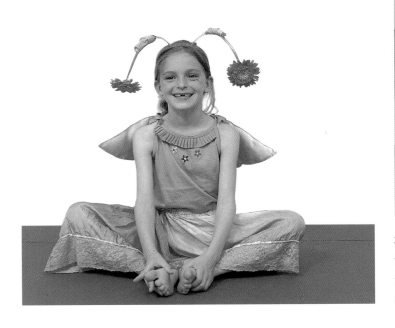

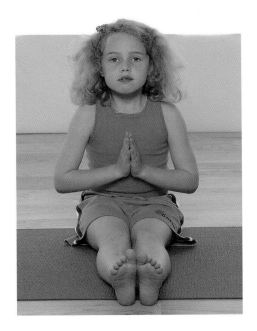

1 Sit on the floor with both legs outstretched in front of you and your feet together. Hold your hands in Prayer position (Namaste). Look straight ahead.

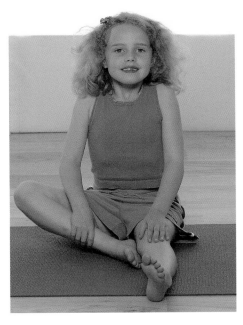

2 Bend your right leg and bring the sole of the foot into the inside of your left thigh. Hold the position.

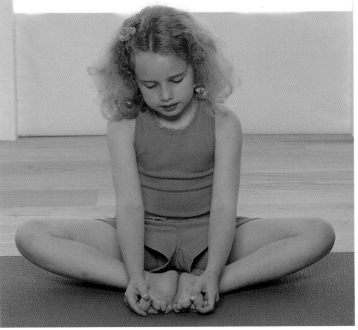

3 Then bring the left leg in so that the soles of your feet are together. You will be able to feel a gentle stretch of your inner thighs. Try opening your feet with your hands like the covers of a book. This will help your knees to drop open a little more.

4 Then interlace your fingers and place them under the outer edges of your feet. Sit up tall, with your back nice and straight.

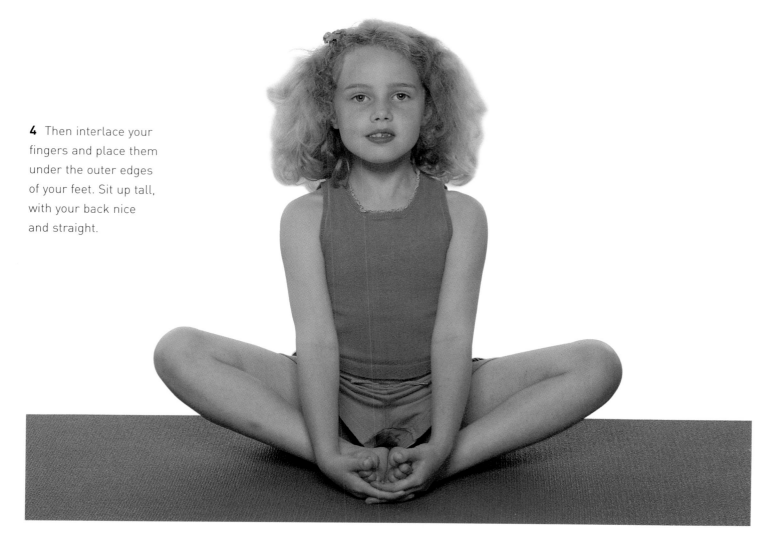

A summary of the movements

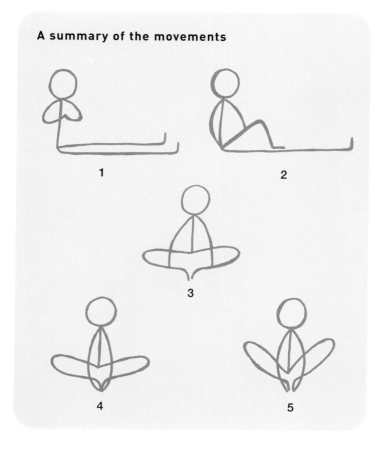

1

2

3

4

5

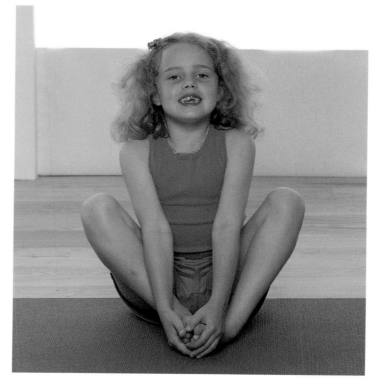

5 Gently lift and lower your knees as if you are a butterfly flapping its delicate, colourful wings. Relax.

Pigeon
KAPOTASANA

Homing pigeons have an in-built compass that allows them to navigate their way home, no matter how far they have flown.

Benefits

Pigeon pose will give a deep, long stretch to your buttock muscles. The forward bending stage of this pose is particularly good at helping to calm an agitated mind.

When to do the pose

Pigeon energizes the body after a busy day or after a series of strong standing poses, such as Warrior and Triangle.

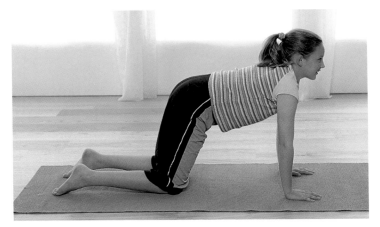

1 Get down on your hands and knees in Cat pose.

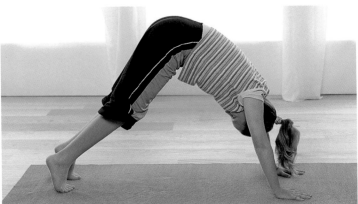

2 Now tuck under your toes, lift your knees and come into Dog pose. Take a moment to stretch out your legs.

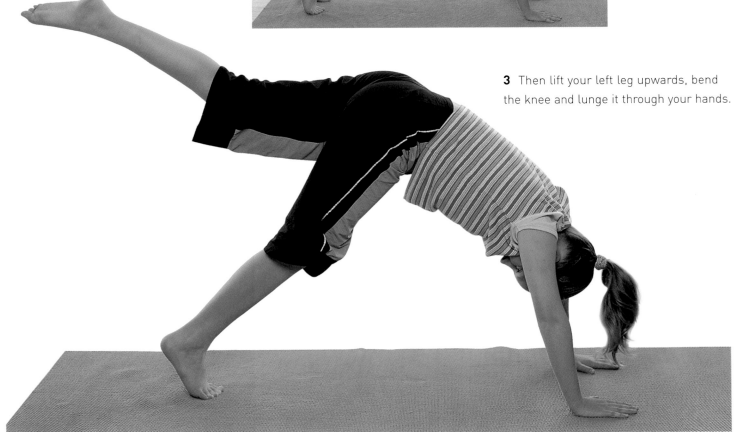

3 Then lift your left leg upwards, bend the knee and lunge it through your hands.

A summary of the movements

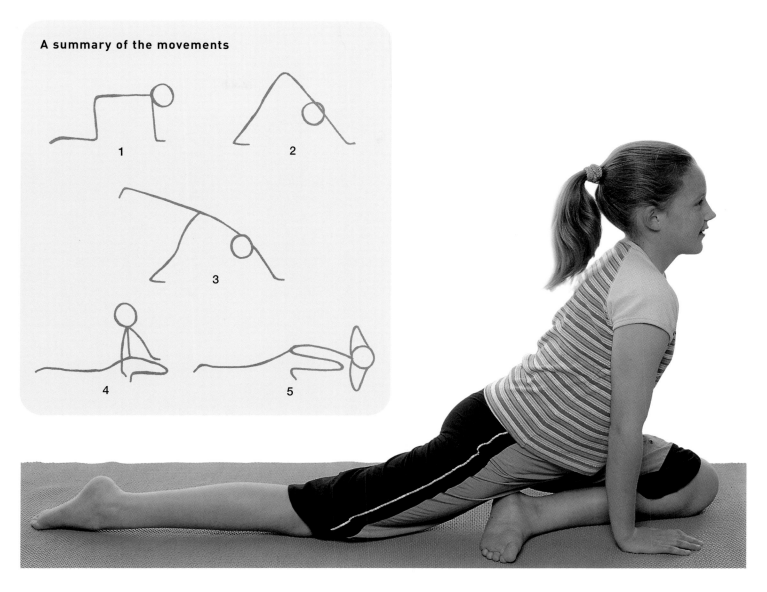

4 above Place the knee on the floor and bring the heel to the right. Sit to the outside of your left knee. Let the back of your left thigh release on to the floor. Stretch out your right leg and prop yourself up with your hands.

5 below Breathe steadily and, as you exhale, lean your chest forwards over your knee. Make a pillow with your hands and relax. Close your eyes for a few minutes. Release and rest in Child's pose, then change sides.

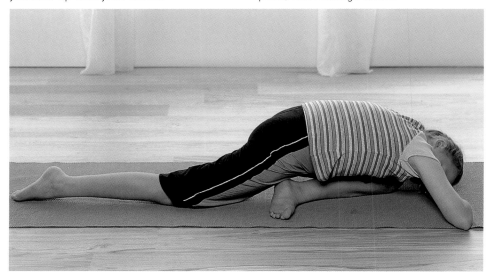

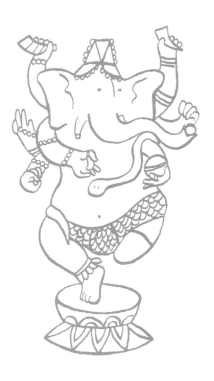

Tortoise
KOORMASANA

This gentle seated pose will help you to feel the quiet and calmness of a tortoise who knows he is protected by his strong shell. A famous Indian fable called the Bhagavad Gita states that if you can stay safe and calm inside your body, without reacting to danger or difficulty, then, like the tortoise safely inside his protective shell, you will become mighty and wise. This is a useful piece of advice!

1 Sit on the floor, legs wide apart and bent at the knees. The soles of your feet should be flat on the floor. Your hands can be held in Prayer position (Namaste). Breathe steadily.

2 As you breathe in, reach up with your right arm, keeping your fingers stretched. Breathe out and feed your right arm underneath your right knee. Hold it there.

Benefits
Tortoise pose will make you feel calm and secure because you will imagine yourself protected by a strong shell. This pose will also provide your back and legs with a long stretch.

When to do the pose
Practise Tortoise when you want to feel safe and quiet. It will also help to release your back after a bending pose.

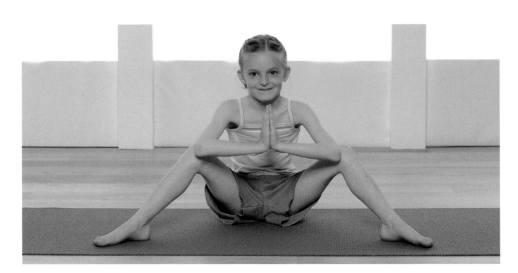

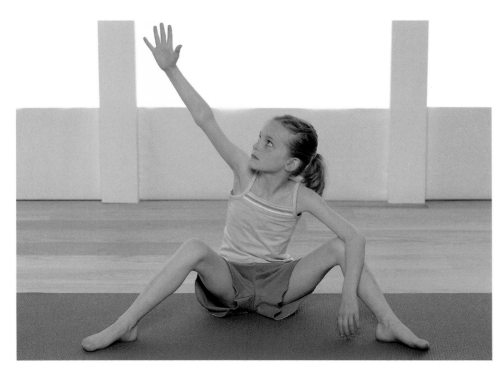

A summary of the movements

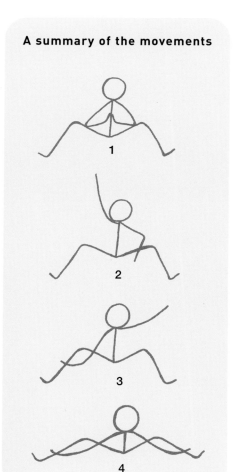

1

2

3

4

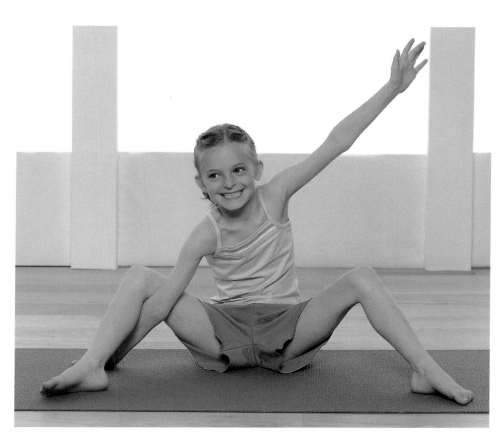

3 Now do the same with your left arm, reaching up and feeding it under your left knee. Breathe steadily.

4 Gradually lower your chest towards the floor as you walk your fingers and hands in the opposite direction to your feet. With practice you may be able to place your chin and chest on the floor in front of you, and straighten your legs on the floor. Slowly release yourself from the position and relax. Have a friend or parent close by to help you unravel yourself from the position.

Locust
SHALABHASANA

A locust is a tropical grasshopper, with long, strong legs with special springy knees that launch its body into flight. It can jump the equivalent of you jumping over your house! This is a very strong back bend and it may prove too difficult for younger children to hold both legs off the floor. With regular practice it will get easier, but begin by lifting one leg at a time. If you find it too uncomfortable lying on your arms, rest your arms by your sides and rest your forehead on the floor. You can lift your legs in this position too.

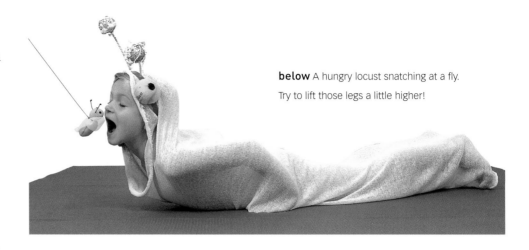

below A hungry locust snatching at a fly. Try to lift those legs a little higher!

Benefits

Locust is a challenging pose that strengthens the back muscles. Like other back bends it will also boost your natural energy.

When to do the pose

Practise Locust after you have got the hang of Cobra pose – this will make it easier for you. Follow Locust with a relaxing forward bend such as Child's pose or Sandwich.

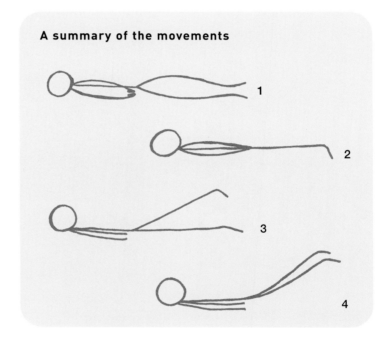

A summary of the movements

1

2

3

4

1 Lie on your side in a straight line with your arms extended in front of you. Wrap your fingers round the thumb of each hand to make a fist. Bring both of your fists side by side.

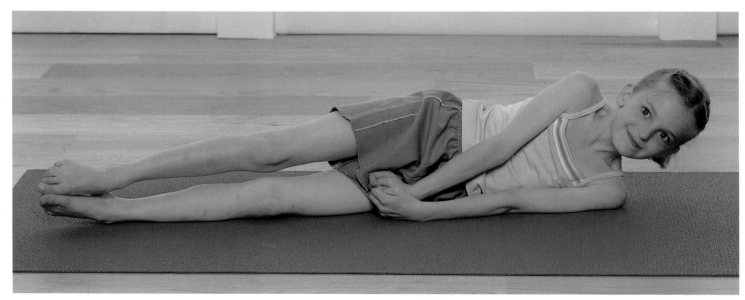

2 Roll gently on to your front so that you are lying on your arms. Wriggle them down as far as you can towards your feet. Let your chin rest on the floor, close your eyes and breathe steadily and deeply to prepare yourself.

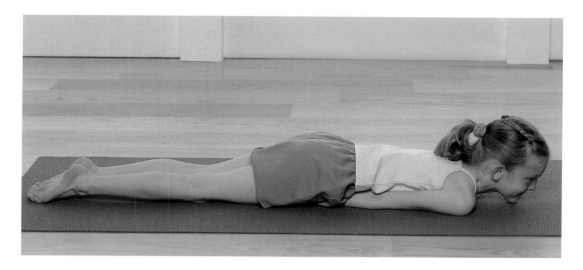

3 Breathe in and lift your right leg off the floor. Push your fists into the ground to help lever the leg upwards. Lower the right leg and, on another breath in, repeat with the left leg. Breathe and hold. Lower the left leg and give yourself a rest.

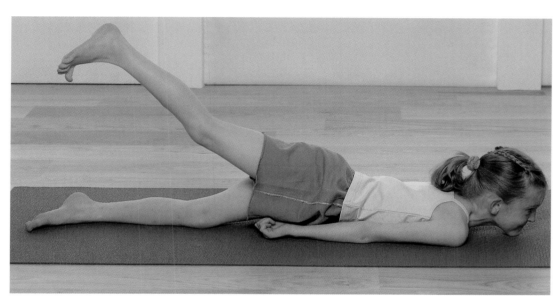

4 When you are ready, take a big breath in and try to lift both legs off the ground. Hold for as long as you can. Gently lower your legs, and come into Child's pose on your knees to relax your back. Well done!

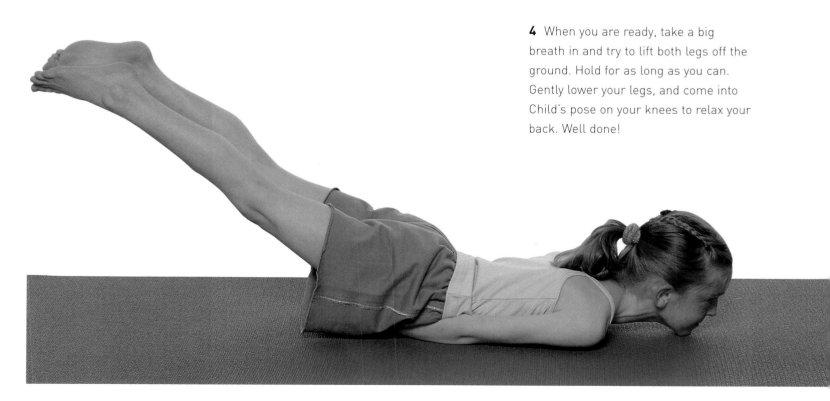

Dragonfly
SARVANGASANA

This is a wonderful variation of the classic Shoulder Stand pose. It is known as the queen of yoga postures because of its many physical and holistic qualities. It may look quite hard but when you get into it and have practised a few times you will find that it isn't all that difficult. Resting your knee on your forehead will help you to keep your balance.

Benefits of the pose

The Dragonfly pose helps to develop patience and emotional stability. It gives the heart a temporary rest from the effects of gravity, and it feels really wonderful if your legs are heavy and tired. The increased blood flow to your face helps to refresh your brain, and you will find it gives you a big burst of energy.

When to do the pose

Dragonfly is just the thing to do when you come home from a tiring day at school and you feel physically and mentally exhausted and a little bit sluggish. It is good to practise Dragonfly before a dream time sequence, and it can help you to feel emotionally calm and quiet before you go to bed at night.

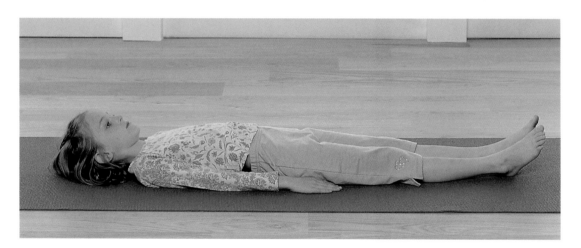

1 Lie flat on your back in Dead Man pose (Savasana), with the feet hip-width apart, the arms away from the body and the eyes closed. Breathe steadily.

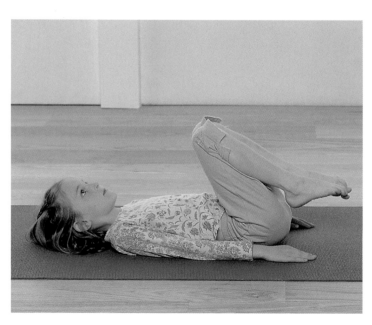

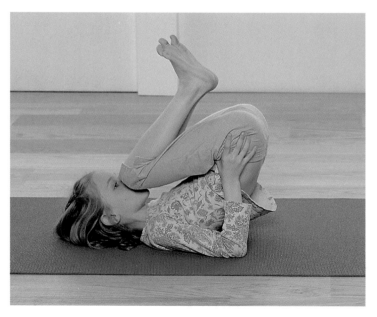

2 Slowly bring your knees in towards your chest, keeping your arms in position at your sides. Continue to breathe steadily.

3 Then slowly draw your knees in towards your forehead by pushing your hips and lower back towards you. Use your hands to guide you, then support your back with your flat palms.

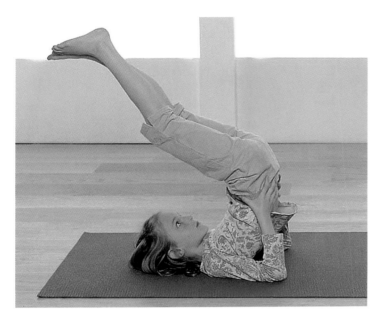

4 Still supporting your lower back, extend your legs upwards so that your toes are directly above you. Hold here and breathe while you get your balance and get used to being upside down.

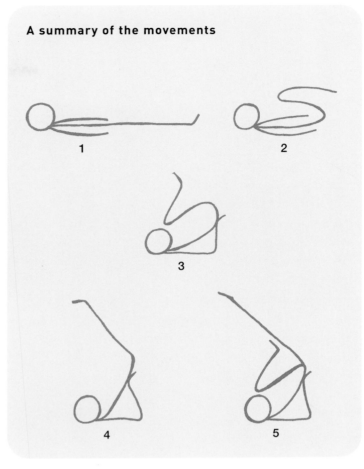

A summary of the movements

1

2

3

4

5

5 Bend your right knee and rest it in the middle of your forehead. Let the front of your left leg rest on the sole of the right foot. Close your eyes and rest in the pose, keeping your breathing quiet and steady. Change legs when you are ready. Then bring both knees in towards your chest and roll back down on to the floor. Extend your legs and rest on your back.

Cow
GOMUKASANA

In India the cow is considered a sacred animal, and is allowed to wander the roads on its own. In this seated pose, your body is supposed to resemble the face of this beloved creature. Your stacked knees form the lips of its face and your raised elbow is one of its ears. Practise the pose in stages, if you like. Begin by sitting with just your legs crossed until you feel comfortable, then practise kneeling with your arms in position. When you are happy to sit like this you can move on to the full Cow position.

Benefits

Cow pose will release tight muscles in the area around your hips and bottom. It opens up the chest, which will improve your posture, and can also help to release and realign tight or rounded shoulders.

When to do the pose

This is a great pose to do when your hips and shoulders feel stiff from tiredness, too much sitting or too much exercise. It is a good pose to do when you want to challenge yourself. Because you end up looking like a cow's face, it will also make you laugh.

right Don't tie yourself in knots over Cow pose. Take it easy and build up the positions in stages.

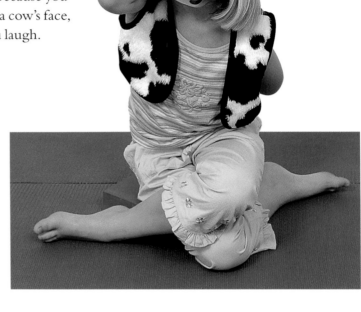

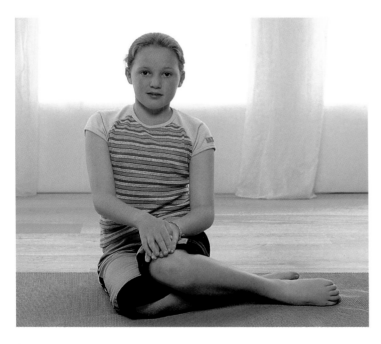

1 Sit down on the floor with your legs folded to the left of you. Hold one hand over the other and rest them on your top knee. Steady your breathing.

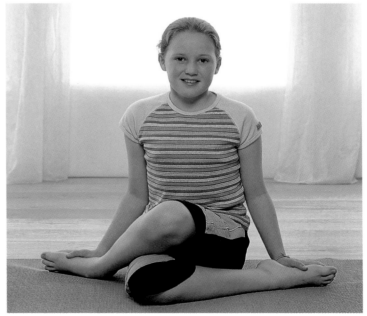

2 Lift up your left leg and cross it over your right knee, so that your knees are now on top of each other. Wriggle your bottom a little so that it is sitting flat on the floor.

below You can give yourself an additional stretch by bending your body forwards over your knees. Breathe deeply and hold for a moment.

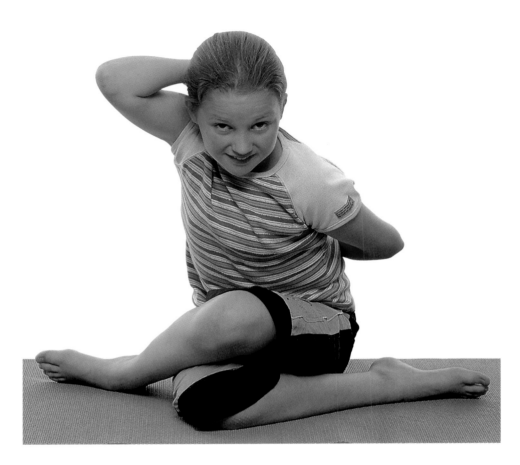

A summary of the movements

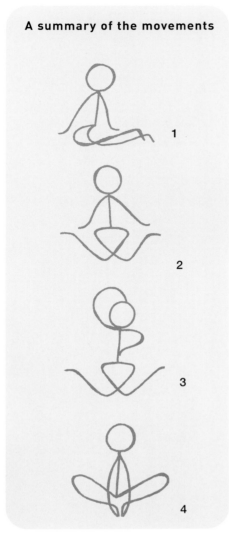

1

2

3

4

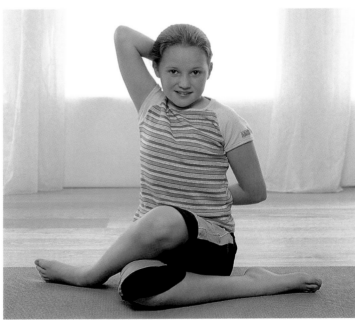

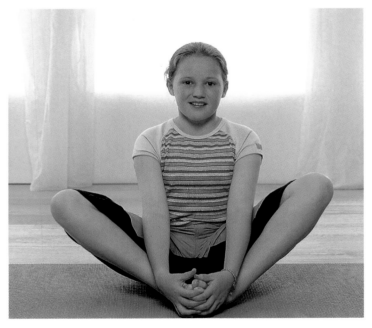

3 Reach up with your right arm and rest your fingers at the base of your neck. Place your left arm behind your back and wriggle it up to meet your other hand. Try to interlink your fingers without rounding your back. Catch hold of your T-shirt if you can't reach. Breathe deeply.

4 Slowly unravel your legs and arms and come into Butterfly pose to relax the muscles. Have a short rest, and change sides whenever you are ready.

Camel
USHTRASANA

This pose is performed on the knees and involves arching carefully backwards so that you make the rounded hump of the camel with your upper body. The arch of the back is particularly important for Camel, so practise getting this part right.

Benefits
Camel pose opens up the chest and the heart, and this helps to correct poor or lazy posture. It can help all children to stand tall and feel proud of who they are. Camel encourages good use of the lungs and aids digestion.

When to do the pose
Camel pose is good when you have been working hard, bent over your desk all day at school. It is also good when you want to wake up your back muscles, and when your energy levels are low and need a boost.

1 Kneel on the floor with your knees hip-width apart. Breathe steadily and deeply for a few minutes.

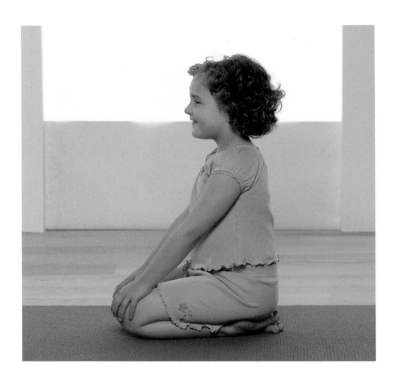

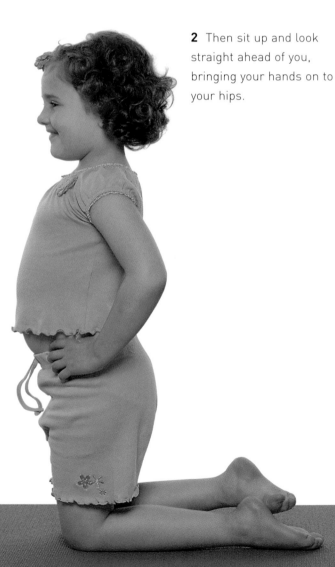

2 Then sit up and look straight ahead of you, bringing your hands on to your hips.

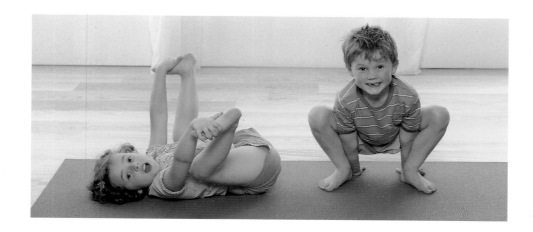

left Beetle and sparrow The upturned beetle, here on the left, must roll out of the way of the hungry chirping sparrow.

below Rag dolls Stand up straight with your feet hip-width apart. Hang your head and let your body and arms fall gently forwards like a drooping flower or a floppy rag doll as it is lifted from the toy box.

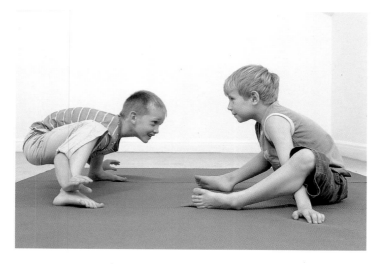

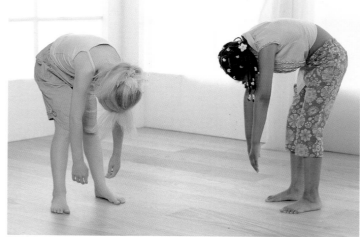

above Animal antics See if you can squat down low like a spider. Which one of you will be the first to collapse?

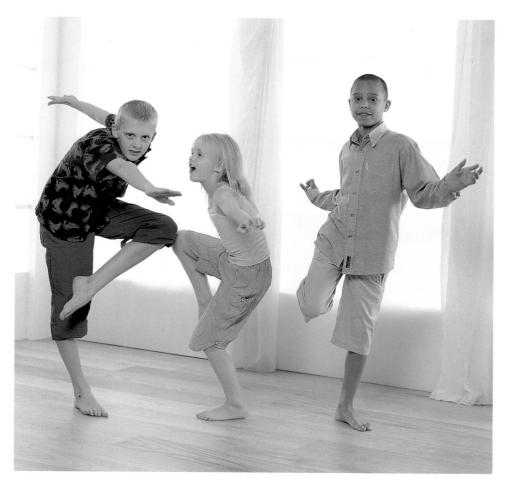

right Cactus plants Stand up straight and lift one knee so that you are balancing on one leg. Angle your arms and legs to make the eerie shapes of prickly cactus plants…but don't touch or it could hurt!

putting it all together

▷

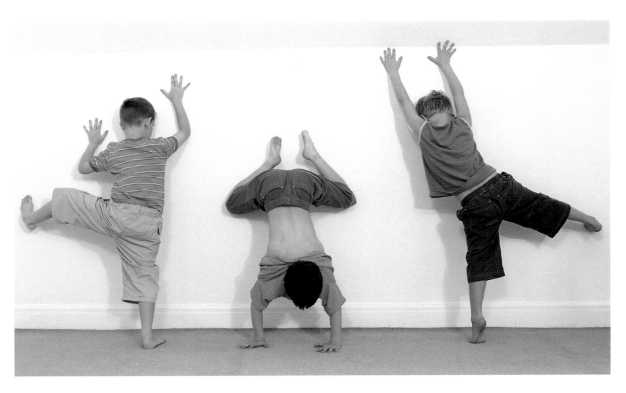

left **Geckos** Use your body to imitate the nimble movements of a gecko – which is a type of lizard – as he clings to a wall. Stretch out your arms and legs, spread your fingers and toes and hang on.

Dragon

This is a pose for two people. As it involves one person carrying the other on their back, it helps if the supporter is an adult. Roaring and fire-breathing are optional!

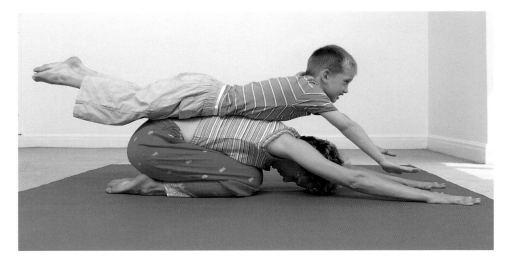

1 The supporter sits on her knees with her forehead on the floor and both her arms stretched out in front. The child lies across her back, and stretches out his arms and legs. It may take a few attempts for you both to find your balance and hold the position.

2 The child on top takes hold of his partner's arms and holds on tight. The supporter tucks her toes under and lifts her back. The dragon then stretches out his legs and gets a wonderful ride, while the supporter strengthens her arms, wrists and legs. Hold still, or lower and lift as many times as you can while the dragon roars. Relax.

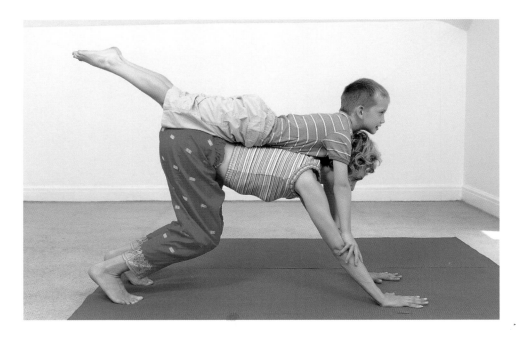

Elephant walk

The more of you the merrier for this one as you imitate the lumbering, trunk-swinging swagger of a herd of elephants.

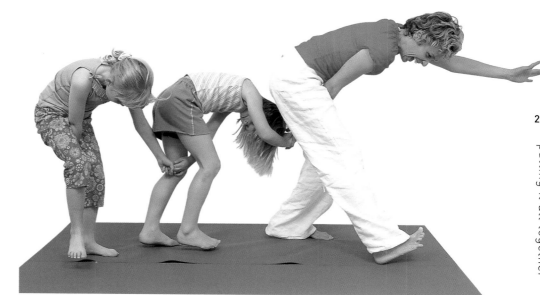

1 Stand in line, one behind the other. All of you now reach forwards. Put one arm between your legs to make a tail and grasp the hand of the elephant behind you. Hold out your other arm in front of you to make a trunk and grasp the hand of the elephant in front.

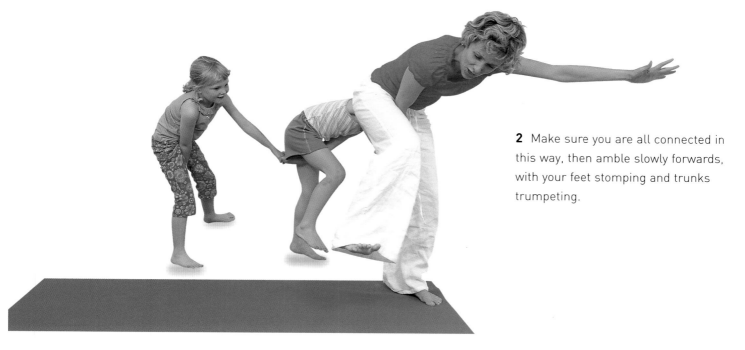

2 Make sure you are all connected in this way, then amble slowly forwards, with your feet stomping and trunks trumpeting.

3 Continue stomping and trumpeting your way around and around the room or the garden. Release your hands and and relax, straightening up your back and stretching your arms up above your head.

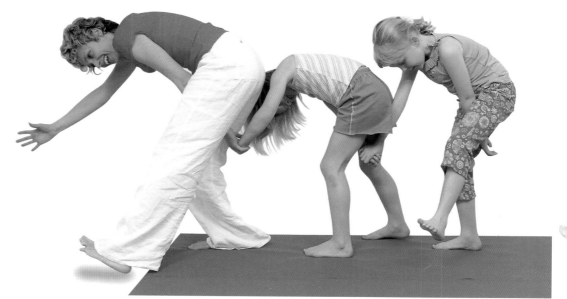

I Am Strong

Developing stamina and strength helps us to feel the amazing power of our physical body. We have all felt the sense of elation that follows physical activity. These poses are empowering, and are designed to build confidence.

Give it some muscle!

It is through our musculoskeletal system that we experience the physical potential of our bodies. It also gives us the sense of how strong we judge ourselves to be. This system of muscles and bones works as a team to give us an extraordinary range of movement and a sense of inner power.

Strong yoga poses – particularly those that support our body weight on either our feet or hands – keep muscles and bones in peak condition. Bones renew themselves and continue to grow only in response to such weight-bearing activity. Muscles like to be stretched gently and smoothly and supplied with as much oxygen as possible. Coming into these poses slowly, and breathing deeply and steadily as you hold them, allows the body to move in a natural way. This gives your muscles a lovely slow, non-violent stretch, and builds solidity and strength in your bones.

Emotional strength

It's important to have emotional strength too. It means that we can stand on our own two feet and deal with the knocks of life and still come up smiling. The drive to succeed and persevere is rooted in a natural instinct for survival deep inside us. These strong poses can help children to access this instinct and deepen their inner conviction and drive.

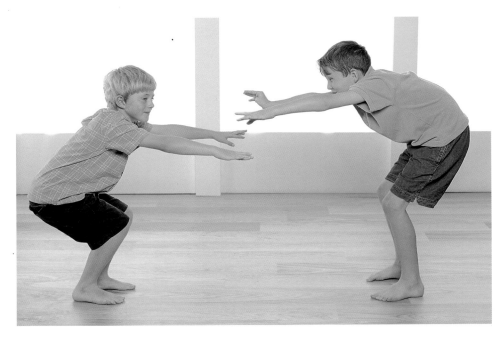

above Chair or fierce pose Stand with your legs together, feet firm. Exhale and bend your knees as if you were sitting on an invisible chair, arms down by your side. Breathe in and lift your arms out in front of you at shoulder height. Hold the position and breathe. To release, roll your body forwards into the Rag Doll pose.

Woodchopper

This pose is fun and will quickly fill you with energy. You can also do it when you are in need of some inspiration. Repeat three or four times until you feel full of energy.

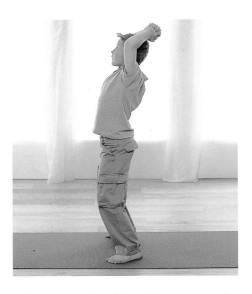

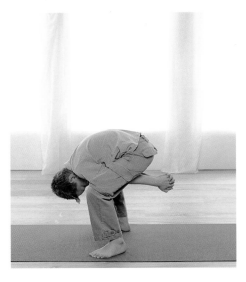

1 Stand with feet hip-width apart, and your knees gently bent. Make a strong fist with both of your hands together, and as you breathe in, lift the fist over your head.

2 Swing the axe through your legs, keeping your knees bent, and exhale through your mouth with a loud "Haaa!". Breathe in and lift your hands over your head again. Repeat.

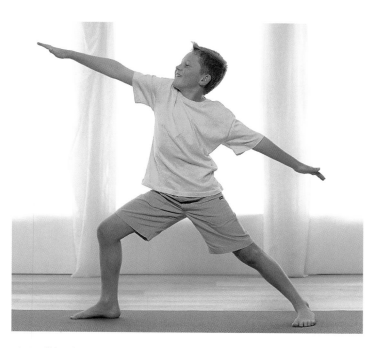

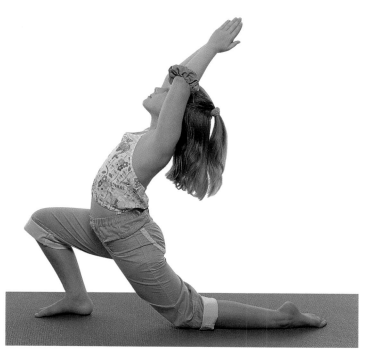

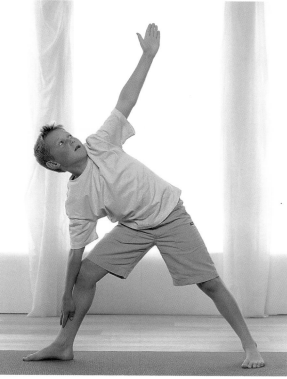

above Warrior Step your feet wide apart and bend your front knee over your ankle, with the front foot facing forwards and the back foot turned away by 30 degrees. Breathe in and lift both arms to the sides. Breathe out and bend your front knee a little more. Look at your front hand. Feel strength growing in your legs. Release and change sides.

right Triangle Position your feet in the same way as for Warrior and stand sideways, this time with both legs straight. Lift your arms to the side as you breathe in and, as you breathe out, reach as far over your front foot as you can. Inhale, then drop your hand down to touch your lower leg as you breathe out. Look up at your other hand and hold for a few deep breaths. Release and change sides. It may be easier for little children to think of this pose as a teapot.

above Crescent moon Kneel on the floor with your bottom off your heels and your back straight. Step your right foot forwards at a right angle to your left leg. Inhale and, as you exhale, push your right knee upright over your right foot. Inhale again and lift your arms over your head into Prayer position. As you breathe out, arch your back to make a lovely curved C-shape from your fingers to your toes. Push your back foot into the floor to keep you steady, and hold. Slowly release and change sides. Rest for a few minutes in Child's pose to rebalance your body, bending forwards over your knees.

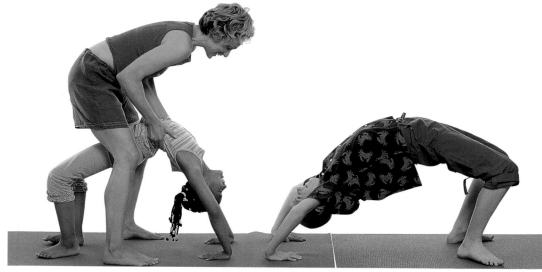

left Wheel Lie on your back with your knees bent and your feet hip-width apart. Raise your arms behind your head, bend them and place your palms flat on the floor with your fingertips tucking in below your shoulders. Take a deep breath and exhale with an "Aahh!" sound as you push into your hands and lift your bottom off the floor. Take a few deep breaths. Lower your back to the floor. Relax and hug your knees.

Jungle Walk

Setting your yoga session in an imaginary location such as the jungle gives you plenty of scope for having fun, as everyone can become the wild creatures and characters they might find there.

First you need to prepare for your jungle journey, shrugging and rolling your shoulders as if to put on imaginary rucksacks, and flexing and pointing your toes to put on your big, strong jungle boots.

Walk through the trees, scanning the horizon for wild animals. Walk on tiptoe to look over the tall grass, and stomp through muddy swamps. Introduce an array of animals and spend some time imitating each one.

1 Lunge forwards as you set off and look all around you. Who knows what creatures may be hiding in the trees!

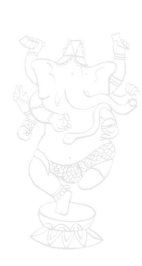

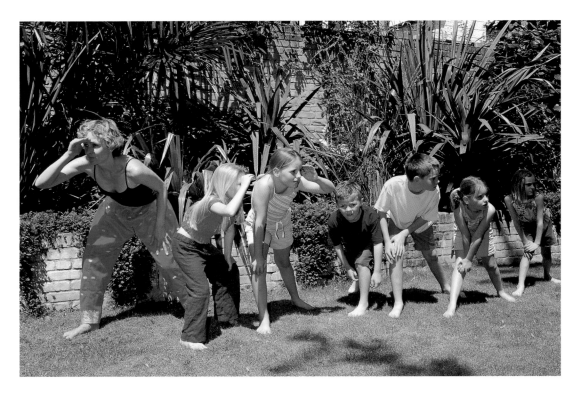

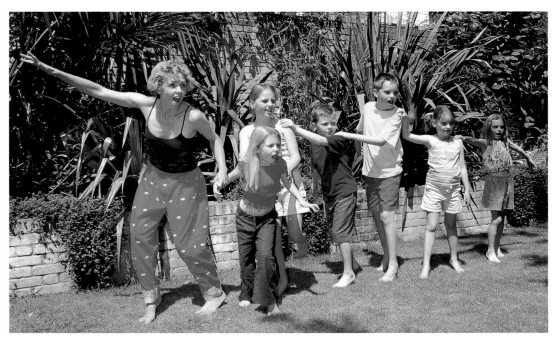

2 Tiptoe quietly through the tall grass. Keep a hand on the shoulder of the person in front of you to make sure no one gets left behind.

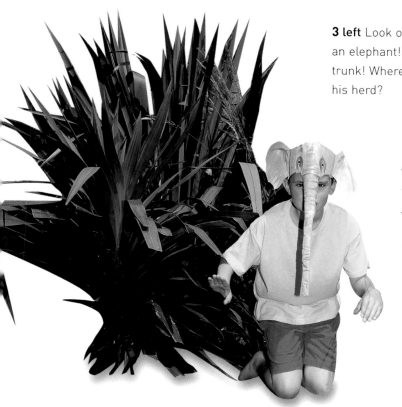

3 left Look over there, there's an elephant! See his long trunk! Where is the rest of his herd?

4 right Now strike a pose as a fierce jungle warrior to make yourself feel more brave.

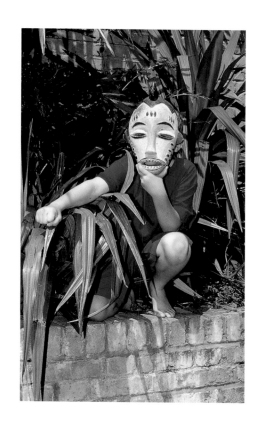

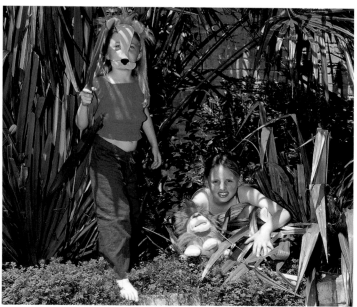

5 Watch out everyone! Over there in the trees are a couple of lions. Let's hope they aren't hungry!

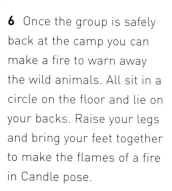

6 Once the group is safely back at the camp you can make a fire to warn away the wild animals. All sit in a circle on the floor and lie on your backs. Raise your legs and bring your feet together to make the flames of a fire in Candle pose.

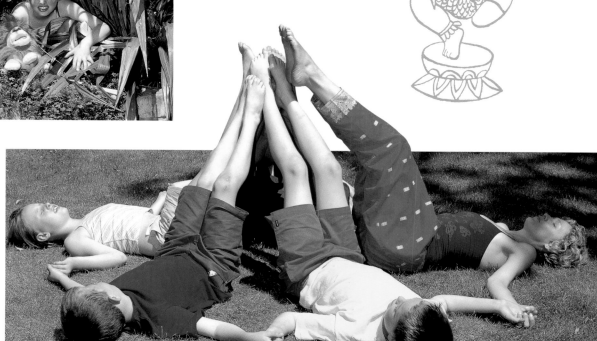

Yoga Games

Yoga postures can be very easily incorporated into many traditional children's games. All that is called for is a little imagination and modification. Using games in this way is a clever way of keeping enthusiasm for yoga practice alive.

Games are also an ideal activity for when friends come round to play, and in fact, the more children the better.

You may recognize the classic games that have been adapted in this section. Copy Me is a version of Simon Says and the idea for Wise Man Walk has come from Grandmother's Footsteps.

Copy me

Appoint a leader to call out the yoga poses. The group must perform the posture only when the leader says "Copy me!" followed by the name of the pose. Anyone who makes three mistakes is out of the game.

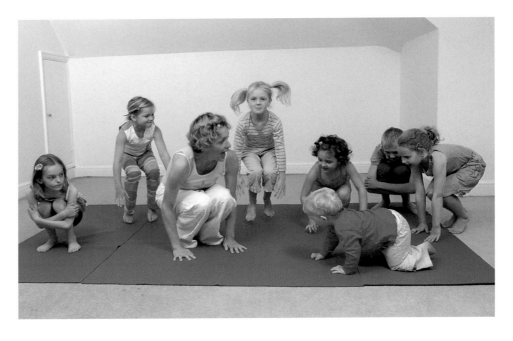

1 Copy me and squat like a rabbit! Everyone squat on the floor and hop up and down.

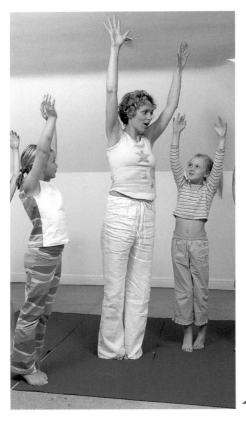

2 left Copy me and be as tall as a mountain! Everyone put your arms in the air and stretch out your fingers to make yourself tall.

3 below Copy me and hoot like an owl! Form "O" shapes with your fingers to make big, wide owl eyes.

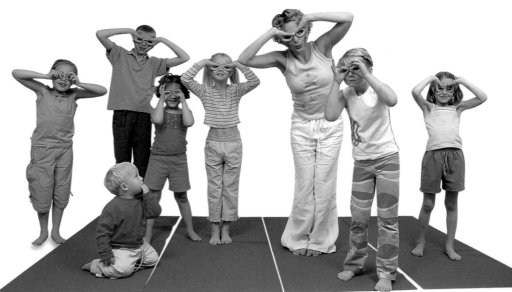

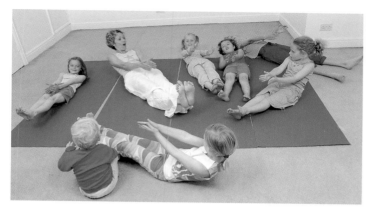

4 Copy me and be a seal! Everyone sit down on the floor and stretch out your legs, lifting them slightly off the floor to make your tail. Extend your arms in front of you to make your flippers.

5 Copy me and be a tall ship! Now all lean back, and hold your legs out wide to make the sails of your ship. Feel the wind in your sails as you try to keep your balance.

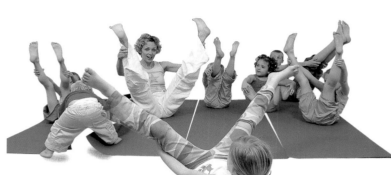

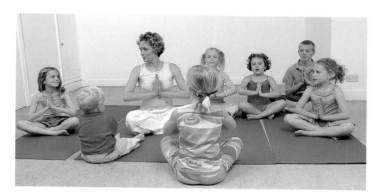

6 Copy me and be a Little Buddha! Everyone sit with their legs crossed and their hands in prayer position, with palms flat together. Try to keep those backs straight!

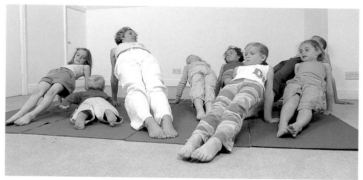

7 Copy me and be a slippery slide! Now everyone stretch out your legs and point your toes. Push up with your hands to lift your bottoms off the floor.

8 left Copy me and stand in Mountain pose. Then squat down slowly to the floor. Uh-oh, out you go!

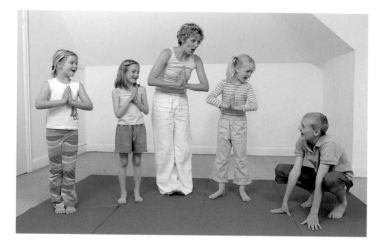

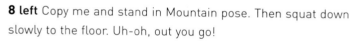

9 left Copy me and be a snake! Lie on your front with your legs stretched behind you. Push down into your hands and lift your chest and head strongly upwards.

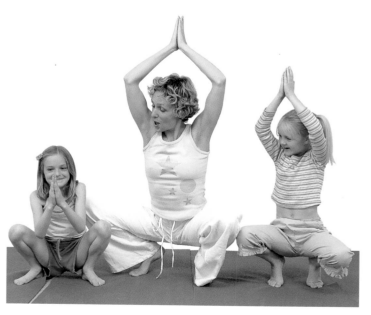

10 Copy me and jump up into squatting! Squat down on the balls of your feet and lift your hands up above your head, with your palms together in prayer position. Oh no, you're out!

▷

Snap and snack

This group game involves a cluster of crocodiles lying side by side. Choose an intrepid explorer to step gingerly over the sleepy crocodiles without touching them. If he or she fails, the crocodiles arch up with tails swishing and teeth snapping and the explorer is out. Try this game as seals too, lying on your backs.

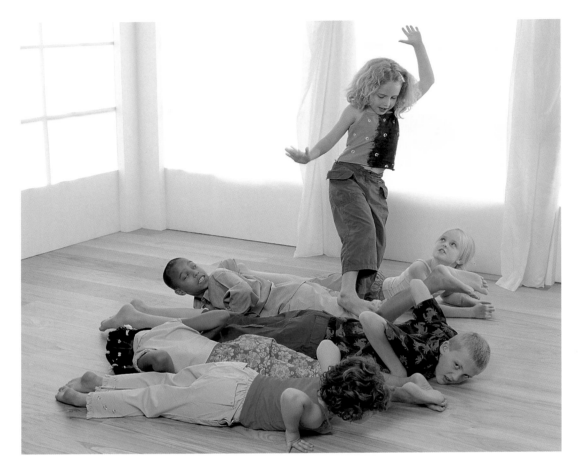

left Crocodiles Come into Crocodile pose by lying on your front and bringing your legs together to make the heavy tail. Bring your hands underneath your shoulders and place your palms flat on the floor. These are your clawed feet. Look out for that unwanted visitor. SNAP!

right Seals These lazy snoozing seals will soon let you know if you've woken them up. Watch out for their noisy barking and flapping fins if you touch them.

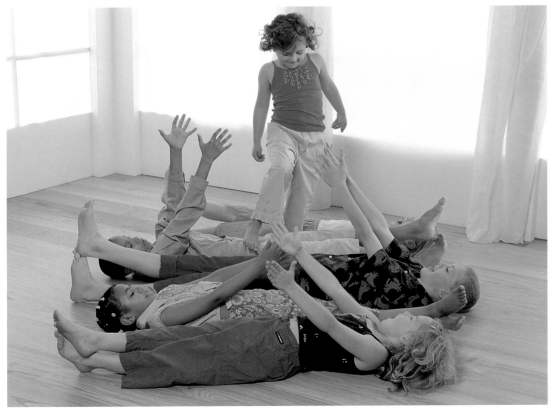

Wise man walk

This involves a group of wise men and a watcher, who stands with his back to the group. The wise men can move only when they are not being watched, and must freeze in a posture when the watcher turns round. If anyone moves when the watcher turns, the whole group goes back to the start.

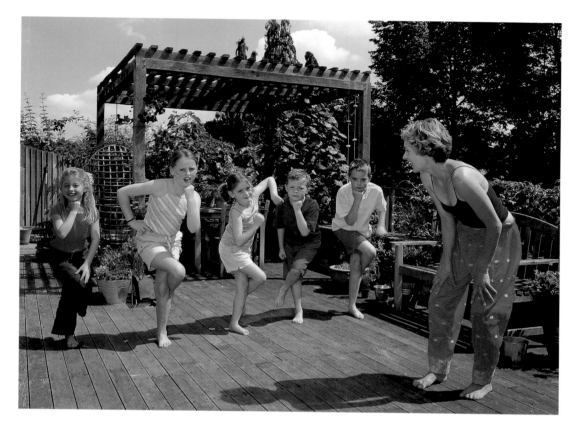

1 Offer a choice of postures before the game starts. When the group is ready, the watcher shouts out, "Everybody become an eagle!" The group of wise men now have to take up the posture. From a standing position, bend your knees and cross one leg over the other. Make a fist and place it under your chin. Support your elbow with the palm of your other hand, and try to balance.

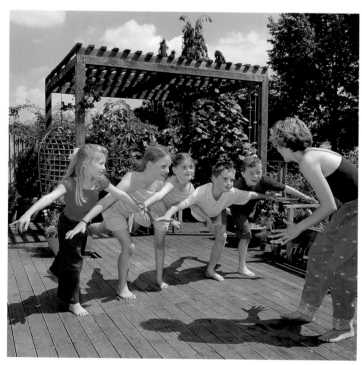

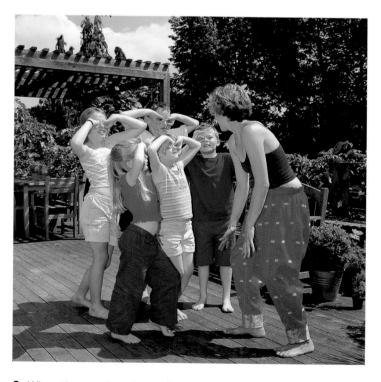

2 When the watcher shouts "Everybody become an aeroplane!", stand up tall and breathe in. As you breathe out, balance on one leg and lift one leg behind you. Spread your arms out to the sides (for the aeroplane's wings) and drop your chest towards your front knee.

3 When the watcher shouts "Everybody become a wise old owl!", point your elbows in the air, make circles with your middle finger and thumb, and place over your eyes. The first wise man to touch the watcher is the winner and becomes the watcher for the next round.

Bunny hopping

This relay race is great fun. Organize your guests into two teams (a minimum of three in each). Each child holds a balloon between their legs and must hop with a carrot baton in their mouth to the next child in the team. The baton is handed over and the next child sets off at full hop.

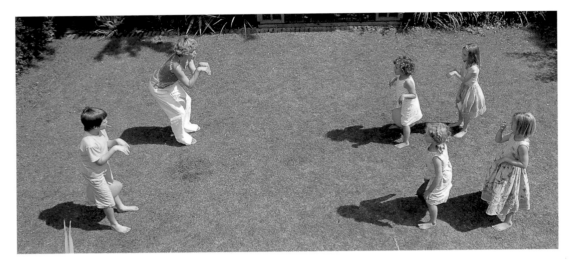

1 Take your positions with the two teams side by side. One bunny from each team stands facing their team at the other end of the garden. Make sure everyone has an inflated balloon between their knees. The first bunny in the line-up has the carrot baton in their mouth. On your marks, get set and GO! The first bunny sets off, hopping over to their opposite bunny team member.

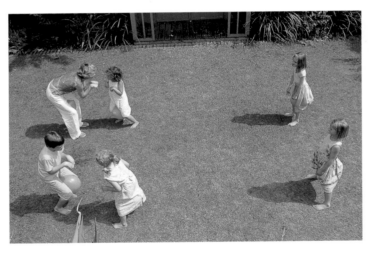

2 The first bunny of each team hops right across the garden towards the opposite bunny and makes the first exchange of the carrot baton. Take care not to let the balloons slip!

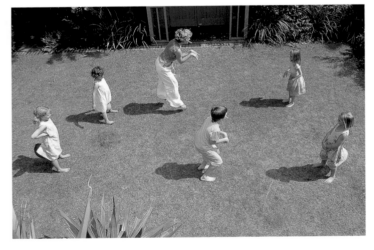

3 The first bunnies now stay where they are while the second bunnies set off hopping back across the garden to the rest of the team line-up, keeping the carrot batons in their mouths.

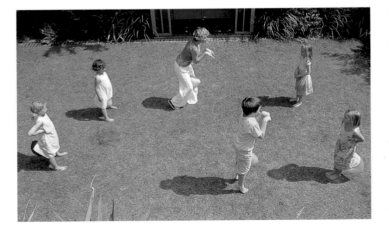

4 Keep those legs springy and hold your hands up like rabbit paws as you hop across the garden.

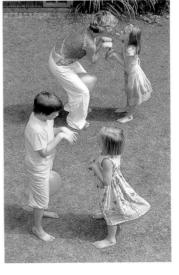

5 As the second bunnies reach the rest of their team they hand over the carrot baton for the final lap of the race.

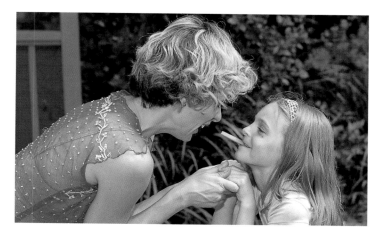

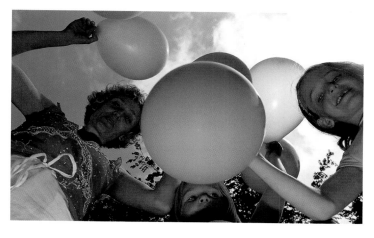

6 After exchanging batons, the third bunnies in the line-up now hop over to their opposite team members. The first team to hand over the carrot baton is the winner!

7 Wave your balloons in the air as the winning bunnies celebrate!

Party poppers

If your guests are still full of energy, get them to be party poppers, crouching down small to begin with, and preparing to spring up into the air with a high-energy burst. This should help to build up an appetite ready for the party food.

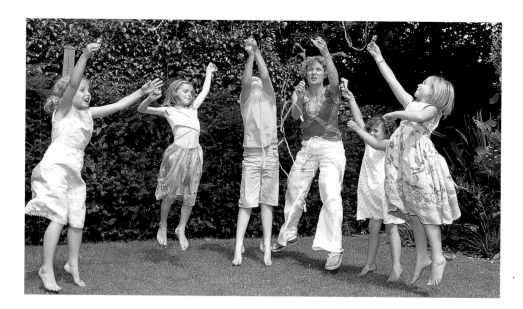

1 All crouch down small together and imagine you are a party popper filled with streamers and confetti and ready to explode. On a count of "1, 2, 3!" leap up into the air, stretching your arms as high as you can. If you like, you could let off party streamers as you jump up.

2 Come back down and repeat your leap all over again. Keep stretching your arms up high. Repeat as many times as you like until you can explode no more. Then all of you flop down together and rest.

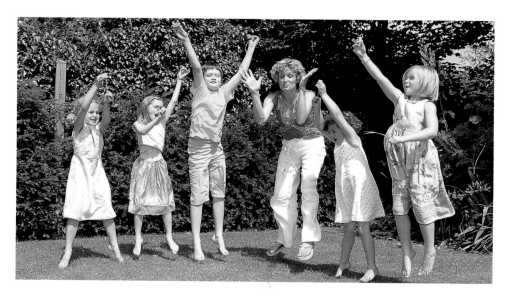

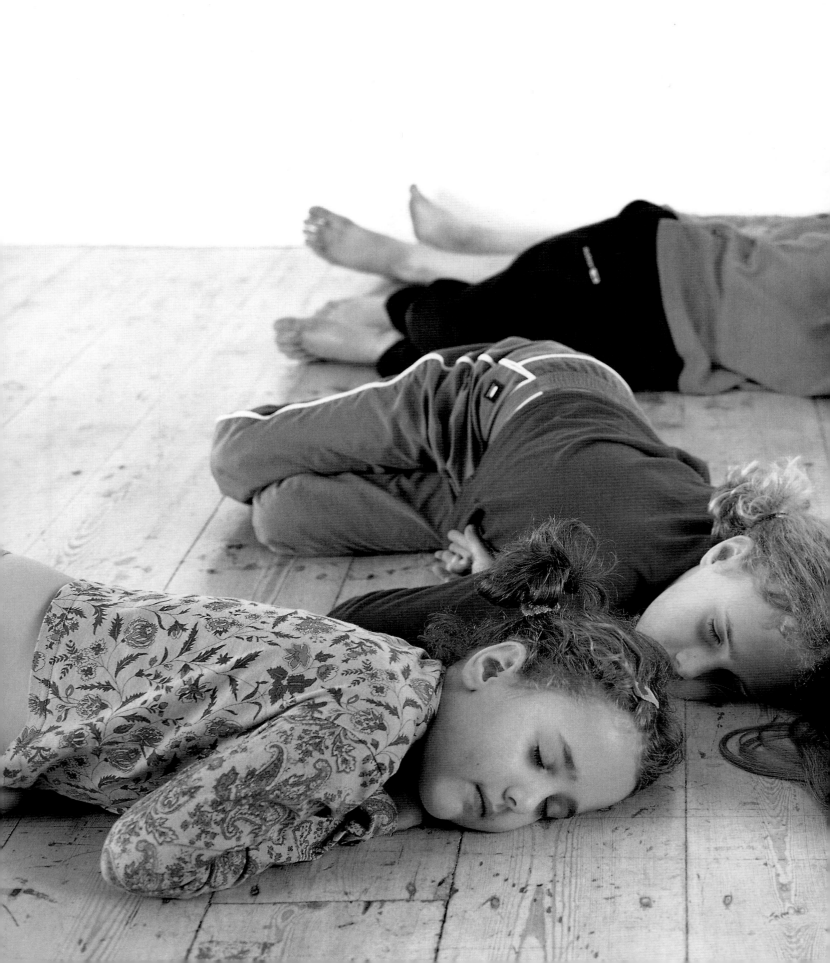

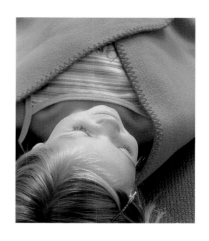

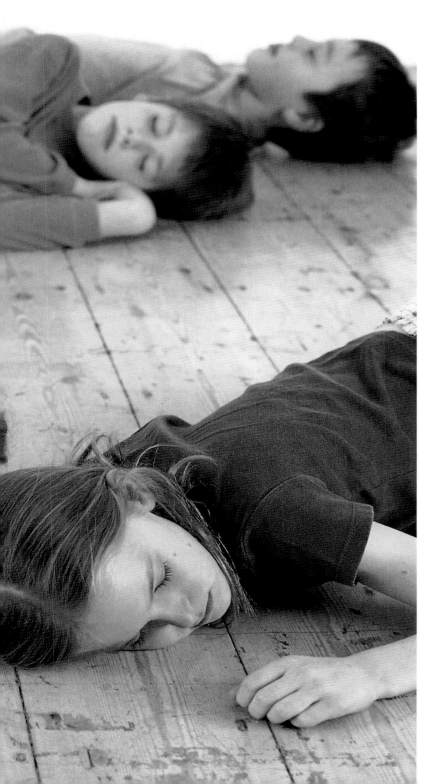

quiet Time

The appreciation of peace and quiet, the notion of being rather than doing, and the ability to jump off the merry-go-round of life and take time out are valuable life skills that we all find beneficial. You can enjoy these tranquil yoga postures when energy levels are low and you are in need of emotional nourishment. Learn how to appease everyday problems with simple, specially chosen postures.

Being Quiet

Cultivating quiet time in our busy lives should be a weekly if not daily priority. Yoga teaches children to rediscover the joy of stillness and silence, and to see that being able to relax is just as important to health and well-being as exercise and activity.

These are a few simple exercises that can reconnect us with our breathing and encourage us to explore our senses. Being able to spend time in this contemplative state is a very important life skill, making us less reliant on external distractions, such as the television, and helping us to keep calm when life becomes frenetic.

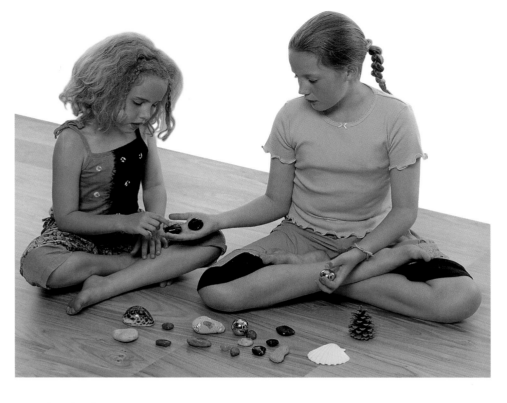

Tummy breathing

Lie down in a quiet room in Dead Man's pose (Savasana). Place your hands or a soft toy on your tummy so that you can feel where your breath is and how it moves. Breathe deeply so that your tummy rises as you breathe in and falls as you breathe out. After about 5 minutes, roll to one side and slowly come up to a sitting position.

Touchy feely

Our skin is a powerful sense organ. Simply touching objects with a pleasant surface can engender feelings of well-being. Stroking a pet, cuddling a soft teddy bear or exploring the surface of a pebble or sea shell encourages sensory awareness and a calm, contended state of mind.

above Re-acquainting yourself with special objects or treasures helps to rekindle happy memories and encourages contemplation.

Mala beads are used in traditional yoga practice to encourage inner contentment and mindfulness. The beads are held in the right hand and each bead is rolled between thumb and middle finger while a mantra (a special phrase or syllable) is repeated. You can use any string of beads instead of mala beads. Choose two words that are relevant to you. Sitting cross-legged with eyes closed, the beads can be rolled through the fingers while you repeat the word "Peace" on the in breath and "Calm" on the outward breath.

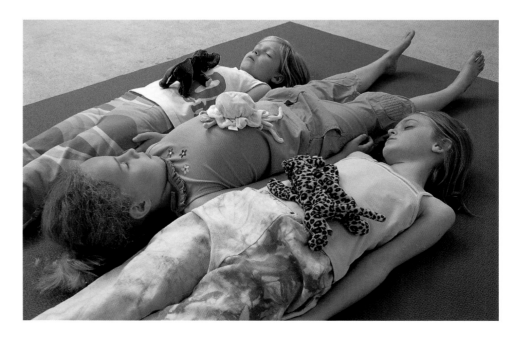

left Letting your mind rest on the ebb and flow of your natural breath is soothing and encourages physical stillness, which to a child can be the most challenging of all activities. Using a toy as a prop makes relaxation more fun.

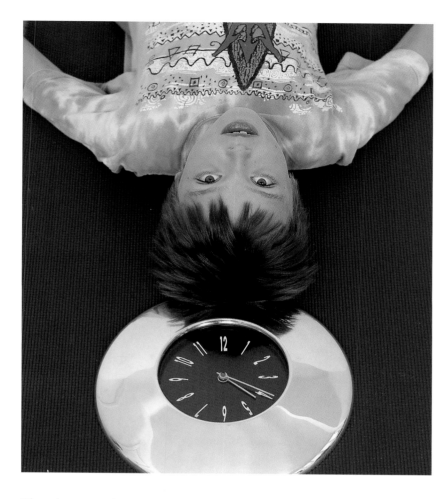

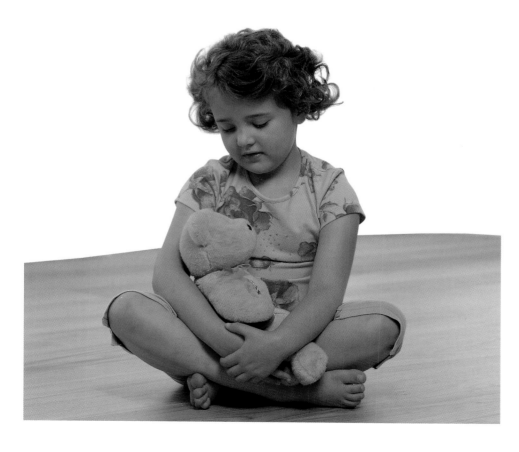

"Concentrate on silence. When it comes, dwell on what it sounds like. Then strive to carry that quiet wherever you go."

below Spend time encouraging connectedness. Caring for special things at a young age can develop a child's ability to care for others later on in life, as well as showing her the pleasures to be found in modest possessions.

Simple sounds

Relaxing music is used instead of medication in the treatment of some stress-related illnesses and problems, and often with tremendous success. This testifies to the power of sound and its effects on our well-being. On the other hand, the wrong type of sound can be damaging to our health. The rumble of traffic in our cities, constant background music piped into shopping centres and the ringing of phones both inside and outside the home, can wear us down.

A breaking glass can shatter nerves whereas bird song or the chiming of bells can elicit positive feelings of peace and joy. Everyday sounds, such as the simple ticking of a clock, engage our minds and, in turn, can improve our ability to concentrate. As our mind tunes in, our body gets a chance to "chill out" for a while. Try writing a list of the sounds you like, along with another list of the sounds that make you feel edgy or cross.

above The gentle repetition of a pleasant and familiar sound, such as a ticking wall clock, can help to still a busy mind.

Peaceful Postures

Poses that bring calm and tranquillity are restorative and rejuvenating to mind, body and soul. They are lovely to practise after a busy day or when you just feel like being quiet. You can practise them to wind yourself down after the energizing animal poses in the Animal Parade chapter, and done before bedtime they will ensure you get a sound and restful night's sleep.

Peaceful postures help to conserve your energy, rather than drain it out of your system. Even though you may feel you are doing very little as you practise them, you are actually doing something extremely powerful. You are recharging your internal batteries, rekindling your life force or prana, and this is what will keep you feeling full of energy, alive and well.

Many of the poses that bring a sense of peace to the body are done lying or sitting down with the eyes closed. The exceptions are the standing poses such as Tree pose, Mountain pose and Dancer. Concentration is needed to stand completely still. In doing so, we encourage our mind's internal chattering to fade away softly into the background.

below Tree Stand on one foot and lift the other up, placing the sole of your foot against your inner thigh. Bring your hands into Prayer position (Namaste) in front of you and steady yourself. Begin to feel your supporting foot spreading into the floor like imaginary roots growing down deep into the earth. Focus on a stationary point in front of you. Gently lift your arms above your head to form the branches of your tree. Feel strong and silent like a magnificent oak. Hold for a few deep breaths, then slowly release and change sides.

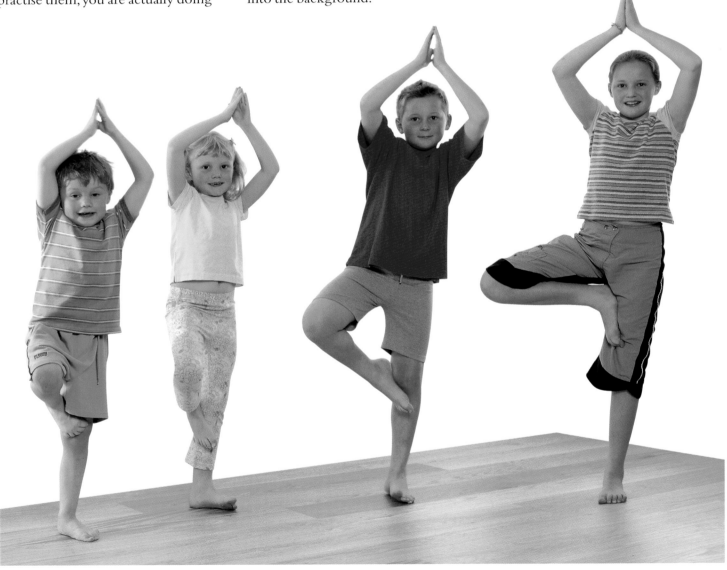

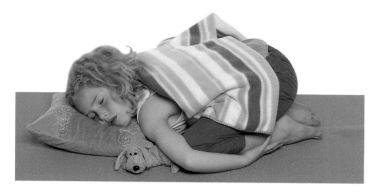

above Child's pose Rest on your knees with your forehead on the floor or a cushion in front of you, arms by your sides. Picture a mouse curled up small and still, or a pebble on the beach, made smooth by the sea and warmed by the sun.

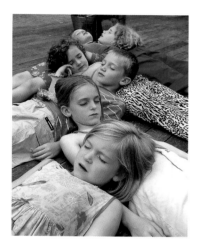

left Sleeping snake This is a lovely exercise for a group of friends. Lie down, one by one, with your head on the stomach of the person beneath you, forming a herringbone pattern. When assembled, close your eyes and feel your head gently lifting and dropping as the person you are resting on breathes in and out.

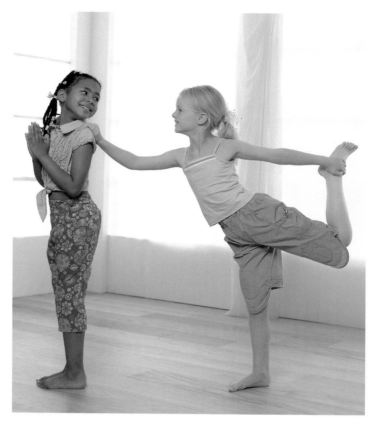

above Mountain and Dancer Feel as motionless as a mountain (left), with feet firm and an imaginary cord from the crown of your head helping you stand tall and proud. Face straight ahead to hold the position correctly. Dancer pose (right) requires a firm foot and an elegant grace.

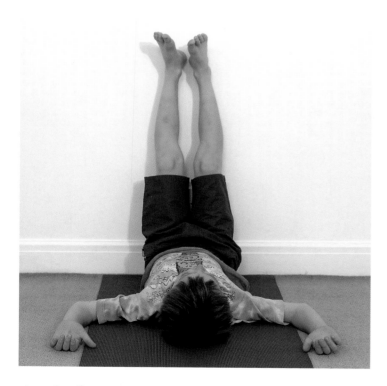

above Candle Lying flat on your back with your legs up the wall, like a tall candle, gives legs a rest from the effects of gravity. Stretch your arms above your head, close your eyes and breathe deeply. Imagine a cool waterfall refreshing your legs and whole body.

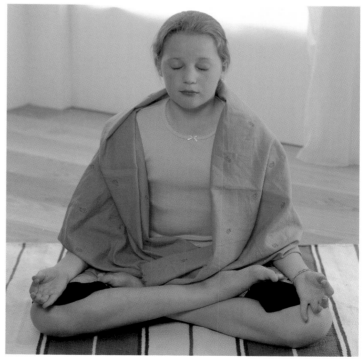

above Little Buddha Sitting with the legs crossed ensures your spine is anchored and that you are able to sit tall and straight. With your hands in your lap or resting on the knees you can feel strength and wisdom growing inside you. This is a classic pose for meditation.

Dream Time

Dream time is simply deep relaxation for children. This is a time when you lie completely still, allowing your body to relax and switch off for a while. With regular practice and encouragement, you will come to look forward to this part of your yoga session, particularly if you aim to make it special.

Preparation

To make the dream time session more fun, put some thought into getting ready. Think about the music you would like to listen to and allow yourself one special toy that can lie down with you while you dream.

Select a favourite cushion or blanket and make yourself feel as warm and comfortable as possible. The best time for dream time is towards the end of the day, when your energy levels are naturally low, and fading light and the prospect of bedtime makes you want to feel cosy and snug. You can either practise dream time after your active yoga poses or on its own as an extra special dream session, especially if you are feeling tired.

The rewards of stillness

Children can be offered a simple reward for stillness if they are unable to concentrate on being quiet –

for example, a pretty pebble, shell, wild flower, feather or crystal. Younger children can be told that a visiting fairy or elf will place something nice in their hands but only when they are completely still and quiet. This small incentive can work wonders.

Dead Man pose

The classic yoga relaxation pose is Savasana, also known as Corpse pose or Dead Man pose. The body lies still, with the feet hip-width apart, the arms away from the body and the eyes closed. Resting in Savasana allows the body to rest and recharge depleted energy stores.

Sweet dreams

• Choose a quiet room, turn off the lights and light a few candles (but do not leave these burning unattended). Make the children comfortable with cushions, pillows, blankets and any toys or props.
• Put on some soothing music – natural sounds such as bird song, waves or rainfall, soft drums or pipes usually work best.
• As they lie on their backs, ask the children to feel really heavy. As gravity gently draws them down into the ground, let them feel their body melting like ice cream.
• Do the "spaghetti" test. Gently go round to each child and lift one leg or arm at a time and tell them to make it feel really heavy. This will show that they are starting to relax. Rock the limb gently from side to side, then place it carefully back on the floor.

• Ask the child to think about their breathing and whereabouts in their bodies their breath is. Ask them to feel their tummies moving up and down as they breathe in and out. They could try to imagine a tiny boat at sea, bobbing up and down gently on the ocean waves.
• Tell them to relax their feet, repeating, "Relax my feet, my feet are heavy and r-e-l-a-x-e-d", and continue for each part of the body right up to their head.
• Tell them how difficult it is to be still and how clever they are to resist moving. Remind them that their ability to relax is a special gift.
• Visually guide them on a special journey. Let their yoga mat become a flying carpet gliding over a tropical rainforest or a soft cloud passing through a rainbow. Or take them to a golden beach where they can feel the warm yellow sand underneath their feet, and

hear the playful call of dolphins inviting them to come and swim. Choose a theme, using your imagination, and keep the language simple. Allow time for them to explore their "dream".
• When the children look relaxed and still, introduce a simple affirmation or resolve, such as "I feel free and happy!". Ask them to repeat it to themselves three times. Pause for a moment and then gently guide them back to reality. Tell them they are waking up in bed and ask them to gently stretch and yawn.
• When they are ready, ask them to talk about their dream and share it with you.

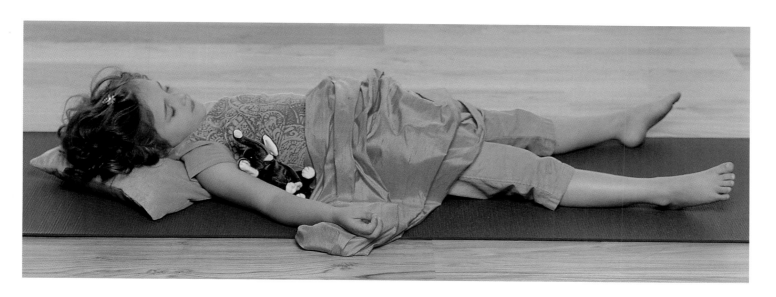

above Savasana Praise your child for lying motionless and resisting the urge to move. Tell her that in doing so her mind is being taken on a wonderful holiday.

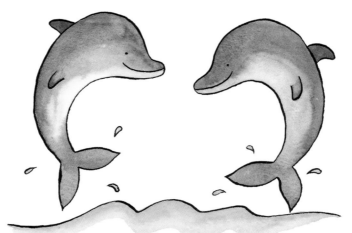

left The magical image of a dolphin is an old favourite with young children and it is easy for them to relate to.

Special time

Many important physiological changes take place in Savasana. Respiration levels are lowered, strain on the heart is reduced and the vital life energy, or prana, that has been created in posture work can be assimilated into the body. As the breath quietens and softens, the mind becomes clear and detached. It is then receptive to any positive images or sounds you may hear.

Making an affirmation

Relaxation encourages the mind to be open and receptive. It is therefore a wonderful time to be introduced to positive ideas and images in the form of affirmations or *sankalpa*. These little seeds of hope will embed themselves in your consciousness over time, and can help you to feel good about yourself. Affirmations should only ever be simple, even for older

children and adults, and negative words and images should be avoided as these can be counterproductive. Choose one affirmation for the session, and repeat it in your head three times.

below If you are talking a child through their dream, keep the images and words that you use light, sunny and positive.

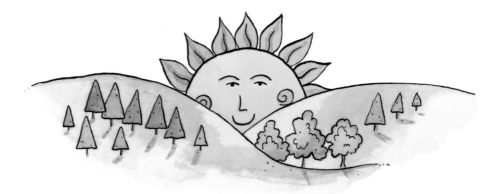

Sounding It Out

Sound is an invisible yet powerful form of energy created by the vibration of molecules. Adding sound to your practice encourages self–expression and develops good communications skills. Sighing, humming or chanting also helps to put us in touch with the quiet place inside us, where new sensations and emotions can be experienced.

Animal antics

Everyone will enjoy panting like a dog, sniffing like a rabbit, hissing like a snake or roaring like a lion as they practise the animal poses in the Animal Parade chapter. Get really involved and make sounds and movements to elaborate on the pose.

Humming bee breath

This breath helps to open up the throat chakra, which is the centre of communication. It can help to dissolve the fear of speaking up at school to teachers, and will help when speaking to new friends. To do the Humming Bee Breath, sit in Little Buddha pose with your eyes closed. Breathe in and as you breathe out through your mouth, gently hum at the same time. Feel the sound gently vibrating in your throat.

Try putting your fingers in your ears as you hum to really help you concentrate and feel the sound resonating deep within you.

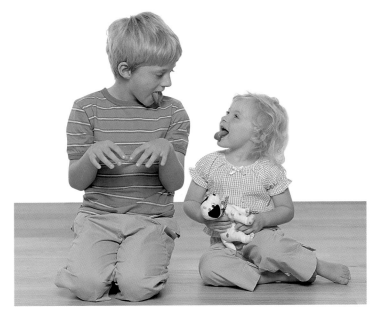

left Imitating animals and the sounds they make is a fun and creative part of your yoga practice.

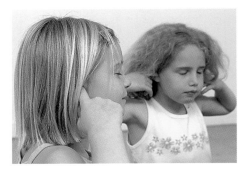

above and below Removing the distractions of external noises by putting fingers in your ears can help to put you in touch with your inner world.

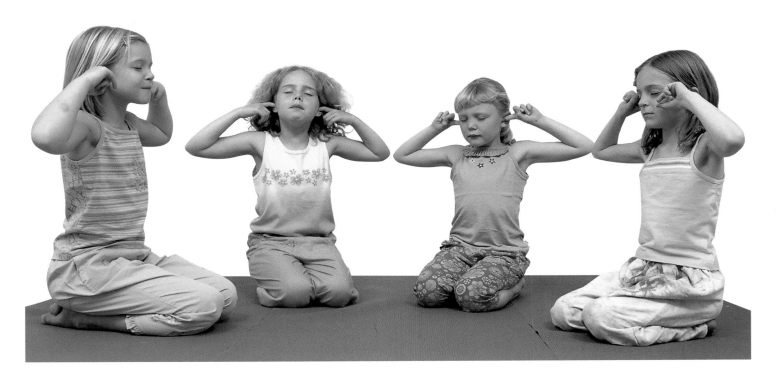

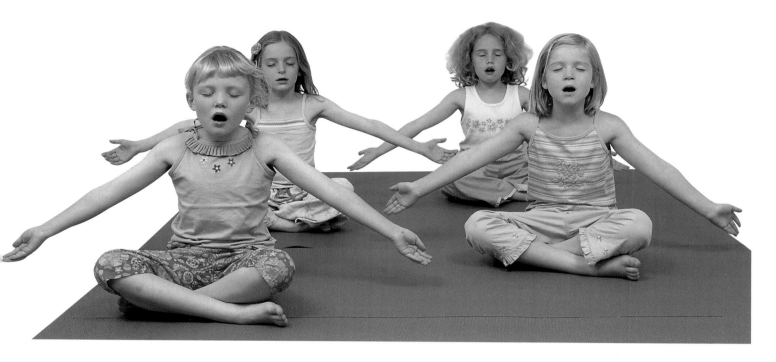

Sighing breath

This breath helps you to let go of stresses and strains at the end of a busy day. First breathe in deeply, then sigh the breath out of your mouth with a lovely strong "Aaaahh!" sound. Repeat a few times and now visualize anything that has made you cross or sad floating out with your breath and up and away into space.

Chanting

Yogic chanting is a form of singing or humming and produces special vibrations that soothe body, mind and soul. A mantra is a special word that can be hummed as you chant.

"Om" is the classic yoga mantra – meaning absolute peace. The wise yogis believed that we should "live in Om". In other words, we should live our lives in total peace and harmony.

Begin by repeating Om in your head, breaking it down into three sections. Start with an "Ah" sound, then an "Oh" sound then "Mmmm". Then breathe in and, as you breathe

out, hum the Om out nice and loudly, visualizing each syllable as a little bubble of energy growing inside you and floating up into the sky. Try lifting your arms up slowly as you hum it to help your energy bubbles float upwards. Pause after each repetition and see if you can hear or feel the echo of Om in your mind, and maybe in your body, too, as the sound waves keep on vibrating through you.

above Chanting "Om" with your friends bonds you together. It makes you feel good about yourselves and makes friendships stronger.

You can also make up your own mantras, choosing a word relevant to how you are feeling. Evocative words such as "Peace", "Calm" or "Love" work very well. Let their soothing tones suffuse every molecule of your body.

right Sighing out through the mouth brings a sense of relief and helps you let go of unwanted feelings.

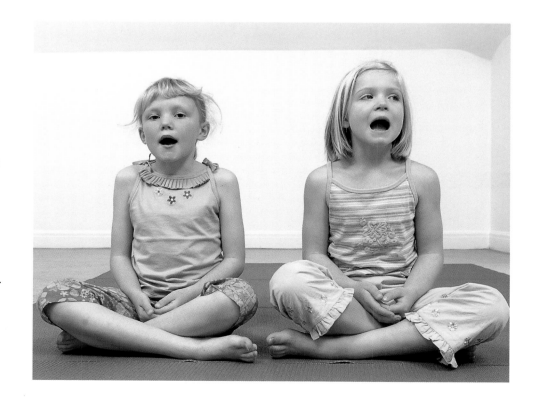

The Wise Yogi

Yoga is often referred to as "skill in action". This defines not just the physical skills that yoga provides us with, but also the mental skills that teach us control of our mind and our emotions.

Establishing these skills helps us to understand our true nature, and this gives us more control over our lives. Getting to know and accept our strengths and weaknesses gives us a sort of inner power and equips us with a code for living. This helps us to manage the up and downs of daily life more easily and with confidence.

Being able to help yourself and the rest of your family overcome everyday ailments and upsets is a wonderful example of how yoga gives us better control over our lives. In addition to the physical advantages of yoga practice, you can learn how to use the postures therapeutically and holistically to make yourself feel better.

below Wheel Prepare your back by doing Blue Whale pose a few times. Then lie in the same starting position tuck your flat palms under your shoulders. Breathe deeply and on a breath out, push strongly into your hands and lift your bottom and head off the floor. Hold for a few breaths, then release and hug your knees.

Headaches

Forward bends can help to relieve everyday headaches. The act of leaning forwards also helps to still the mind and lessen the load on the heart. In a darkened room, try Child's pose with your head on a cushion, or a Forward Bend supporting your head and arms with a chair. Close your eyes and breathe calmly for 5–10 minutes.

Low energy

Back bends are energizing as they open the heart and lungs, allowing us to breathe deeply. They also strengthen the nervous system and stimulate the digestive organs, improving the elimination of waste products. Try Cobra, Fish or Locust poses, or simply lie over a bean bag, arching your back. Take long breaths. For a really strong back bend, try doing Wheel pose.

Stiffness and tension

Aches in the lower back can be caused by many things from slouching to carrying heavy loads, or strenuous physical activity. You can find relief by lying on your back and hugging your knees tightly to your chest. Rocking forwards and backwards helps massage the back muscles, "ironing" away strain and tension. Child's pose, Beetle and Blue Whale are also very effective. To maintain spinal mobility and strength, practise Sunshine Stretch and Cat, Dog, Snake and Mouse.

Tummy ache

Lie on your front allowing the floor to gently cushion your tummy. Breathe deep breaths to let your tummy relax.

Sore throat

Roaring Lion is good for keeping sore throats at bay. It is also guaranteed to bring a smile to the face of anyone in a bad mood. Practised in a group, it encourages teamwork.

Nerves

Woodchopper pose or Roaring Lion help to release pent up energy and nervousness, particularly before an important event.

> "Yoga helps to cure what need not be endured and to endure what cannot be cured"

Asthma

With commitment, yoga can help you to manage and even control the symptoms of bronchial asthma. Regular practice strengthens the respiratory system, drains mucus from the lungs, promotes breath awareness and control, and relaxes tense chest muscles. Gentle movements, which encourage rhythmic breathing, are good for asthma sufferers; aggressive movements may over-stimulate the lungs. Try Sunshine Stretch to get the whole body moving, and gentle back bends to relax the chest.

A breathing exercise such as Sniffing Breath can be useful. Sit quietly with crossed legs. Bring your mind to your breath and breathe naturally for a few moments. Then begin to sniff as you breathe in, taking two or three short sniffing breaths until the lungs are full, then a long breath out. Repeat until your chest feels open and relaxed. This also helps if you have been upset or crying.

Hyperactivity

Strong poses and animal postures with accompanying noises will use up excess energy and disperse physical tension. Follow with some of the breathing techniques, such as Sighing Breath or Humming Bee Breath, to soothe and relax you.

below Supported back bend Arching your body backwards over an exercise ball or bean bag makes you feel wide awake. Not having to support your own weight means you can relax and hold the pose for longer.

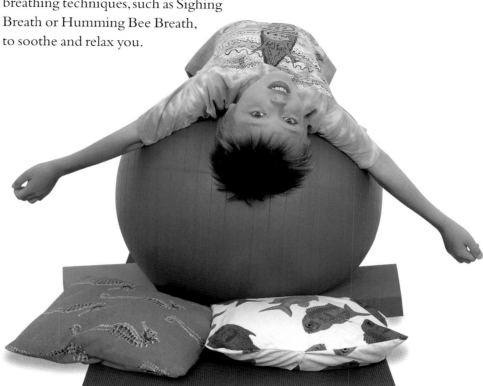

Shoulder stand

This calming pose revives you after a busy day and reverses the effects of gravity on the legs and heart. Close your eyes and visualize a refreshing mountain waterfall pouring energy back into your legs. For a milder version, lie sideways against a wall, and extend your legs so that they rest against the wall. Take your arms to the floor behind your head and relax completely for 5 minutes.

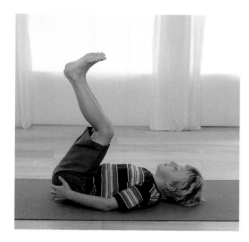

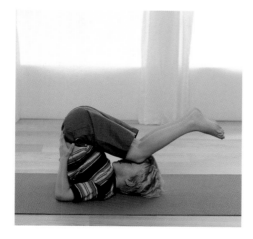

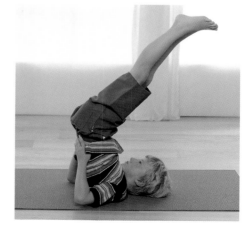

1 Lie on your back on the floor and lift your legs upwards, with your knees bent. Keep your chin tucked in towards your chest to protect your neck.

2 With your hands on your lower back, drop your knees down towards your face. This will allow your back to peel off the floor. You can support your back with your hands.

3 Lift your legs upwards as you push your lower back towards your face with your hands. Close your eyes and breathe. Roll your back down on to the floor. Hug your knees.

▷

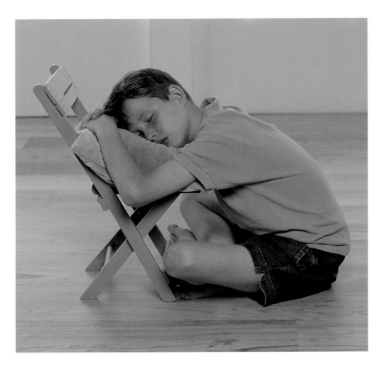

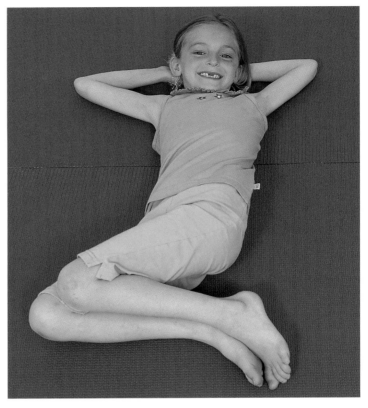

above Forward bend with chair This lovely relaxing pose requires no effort and helps to quieten a busy mind or an aching head.

below Canny cat Cat pose is a very versatile pose and it is fun and easy to do. Get down on your hands and knees and roar like a big cat or tuck your toes under, lift up your bottom and become a dog. Become a cat again, then sit on your heels and be quiet again in Child's pose.

above Easy twist To ease a strained or aching back, lie on your back, knees bent and feet flat on the floor. Interlace your fingers under your head and, as you breathe out, let your knees drop to one side. Hold for five deep breaths and change sides. Feel your back waking up.

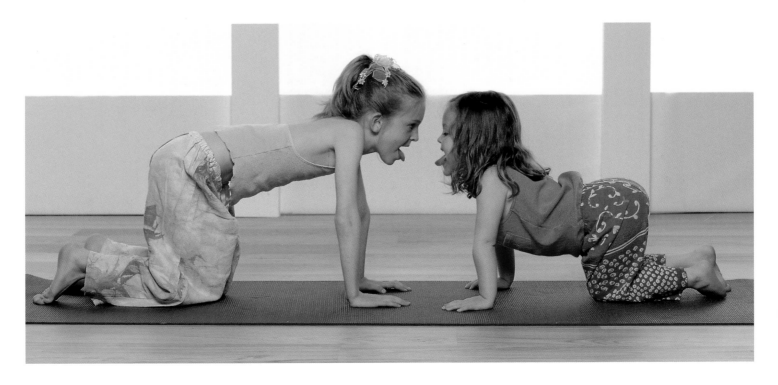

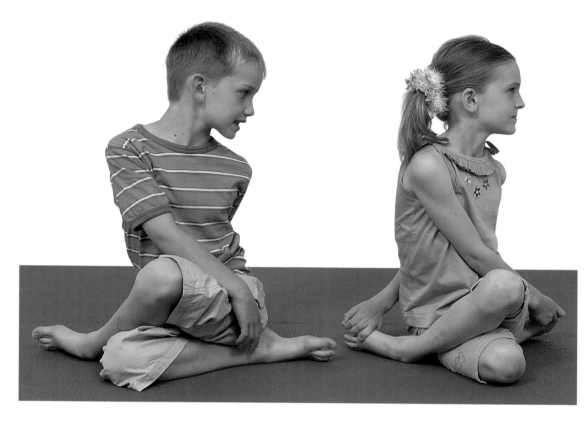

left Seated twist Twisting poses help to unravel knots or tight bits in your back and, according to yoga therapists, any knots or problems in your head too. Sit cross-legged with your left leg on the top. Slide this leg over so that your knees are almost on top of one another and your left heel is by your right thigh. Breathe in and lift your chest. Then breathe out and turn your body to the left. Let your spine spiral round, from the bottom upwards. Place your right arm on your left thigh and try to catch your left toes with your left hand. Change sides after a few deep breaths.

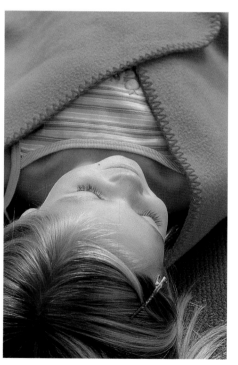

right Sweet dreams The yogis believed that stilling the eyes and focusing the gaze, or *drushti*, would help to focus the mind. Learn to relax with a prop. A soothing, lavender eye bag or silk scarf will help you to keep inquisitive, seaching eyes closed.

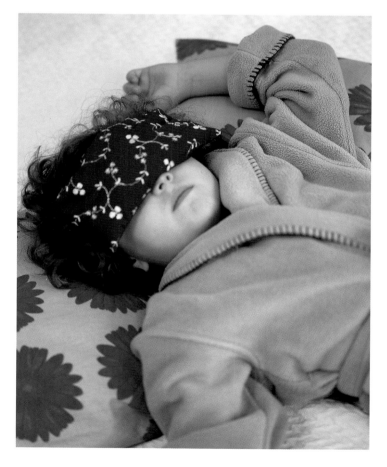

above Savasana "I closed my eyes so I could see". Just a few quiet moments lying down wrapped in a cosy blanket can help you to feel calm and good about yourself again.

Index

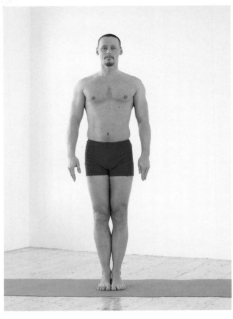

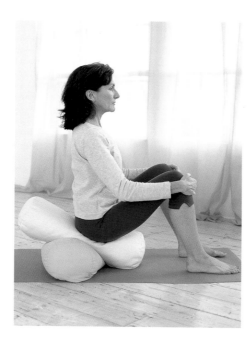

index

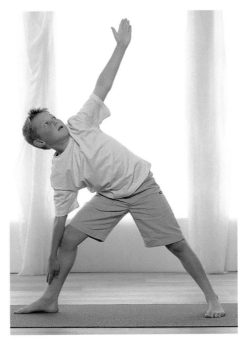

ACKNOWLEDGEMENTS

Extracts from The Yoga Sutras of Patanjali by Alistair Shearer published by Rider. Used by permission of the Random House Group Limited. For editions sold in the US and Canada: Extracts appear from The Yoga Sutras of Patanjali by Patanjali, translated by Alistair Shearer, copyright © 1982 by Alistair Shearer. Used by permission of Bell Tower, a division of Random House, Inc.

Thanks to the following agencies and individuals for permission to reproduce their images:
t=top, b=bottom, r=right; l=left: p17 (both) Gerry Clist and Michael Rabe; p149tr and br Craig Knowles; p159br Alistair Hughes; p163bl Don Last; p169t Fiona Pragoff.